What's Behind the Symptom?

THEORY AND PRACTICE IN MEDICAL ANTHROPOLOGY AND INTERNATIONAL HEALTH

A series edited by

Susan M. DiGiacomo
University of Massachusetts, Amherst

Editorial Board

H. Kris Heggenhougen
Harvard University
Cambridge, Massachusetts

Daniel E. Moerman
University of Michigan, Dearborn

R. Brooke Thomas
University of Massachusetts, Amherst

International Advisory Board

George Armelagos, Hans Baer, Peter Brown, Xòchitl Castaneda, Deborah Gordon, Xòchitl Herrera, Judith Justice, Montasser Kamal, Charles Leslie, Shirley Lindenbaum, Margaret Lock, Setha Low, Mark Nichter, Duncan Pedersen, Thomas Ots, Nancy Scheper-Hughes, Merrill Singer

Founding Editor

Libbet Crandon-Malamud†

Volume 1
**Hippocrates' Latin American Legacy:
Humoral Medicine in the New World**
George M. Foster

Volume 2
**Forbidden Narratives:
Critical Autobiography as Social Science**
Kathryn Church

Volume 3
**Anthropology and International Health:
Asian Case Studies**
Mark Nichter and Mimi Nichter

Volume 4
**The Anthropology of Infectious Disease:
International Health Perspectives**
Edited by *Marcia C. Inhorn and Peter J. Brown*

See the back of this book for other titles in Theory and Practice in Medical Anthropology and International Health.

What's Behind the Symptom?

On Psychiatric Observation and Anthropological Understanding

Angel Martínez-Hernáez

Translated by
Susan M. DiGiacomo and John Bates

Foreword by Arthur M. Kleinman

 harwood academic publishers

Australia Canada France Germany India
Japan Luxembourg Malaysia The Netherlands
Russia Singapore Switzerland

Amsteldijk 166
1st Floor
1079 LH Amsterdam
The Netherlands

British Library Cataloguing in Publication Data

Martínez-Hernáez, Angel
  What's behind the symptom? : on psychiatric observation and
  anthropological understanding. - (Theory and practice in
  medical anthropology and international health ; v. 6 –
  ISSN 1068-3291)
  1.Symptomatology 2.Medical anthropology 3.Psychiatry
  I.Title
  616'.047

  ISBN 90-5702-612-0

To *my parents*
in memoriam

CONTENTS

INTRODUCTION TO THE SERIES

Theory and Practice in Medical Anthropology and International Health seeks to promote works of direct relevance to anthropologically informed international health issues, practice, and policy. It aims to bridge medical anthropology—both biological and cultural—with international public health, social medicine, and sociomedical sciences. The series' theoretical scope is intentionally flexible, incorporating the most current advances in social science theory, while its topical breadth ranges from specific issues to contemporary debates to practical applications informed by current anthropological theory. The distinguishing characteristic of this new series is its emphasis on cultural aspects of medicine and their links to larger social contexts and concrete applicability of the anthropological endeavor.

PREFACE

La santé est la vie dans le silence des organes.
[Health is life lived in the silence of the organs]

— R. Leriche
De la Santé a la maladie
Encyclopédie française

If health is silence, then this book is about speech, the meaning of complaint, the voice of illness. It is also about the clinical gaze, that peculiar form of scrutiny which lays down the conditions for medical and psychiatric knowledge.

In the context of Western science, the symptom has been an undisputed redoubt of biomedicine. Although medical and psychiatric manuals have differentiated between signs as observed by the professional and symptoms as expressed by the sufferer, symptoms have generally been regarded as physical manifestations, natural realities that acquire meaning only through medical interpretation. The voice of the sufferer is thus silenced. Deprived of legitimacy, the sufferer's words are associated with error and ignorance.

However, in recent years, this traditional perception of symptoms has been challenged. For at least the past two decades, such specialities as medical and psychiatric anthropology have advanced into new ethnographic territories: symptoms, illness, the body and suffering. Kluckhohn's characterization of anthropology as an intellectual poaching license, taken up by Clifford Geertz in "Blurred Genres" (1983, p.21), has become unexpectedly relevant in the terrain of illness and its forms of expression. As a result, anthropology has been able to mobilize its well-known sensitivity to lay and local discourses against the naturalism of totalizing biomedical interpretations. This book is another move in this game of confrontations and poaching activities.

Following chapter 1, the book is divided into two parts addressing different ways of viewing symptoms: as organic manifestations and as symbolic constructions.

In the first part, I develop a critique of the perception of symptoms as simple pathophysiological phenomena, focusing in particular on the hegemonic paradigm of contemporary psychiatry: neo-Kraepelinism. The aim of this section is, then, not to review various psychiatric trends and their ways of conceptualizing symptoms, but to examine in depth one particular trend and one particular conceptualization. This does not prevent me, however, from making a brief foray into classical psychoanalysis as a counterpoint to Kraepelinism. Nor does it mean that my critique is limited to psychiatry; much of it is also applicable to biomedicine in general.

In the second part, I approach symptoms as symbolic and cultural forms of expression. Here also my efforts are restricted to one particular theoretical domain: that of an interpretive or hermeneutic psychiatric anthropology. I support this approach with my own ethnographic data as well as an incursion into the field of semiotics.

My purpose here is to envision symptoms as an open process, a communicative act, the result of a creative interplay of values and discourses, everyday experience, local knowledge and forms of oppression. It is an attempt to return to symptoms their meaningful dimension, to rescue their oft-denied semiotic and cultural nature. Nevertheless, alongside this general aim there are other, more specific ones. I hope to show that contemporary psychiatry treats winks as twitches; that this approach places serious limitations on both clinical practice and epidemiology; that there is a less positivist and more efficient way of perceiving symptoms; that symptoms can also be ethnographic objects; and that Barthes, Foucault and Peirce are mistaken in their approach to symptoms because they fail to take into account the human sender of the message. I could point out several others, but I leave this task to the readers' critical judgment.

Many people have helped to bring this book to completion either directly or indirectly, academically and/or personally. First of all, I would like to thank the two people who were my supervisors when, in November 1994, I publicly presented an earlier version of this book as a doctoral dissertation in the Department of Anthropology of the University of Barcelona: namely, Professors Claudio Esteva Fabregat and Josep Maria Comelles. In many conversations both formal and informal, the first has shared with me the rich harvest of a professional lifetime, a wealth of insight from which I have benefited, I suspect, much more than I am consciously aware. The second has been a demanding critic, an excellent friend and a generous teacher.

I am also grateful for critical comments, help and inspiration from Joan Frigolé, Joan Bestard, José Luís García, Marcial Gondar, Joan Obiols and Ignasi Terrades. The first was my tutor, while the rest were members of the examining board of my doctoral dissertation. Other scholars—Carole Browner (UCLA), María J. Buxó (University of Barcelona), Dolors Comas (Roviri i Virgili University), Jesús Contreras (University of Barcelona), Aurora González (Universidad Autónoma de Barcelona), Carl Kendall (Tulane University), Arthur Kleinman (Harvard University), Lluís Mallart (University of Paris X), Eduardo Menéndez (CIESAS-Mexico), Rafael Pérez

Taylor (UNAM-Mexico), Joan Prat, Juanjo Pujadas and Oriol Romaní (Rovira i Virgili University) and Tullio Seppilli (University of Perugia)—read and commented on part or the whole of the manuscript. They too deserve my thanks.

Susan DiGiacomo's invaluable help is worthy of special mention. She is not only responsible for the English translation of this book, together with John Bates, but is also a valiant scholar who knows how to speak the truth to academic power and reveal its mystifications.

I would also like to thank my colleagues from the Departments of Anthropology of the University of Barcelona and of the Rovira i Virgili University for their support. I am grateful to the Department of Anthropology of the University of California at Berkeley for welcoming me as a visiting scholar in 1996, when I rewrote several chapters of this book. I also acknowledge my gratitude to Nancy Scheper-Hughes for facilitating my stay in the department, and particularly to Stanley Brandes for his *savoir faire* as an advisor.

I should also mention the Department of Psychiatry of the University of Barcelona and the Clinical Section of Barcelona-Department of Psychoanalysis (University of Paris VIII), where I learned much of what I know about psychiatry and psychoanalysis.

The mental health care facilities in Barcelona where I did the ethnographic fieldwork that is the source of the case examples used in Chapters 1, 10 and 11 should not go unmentioned: the *Hospital Clínic* of Barcelona, the *Instituto Frenopático*, ARI and the Center for Psychosocial Rehabilitation for chronic psychotics of the ARAPDIS Foundation.

Likewise, I am grateful to all my informants. Although at first it was not easy for me to develop empathic relations with them, I believe that, with time, I became a familiar character in their daily lives. Proof of this came one day when a new patient arrived at the center for psychosocial rehabilitation, the ARI, where I was carrying out my fieldwork. Seeing the familiarity with which the others treated me, he asked, "Have you been here long?" I replied that I was an anthropologist, and explained that I was doing research and was very interested in what they residents did and thought. To my surprise he shot back, "Is that so! And how long have you been feeling like this?"

My research was possible thanks to funding provided by the *Programa Sectorial de Formación de Profesorado Universitario y Personal Investigador* (Program for the Training of University Teachers and Researchers) of the Spanish Ministry of Education and Science (reference AP92 40978896) and by the *Direcció General de Recerca de la Generalitat de Catalunya* (Research Office of the Autonomous Government of Catalonia; reference

1996BEAI300384). The translation of the text into English was financed thanks to the help of two of my colleagues at the Rovira i Virgili University, Dolors Comas and Juanjo Pujadas.

Many people have contributed to the making of this book in a less academic fashion. Montse, my wife, has made valuable suggestions and criticisms. The comments of Pere and Charo have enriched my brief incursion into Freud's work. I am indebted to Isabel and Hugo for the pleasure of long conversations on these topics which sometimes went on for days. The wholehearted support of Montse, Tomás, Gabi, Isabel, Pilar, Jordi, Felicitas, Carmen, Gabriel, Carmelo, Inés and Mishin as well as Irene, Enzo and Andrea has been of incalculable value.

I do not want to end this preface without mentioning my parents, who passed away while still young. This book is dedicated to their memory. Had I not lost them as I did, I would have written a very different book. They introduced me to suffering and loss, but also to the wholeness of life in the face of human limitation.

FOREWORD

Angel Martínez-Hernáez's great contribution in this intriguing volume is to use the image of the "what" that stands behind the symptom as a means of canvassing much that really matters in contemporary medical anthropology and psychiatry. Symptoms, as the author invokes them, inform the reader as much about anthropology and medicine as about patients and illnesses. *What's Behind the Symptom?* is the most thorough elaboration of the semiotics of psychiatry in our era. Commencing with the seemingly secure relation of symptoms and signs and a disarming—if soon to be ensnaring—definition of his own making, the author draws the reader deeper and deeper into the many confusions, arresting distortions, and creative misunderstandings that confound the work of meaning in medicine and anthropology. His prose is simple and direct, but his goal is anything but. Rather, like a master magician, Martínez-Hernáez conjures up the very reality he seeks to analyze by turning the analysis, as it were, into a simulacrum of the problem itself. This is a major achievement.

So, when all is said and done, what does lie behind symptoms? What looms large in the background of words and categories? What small or vast presence lies hidden beneath the sounds and complaints? A tangle of symbol systems, biology, and the political and economic processes of everyday social experience form this deeper presence. This sociosomatic ganglion connects the subjective with the collective in the context of pathology and in normality too. Psychiatric disorder makes it unavoidable that psychological processes —memory, affect, self—also receive their due in this contextual world of felt signs and storied, signifying lives.

A model of the text may advance the hermeneutics of signs and symptoms, as the author avers, but this comfortable (and comforting) image of the book, the page, the sentence now seems to me simply too intellectualist, too redolent of the security of the library to be a useful key to overheated or frigid worlds where danger is at the heart of things, uncertainty is everywhere and action, even when it so clearly falls short or worsens things, still must take place. Local worlds are places of overwhelming practicality. They are no more texts than they are games. So what are they? One wants to say they are the very stuff of lived experience, the moral entanglement of collective and individual experience. But what is experience and how does it relate to signs and symptoms? Is experience to psychiatry as symptom is to anthropology? Or is it the other way round?

There are destabilizing thoughts galore here that Martínez-Hernáez draws into a scholarly account that unsettles conventional understandings. Medical anthropology seems more the product of the Hedgehog than the Fox we usually take it to be. Signs and symptoms run like a golden thread as the core knowledge of a discipline that is shown to have accumulated a trove of concepts and findings that illumine this subject. With close readings of Freud, Kraepelin, and a generation of psychiatric anthropologists, Martínez-Hernáez tells, along the way, several different stories, including those of anthropology, psychiatry, psychiatric epidemiology, and semiotics. But above all this is the story of the symptom in medical anthropology.

It must be extraordinary that cries of pain and other human complaints are formulated by psychiatry and anthroplogy primarily as epistemological debates over the kind of knowledge we have of them and the kind of knowledge they represent. The question of the ontology of symptoms as forms of living in the world—even with all the interest in phenomenology —is a decidedly secondary interest in psychiatric anthropology, and in psychiatry. The ethical question of what good this knowledge is for—seems equally secondary. This must be telling us something about the disciplines. Psychiatric anthropology, like psychiatry itself, begins not at all with the ethical act of affirming the patient's experience of suffering, acknowledging the pain and tribulation. In that sense, symptoms and signs lose a crucial significance. Whether deconstructed by clinicians or ethnographers the action seems to be a search for something else (the disease state, the political economy, the embodied symbol). Something else—usually said to be deeper, hidden, more significant—replaces the human voice and sentiment. Interpretation can annul the human project itself when it avoids the *prima facie* expression of suffering. Medicine misconceives what is at stake when it emphasizes "First, do no harm." Anthropology does the same when interpretation precedes acknowledgment. Symptoms and signs, to paraphrase Emmanuel Levinas, are useless in themselves. They become humanly useful when they draw attention to the injured, to the disabled, so they can be seen, heard, engaged, and helped. Where is this utterly human ethical project amidst the icons, indexes and other vehicles of meaning that preoccupy the scholars in today's psychiatric anthropology? What about the symptoms of social injustice and health inequalities as a *raison d'être* for moving psychiatric anthropology toward policies and programs? This has become a major feature of the anthropology of infectious disease. Shouldn't it be a serious focus in psychiatric anthropology as well?

—Arthur Kleinman

CHAPTER 1

What Is Behind The Symptom?

Car l'exactitude se distingue de la verité, et la conjecture n'exclut pas la rigueur. [For exactness is distinct from truth, and conjecture does not exclude rigor.]

—Jacques Lacan, *Écrits*

In *The Vital Balance*, the American psychiatrist Karl Menninger posed a question that, despite its apparent simplicity, has been of great importance in the history of psychiatry: "What is behind the symptom?" (1963, p. 325). He was seeking what was, in his opinion, the ultimate meaning of symptoms for, in his words, "no man steals a watch for the sole purpose of obtaining a timepiece. No man cuts his throat merely in order to die." "Human motivation is not that simple," but the result of a multitude of pressures and events that the therapist must discover and describe (p. 326).

From the end of the 18th century, when psychiatry was taking its first steps as "special Medicine" (Castel, 1980, p. 109), to the period in which Menninger formulated his theory on the importance of environmental pressures on mental imbalance (1963), the problem of the nature of the symptom has been at the center of a series of psychological and psychiatric debates. Even in the biologicist period in which we are immersed at present, the question of the nature and content of the symptom has become common ground for psychiatric reflection (Jackson, 1992; Wilson, 1993). In fact, we are faced with one of those fundamental scientific questions that transcends fashions and trends, since it addresses the very purpose of the discipline: the study and alleviation of mental dysfunction.

1

Precisely because of the key importance of the problem of symptom for psychiatry, some situations may at first glance seem to be paradoxical. I am thinking, in particular, of the interest that has recently been generated in disciplines with no therapeutic aims, such as anthropology, by questions about symptoms, illness complaints, idioms of distress and expressions of affliction. In a short time, what had been understood by psychiatry to be a pathophysiological, or at least a psychological, reality has been understood to be a cultural manifestation, a highly suggestive metaphor, a symbol which condenses social and political-economic contradictions. I believe that in spite of the disparity of opinions in anthropology, most authors will agree with this, from Mary-Jo DelVecchio Good and Byron Good (1981) to Margaret Lock (1991), from Arthur Kleinman (1988a) to Scheper-Hughes (1992), from Mariella Pandolfi (1990) to the caustic Michael Taussig (1980).

In this intellectual context in which psychiatry and anthropology meet, the question about the nature of symptoms seems to have acquired greater complexity. What is a symptom? A pathophysiological reality or a cultural manifestation? What is behind the symptom? An intrapsychic conflict or the complex structures of political economy? And just as importantly, how can we explain a symptom? Using an interpretive approach or a natural-science one? By clinical inference or ethnographic interpretation? The issue demands some sort of clarification.

ANTHROPOLOGY OR PSYCHIATRY?

During the last two decades, the problem of symptom has attracted the attention of those anthropologists who, from interpretive, critical-interpretive, semiotic or hermeneutic perspectives, have attempted to construct an ethnographic approach to illness and its expressions within so-called medical anthropology, psychiatric anthropology, anthropology of health and illness and, in other national traditions, *anthropologie médicale* (France), *antropología de la medicina* (Spain and Latin America) or *antropologia medica* (Italy).

Most studies of this sort are to be found in the United States, although this by no means implies that there is a homogeneity of approaches. Some authors, for example, have avoided the atheoretical empiricism of the North American culturalist and sociological approach in an attempt to combine theory and ethnographic practice (Kleinman, 1980, 1995; Good, 1977, 1994). Other authors, in line with these theoreticians, have developed a pragmatic approach called "clinically applied anthropology,"[1] the main focus of which is not so much illness and symptoms but the problems which derive from the practice of Western medicine (Chrisman & Maretzki, 1982; Chrisman & Johnson, 1990). As was to be expected, some authors have been quick to criticize this excess of concessions to the medical sciences and have developed a more independent and critical position grounded in Marxist and neo-Marxist perspectives which has come to be called "critical medical anthropology" (Baer, Singer & Johnsen, 1986; Singer, Baer & Lazarus, 1990; Singer, 1990, 1995). The materialistic orientation of this tendency has not given much attention to the semiotic and hermeneutic approaches. However, its criticisms have given rise to new theories, for instance the approach known as "critically applied medical anthropology,"[1] (Scheper-Hughes, 1990) or, what is more interesting here, that mixture of interpretivism and historicism, of genealogical thought and embodiment theory which is the "critical-interpretive perspective" (Lock & Scheper-Hughes, 1990).

Despite the enormous variety of tendencies and terminology generated in recent years, we can speak of the existence of an interpretive anthropology of illness which, with greater or lesser critical intent, has approached symptoms as expressive forms which reflect local worlds of meaning (Good, 1977, 1994; Kleinman, 1980; Good & Good, 1981; Scheper-Hughes & Lock, 1987; Lock, 1990; Kirmayer, 1992; Scheper-Hughes, 1992). The ethnographic task here has been to gain access to the cultural domain within which symptoms are experienced, understood, and interpreted. This approach reflects the influences of European hermeneutic philosophy (Gadamer, 1975; Ricoeur, 1969) as well as those of the leading authors in symbolic and interpretive cultural anthropology of the 1960s and 1970s such as Victor Turner and Clifford Geertz. As is well known, these two anthropologists were committed to an approach that focused on an interpretation of symbols, meanings and clusters of meanings more than on the possibility of a causalist and natural-scientific knowledge of sociocultural phenomena. As Geertz put it, they were "looking less for the sort of thing that connects planets and pendulums and more for the sort that connects chrysanthemums and swords"[2] (1983, p. 19).

Whereas in anthropology symptoms have been of interest as meaningful realities, the theoretical path taken in psychiatry has been very different. Following a historical confrontation between biological, psychological, phenomenological, psychosocial and even political-economic approaches, psychiatry opted for a biological orientation which elevated it to the rank of a speciality within Western medicine, sometimes called biomedicine. The old arguments about the role of the sex life, the Oedipus complex, intrapsychic conflicts (psychoanalytical theories), family communication (systemic theories), the State and its institutions (antipsychiatric theories) or existential forms of *being-in-the-world* (phenomenological and existentialist theories)[3] have given way to more biologized principles. As a result, symptoms are understood in terms of organic dysfunction or abnormality. In other words, an attempt has been made to reduce symptoms to the conceptual domain of what in biomedical terminology constitutes signs of disease. Here signs are understood to be objective evidence of disease which can be perceived by a professional, while symptoms, on the other hand, are viewed as more ambiguous and uncertain because they originate in the perception and expression of the patients themselves. Stone, for example, gives the following definition in his *American Psychiatric Glossary* (1988): "Sign: objective evidence of disease or disorder. See also symptom." And: "Symptom: A specific manifestation of a patient, condition indicative of an abnormal or mental state; a subjective perception of illness" (p. 98).[4]

It should be noted that "sign" and "symptom," in their most divergent senses, denote completely different orders of reality. Signs, as defined in psychiatric and biomedical terminology, are closely connected to what has been understood in semiotics as indices or natural signals. In the same way that we infer the presence of fire when we see smoke, disease can also be inferred from medical signs such as fever. Neither fever nor smoke (at least not usually in the latter case) is a meaningful creation based on semiotic or cultural conventions; rather, they are both natural occurrences. Signs, then, are characteristically a part of a natural and self-evident reality which, like the tip of an iceberg, only enter the domain of semiosis[5] (signification) to the extent that they are interpreted, as a particular disease is inferred from the presence of fever.

In contrast, symptoms refer to a "patient's self-report," to "a subjective perception." Without going any deeper into what is meant here by the word "subjective," we can say that symptoms are the patient's interpretation of a series of bodily, psychic and emotional sensations: "I've got a headache," "I feel depressed," "I'm a bundle of nerves." Symptoms are thus verbalized or mimed and, therefore, their construction reflects the expressive needs of the speaker. So they arise not as part of a physical reality or the visible effect of a cause, but as a human expression that embodies meaning.

There is a world of difference between a case of eczema and a statement such as "My heart is upset." It is no accident that symptoms have constituted a problem of immense proportions in psychiatry and medicine. Eczema is always eczema, but a complaint of heart distress is not the same when expressed by an Iranian woman, a character in a European romantic novel, a patient from Barcelona with coronary heart disease, or a Nahuatl native from Hueyapan. For the Iranian woman, the heart is a physiological organ which is vulnerable to the oppression of daily life and the problems of feminine sexuality (Good, 1977); for others, however, it may be the (symbolic) center of emotional life (romantic characters), an organ that does not function as it should (Barcelona patient), or an organ necessary for the digestion of food (the Nahuatls) (Alvarez, 1987).[6]

The distinction between sign and symptom is of greater importance in clinical knowledge and practice than has generally been recognized. Psychoanalysis, for example, has even semioticized some physical signs; that is to say, what at first seemed to be a sign is understood as a symptom. Here I am thinking of the meaning of "simulation of childbirth" which Freud attributes to Dora's fever and perityphlitis in *Fragments of an Analysis of a Case of Hysteria* (1988, p. 87). I am also thinking of Freud's and Breuer's interpretation of Anna O's *tussis nervosa* in *Studies on Hysteria* (Breuer & Freud 1985, p. 48). It is even reasonable to state that any psychoanalyst will understand both fever and eczema to be something more than mere pathophysiological signs.[7] Nevertheless, contemporary psychiatry and biomedicine have more often than not adopted the opposite view. That is to say, symptoms are objectified as if they were physical signs that bespeak a natural, universal and abiographical reality.

As we can deduce from the foregoing discussion, widely differing problems and interests have arisen around symptoms: anthropologists are searching for meanings while psychiatrists are looking for pathologies. What, then, should we make of Geertz's identification of certain similarities between anthropological interpretation and clinical inference?

Clifford Geertz has stated that the common ground of ethnographic interpretation and clinical diagnosis is that both procedures generalize not across cases, but within them. That is to say, laws are not formulated through the collection of individual cases, but by situating the case within an intelligible context. Although Geertz does not speak in these terms, in both types of interpretation the procedure is one of abduction,[8] and up to this point we can agree with him. But if we attempt to go any further with the analogy we run the risk of confusing two approaches which are essentially very different, at least in the context of the type of anthropology and psychiatry with which we are dealing. Let us have a look at what Geertz himself said because, although only tangentially, he provides us with the keys for understanding the limits of his analogy:

> To generalize within cases is usually called, at least in medicine and depth psychology, clinical inference. Rather than beginning with a set of observations and attempting to subsume them under a governing law, such inference begins with a set of (presumptive) signifiers and attempts to place them within an intelligible frame. Measures are matched to theoretical predictions, but symptoms (even when they are measured) are scanned for theoretical peculiarities—that is, they are diagnosed. In the study of culture the signifiers are not symptoms or clusters of symptoms, but symbolic acts or clusters of symbolic acts, and the aim is not therapy but the analysis of social discourse. But the way in which theory is used—to ferret out the unapparent import of things—is the same (1973, p. 26).

Geertz locates the analogical force that joins anthropological and clinical generalization in a parallelism: symbols are assigned to cultural contexts in the same way as symptoms are assigned to pathological categories. If the idea of generalization is understood in its widest sense, the parallel is not at all implausible. Nevertheless, if we try to push the analogy further, differences begin to show up.

A careful reading of the above quotation reveals an idea of only tangential importance to Geertz' argument: the similarity established between symptoms and signifiers. This link reveals one of the main differences between clinical and anthropological generalization, at least when they both attempt to account for the phenomenon of the symptom.[9] That is to say, the former considers the symptoms to be signifiers while the latter interprets them as meanings.[9] In other words, in clinical inference the context of meaning is provided by a medical world view and, for this reason, the symptom is a sort of natural signifier whose meaning depends on the receiver.[10] However, from the perspective of interpretive anthropology, the important thing is the original significance of the symptom as the expression of the informant's distress. And it is not the same thing to interpret this expression—whether it be a verbal complaint or a gesture—in terms of how its content corresponds to a domain of meaning, as it is to regard symptoms as natural or psychophysiological realities.

For example, the auditory hallucinations of a North American Amerind in mourning may be interesting from an ethnographic point of view inasmuch as they reveal a way of viewing the world that brings together a series of elements: the loss of a spouse; a particular conception of how to mourn; and the idea that the spirit of the deceased speaks from another dimension with the individual in question (Kleinman, 1988b, p. 11). Here we are faced with a procedure of generalization within a case which enables us to assign the symptom to a cultural framework. Consequently, the symptom can be seen as a symbol or as a "text"—as a way of fixing or objectifying *something that is said*[11]—interpreted in terms of a "context" that qualifies and filters the polysemic nature of the symptom. This kind of generalization does not involve universalizing the symptom, since it can have other meanings in other contexts, but assigning it to a particular cultural domain.

However, if we respond to an auditory hallucination as if it were a physical sign and we proceed to diagnose and treat it, we are generalizing in a manner that has other connotations. In this case, we attempt to define the phenomenon by reference to the relation this symptom has with other symptoms and signs, as well as to the prognosis, course and duration of the illness. Up to this point in the argument, symptoms can be assigned to the context of a particular psychopathology just as they can be assigned to a particular cultural framework, but with the peculiarity that a universal mechanism of causality is added to the clinical contextualization, making it clearly different from the ethnographic procedure. Thus, the diagnosis will assume that there is a preestablished association between auditory hallucinations and some pathophysiological process such as the hyperactivation of the cerebral dopaminergetic pathways. The diagnosis, in turn, will permit treatment with antipsychotic drugs to block the supposed neurochemical hyperactivation. The result will be, then, very different from the kind of generalization carried out from the ethnographic perspective. The important thing will be to associate the symptom with a series of presumedly universal psychophysiological processes, not with its context of meaning. In other words, and quoting Geertz himself, we shall be operating from supposed laws governing relationships between planets and pendulums (auditory hallucinations and neurochemical disorders) rather than from associations of meaning between chrysanthemums and swords (hearing voices and cultural conceptions about mourning).

What, then, does a symptom involve? In order to apprehend the significance of what appears to be an enigma, whether it arises as a simple complaint or as a complicated set of representations, the question we must ask is: What does it mean? The symptom is thus restored to the epistemological domain of comprehension (*Verstehen*) and, therefore, is understood in relation to a biographical, cultural and historico-cultural context. Thus we find ourselves on ground which, ever since Dilthey, seems to be reserved for the so-called sciences of the spirit (*Geisteswissenschaften*) (Dilthey, 1949; Ricoeur, 1979; Habermas, 1989) and which at present are known as the social and human sciences.

If, on the other hand, our question is formulated as "What are the causes of a symptom?" and "What are the processes and facts involved in an event of this sort?", the answer is caught up in the search for an explanation (*Erklärung*). Here the concept of explanation is understood as a positivist type of knowledge characteristic of the natural-science approach. Obviously, what is taking place here is not a search for meaning, but an inquiry, using causalist logic, into the relation between symptoms and a series of underlying biological and psychobiological processes.

By now, it should be clear that to ask "What does a symptom mean?" is not the same as to ask "What is it caused by?" These questions generate different derivations of knowledge and, therefore, a conflict of interpretations, even though it is not strictly necessary to exclude explanation (*Erklärung*) from the analytic repertoire of the social sciences. For example, Ricoeur, in opposition to the classical Diltheyian identification of comprehension with "sciences of the spirit" and explanation with "natural sciences," has skillfully shown us how it is possible to understand comprehension and explanation as a two-way dialectic moving from comprehension to explanation and vice versa (Ricoeur, 1979)—provided, of course, that this movement takes place within the same sphere of meaningful reality or, to use another image, within the hermeneutic arc or circle (Ricoeur, 1979). Ricoeur's insight directs our attention to a reality which is much more complex than was initially suggested, but which does not discount the possibility of there being a difference between comprehension and explanation, at least in situations of great contrast. Clinical diagnosis, for example, depends on a minimum understanding of the patient's account of symptoms, but for authors such as Popper, this would be a clear case of "causal explanation", because it is subject to laws of prediction or—more correctly in this case—prognosis (Popper, 1985).[12] On the other hand, the structuralism of Lévi-Strauss, which is taken by Ricoeur as a paradigmatic example of the explanation-comprehension dialectic (1979, p. 94), suggests the possibility of a panhuman binary logic and may instead be fully within the domain of explanation (*Erklärung*), but there is no doubt that it has not enabled us even to outline causalities, much less to make predictions. Of course, it is difficult to establish clear differences between comprehension and explanation but, at their extremes, the ambiguities tend to disappear: a) symptom as a natural consequence of psychophysiological processes and b) symptom as a message, text, symbol or discourse. We can go further into this disparity of approaches by using one of Ryle's well-known dilemmas.

WINKS OR TWITCHES?

With the double purpose of defining both the domain of what is culturally significant, and the aim of ethnographic interpretation, in his essay "Thick Description: Toward an Interpretive Theory of Culture" (1973) Clifford Geertz describes one of Ryle's dilemmas. Ryle is a thinker from the Oxford school who is well known for (among other things) attempting to dismantle the Cartesian idea that there is a spirit inhabiting the body—"a ghost in the machine" (Ryle, 1967, p. 19)—and for developing his arguments through dilemmas or logical problems.

The dilemma which concerns us here is the following: two boys quickly contract the eyelid of their right eye. For one of them it is an unintentional action, more specifically a twitch; for the other it is a wink. These actions are quite different, but observed from a phenomenological point of view, in their outward form, they seem to be similar if not identical. Nevertheless, it is clear that a wink is not a twitch. A wink is a meaningful and deliberate action. It is both a movement and a linguistic sign; that is to say, it conveys meaning, and its use is governed by a preexisting socially established code. On the other hand, we can say that a twitch is a psychophysiological movement produced by the involuntary contraction of one or several muscles and which does not form part, at least in any obvious way, of the domain of language.[13]

Geertz (and Ryle) show how some techniques of "thin" description, such as photography and behaviorist models, cannot account for the difference between a wink and a twitch.[14] A photographic image or a behavioral description can only provide evidence of eyelid contraction. Any worthwhile description, then, should introduce a principle which defines the contexts in which this movement acquires meaning, both for the sender and for the receivers of the message; borrowing Ryle's terminology, Geertz characterizes this as "thick" (as opposed to "thin") description.

Thick description is also a complex and often problematic exercise. A wink does not always have the same significance, because the meaning of a communicative action is closely dependent on its context. It is not the same to wink an eye with the aim of conspiring with a friend as with the aim of imitating somebody else who may not have winked with the discretion that is required of a conspiracy. In the same way that we may mistakenly identify a wink with a twitch, we may also mistakenly understand that there is a conspiracy instead of merely parody and ridicule, but this is not all. Things can get even more complicated. Let us suppose that the individual that we are observing is the same as the one who winked his eye to parody someone else whose intention was to conspire, but who is now at home practicing in front of the mirror to perfect his skills. Here also there is a rapid movement of the eyelid and a wink, but the referent is no longer parody but the rehearsal of parody. As is logical, the dilemma can be extended and made infinitely more complex; however, once it has reached this point it has fulfilled its function.

The comparison has the virtue of being extremely versatile. In principle, Geertz's original intention is theoretical: it attempts to define ethnography as thick description in contrast to thin description, in which a twitch, a wink of complicity, parody or rehearsal for parody would be the same. What he is trying to tell us is that we should understand ethnography as the exegesis of complex and hierarchical structures of signification which allow us to sort out the real meaning of a wink. However, the dilemma in question also evokes a set of oppositions: apparent comprehension *versus* deep comprehension, thin description *versus* thick description. This is a clear example of a conflict of interpretations, an opposition in which the different interpretations are tested and their advantages and limitations shown.

On the one hand, analyzing the reality of a purely phenomenal form implies not only recording a wink and a twitch as the same movement, but also the adoption of a specific theoretical position: to focus almost exclusively on what is directly observable and on movement as a merely natural or crude signifier. Here, the movement of the eyelid is treated as a physical sign (as if it were a phenomenon of the same order as eczema, for instance) which does not reflect expressions of a semiosic nature, but whose meaning depends exclusively on the interpreter or receiver.

On the other hand, understanding the movement of the eyelid as a complex and sometimes involved set of meanings assumes that there is a distinction between a wink and a twitch, and reflects a focus on socially constructed meaning and not only on a supposedly natural signifier. In other words, it understands the movement of the eye as potentially codified and intentional, evoking a local world of meanings.

One of the most pressing problems of contemporary psychiatry is precisely the manipulation in clinical practice of symptoms as if they were signs, of winks as if they were twitches which do not reflect a linguistic and cultural logic. In an almost perfect and by no means fortuitous counterpoint, one of the strategies of interpretive medical and psychiatric anthropology is to approach symptoms as winks embodying meanings which bespeak cultural worlds of affliction and suffering. Although we shall later have the chance to go further into this conflict of interpretations, let us pause here to take a look at how it becomes apparent in the analysis of a particular case.

MAL D'OLLO OR PARANOID DISORDER?

During my fieldwork in different psychiatric hospitals in Barcelona (Spain), I had the opportunity to study a case which may be considered to be an example of how clinical and ethnographic interpretations can come into conflict. From the psychiatric point of view, the case was described in the following way:

> Fifty-year-old patient with no previous psychiatric history who was brought to the emergency room by her family because she had had symptoms of paranoia for the previous 48 hours. Her ideas of persecution and harm had caused behavioral disorder. Unstructured ideas of reference which are accompanied by moderate perplexity, psychomotor disturbance and insomnia. The symptoms appear suddenly and with no apparent cause. From what her family says there is no evidence of basic disorders in the area of personality.
>
> Diagnosis: Acute paranoid disorder.

The structure and explanatory style is typical of clinical reports written in biomedical psychiatric institutions. The important thing in the report is the logical grouping of the different symptoms with the aim of producing a diagnosis, whether this might be "delusional (paranoid) disorder," "brief reactive psychosis," or "schizophreniform disorder," which are three diagnostic categories most closely matching the above description. Symptoms such as "ideas of persecution and harm" and "ideas of reference" are related to the patient's previous history, the onset of symptoms, and also to signs arising from a psychophysiological logic which is barely sketched in the clinical report. The reason for this superficial treatment is not a rejection of the possible causal relation between symptoms and pathophysiological processes, but the fact that the causes of these processes are, to date, only hypothetical. As yet there is no biological test which is able to identify an acute paranoid disorder or a persecutory idea as positive realities.

A careful reading of the report also calls our attention to the fact that we know nothing of the meaning of the patient's behavior, symptoms and statements. All we know is that there are ideas of persecution, but not who persecutes or why, and what form this persecution takes from the patient's point of view. The same can be said of the symptom reported as "ideas of reference." Here we can deduce that the patient symbolically constructs the order of events in an egocentric fashion. But we do not know which events are at issue, or what hierarchy of meanings makes sense of this type of experience. And the fact is that special emphasis is given to the formal configuration of the symptoms. In other words, what is important here is not so much to establish the meaningful connections that contextualize a rapid movement of the eyelid or an idea of persecution, but rather to focus on the movement, and the idea, as a natural signifier which reflects a universal psychopathological process.[15]

The priority given to the signifier over the meaning involves a clear reification of the subjective perceptions of the patient: the symptoms. In fact, in the report, there is no noticeable difference in the way signs such as "psychomotor disturbance" and symptoms such as "ideas of reference" are treated, even when we are clearly faced with two different phenomena. Psychomotor disturbance is more easily identifiable with an involuntary movement, a sign lacking an original meaning. It can also be recorded visually, it can be observed. But the idea of reference belongs to the biographical and cultural domain of the patient. In other words, its properties have more in common with those of a wink which, as well as being observed, must also be read and interpreted. However, the report places both signs and symptoms on the same level of reification; ideas of reference can be considered to be "unstructured" in the same way that one can speak of a moderate perplexity. The end result is a psychopathological landscape which seems to have great internal coherence, but which at the same time is isolated from the biographical, historical and cultural framework within which it could acquire a specific meaning. So, the description can be generalized and extrapolated to any cultural and historic framework. But the problem here is that this approach confuses winks and twitches.

For the moment, let us try to distance ourselves from the clinical perspective with its focus on symptomatology and diagnosis, and concentrate on the same case from an ethnographic point of view; that is to say, we shall concentrate on the meanings of symptoms as if they were winks. The following account is taken from my field notes:

> Elvira (our informant) had recently been back to her village, a small hamlet in Galicia (in the northwest of Spain) which she had left some time previously for economic reasons. The reason for her return was a family problem: her mother had died a few months before. As her father, a victim of leukemia, had already been dead for three decades, the death of her mother meant that the inheritance had to be shared out. In Galicia, the inheritance is divided between sons and daughters in a special way: the *casado en casa* or *millorado* (the

married brother or sister who lives at home) receives the *millora* (two thirds of the estate), while the remaining third must be divided in equal parts among all the brothers and sisters (including the *casado en casa*).[16] Although this system is institutionalized, it is generally the cause of serious disagreements. It is hardly surprising, then, that in this case as well there were arguments about how to divide up the land.

On her return to Barcelona, Elvira began to feel strange, as if she were being hounded: "people in the street were looking at me." She started to believe that she was being followed by a group of journalists, and attempted to avoid them by going in and out of different bars. The attitude of passersby seemed to reflect a conspiracy. She also felt that things had changed with her workmates: their voices were different now. On top of all of this was her conviction that she was suffering from leukemia. For our informant, it was a clear case of the evil eye caused by the greed and jealousy of her brothers and sisters who may have been assisted by the village *meiga* or witch.

In Galician culture, the *mal d'ollo* (evil eye) is associated with the idea of harm; for example, the transmission of an illness. In this cultural domain, a person's mere presence, touch, or shadow can cause illnesses such as *o aire, o enganido* or *a sombra*, so Elvira did all she could to keep a prudent distance between herself and her interlocutors. In this case, the evil that could be transmitted to her was "leukemia." Elvira had just turned fifty, the same age as her father when he died of this illness.

This approach in no way resembles the explanatory style of the psychiatric report. Here the case is analyzed in a way which relates symptoms to biography and cultural context through meaning. To borrow Geertz' words, "the said" is central to the description. Let us take, for example, three of the most important symptoms in the clinical description: the ideas of harm, persecution and reference. From the ethnographic point of view, these three symptoms are tightly bound together, not because they reflect a diagnostic category called "brief reactive psychosis" or "delusional (paranoid) disorder," but because they are related in a system of meanings of the following type: "An individual from the Galician cultural domain believes that, because of the greed of her family, she has been subjected to the evil eye, the result of which is the transmission of an illness which will be brought about by the contact or presence of other individuals. For this reason she believes she is being persecuted, she interprets the actions of others in terms of her own fears, and she avoids interpersonal relationships of any sort."

In the same way that the auditory hallucinations of an Amerind can form part of a code of meanings about mourning, or that winks can acquire sense from the context, here the ideas of reference, persecution, and harm also reflect local worlds of meaning. The aim of an ethnographic description such as the one that has just been presented is to reveal these connections. What is important is not to find universal manifestations whose logic reflects psychophysiological processes, but to restore meaning to meaning by assigning symptoms to their context of use. From this point of view, as I have already argued, generalization within a case is very different from clinical-psychiatric generalization, because it is a generalization and also a particularization: a generalization because the cultural domain conceived goes beyond the informant in question, and a particularization because it does not make hasty interpretations of symptoms on the basis of universal criteria.

The limitation to a particular cultural domain is also reflected by the explanatory style. In the clinical report, the concepts and the categories used reflect the researcher's own environment; it speaks of paranoid disorder, persecutory ideas, insomnia, moderate perplexity, psychomotor disturbance, etc. The ethnographic description, however, combines jargon with terms which belong to the environment of the informant such as *millora, casado en casa, mal d'ollo* (the evil eye), *a sombra, o enganido* and *meiga*, among others. And, obviously, it is not the same to speak of the evil eye as of paranoid disorder. In the same way, a description using the diagnostic and symptomatic categories of the observer (dysthymia, generalized anxiety disorder, chronic paranoid schizophrenia, bipolar disorder, etc.) is not the same as a description using terms from the point of view of the informant; that is to say, the evil eye or any other experiences of distress known as folk illnesses or *culture-bound syndromes* such as *chisara-chisara, zuwadanda, empacho, susto, aire, agua, pasmo, bilis, ataque de nervios, celos, mal de pelea, latido, cólera, koro, amok, gila merian, gila talak, gila kena hantu, otak miring, latah, bah-tsi, dhat, shen-k'uei, qissaatuq, pibloktog, quajimaillituq, pa-feng, pa-leng, boxi, wiitiko, inarun, kiesu, giri, hwa-byung, wool-hwa-byung, buduh kedewandewan, dindirin, djukat, afota, abisinwin, aiyiperi, were agba, were alaso, tuyo, wacinko, tabacazo, shin-byung, tripa ida, ruden rupan, zar, womtia* or *espanto*, among many others.[17] The observer's greater or lesser inclination to totalizing explanation is reflected in the categories used to name the object or the phenomenon being observed.

The dichotomy *experience-near/experience-distant*[18] is another way of expressing this. Despite the fact that these two concepts were employed by Geertz for exclusively anthropological purposes, they are on the border between clinical and ethnographic concerns. It is no coincidence that Geertz borrowed them from the psychoanalytical model of Heinz Kohut who, among his other contributions, analyzed the implications of empathy in the therapeutic interview. For this reason, these concepts have a certain potential for demonstrating possible ways of approaching phenomena such as the ones which we are dealing with here. Geertz himself introduces a clinical example to express the relativity of experiential closeness and distance:

> Clearly, the matter is one of degree, not polar opposition: "fear" is experience-nearer than "phobia", and "phobia" experience-nearer than "ego dyssyntonic"...Confinement to experience-near concepts leaves an ethnographer awash in immediacies, as well as entangled in vernacular. Confinement to experience-distant ones leaves him stranded in abstractions and smothered in jargon (Geertz, 1983, p. 57).

The dichotomy is suggestive, because by differentiating fear from phobia it distinguishes the patient from the practitioner, not in a neutral way but in a way in which fear and the patient constitute the criteria on which both the distinction and the epistemiological positions are based. However, the dichotomy is only an abstraction, since neither experience-near nor experience-distant are experiences of patients, subjects or informants themselves, but distinctions generated during clinical and ethnographic work and which, therefore, belong to the field of the researcher. It is experience-distant to speak of phobia, ego dyssyntonic or paranoid syndrome in the same way as it is experience-near to speak of fear or *mal d'ollo*. However, there is still a difference between those who experience fear or who are subject to the evil eye and the "experience-near" itself, since in the final analysis, what this means is that the observer gets closer to the observed in order to understand the experience better. This procedure, even when it may seem limited, does not imply that other experience is ultimately unknowable. Max Weber clarified this point in the following way:

> ... "One need not have been Caesar in order to understand Caesar". "Recapturing experience" is important for accurate understanding, but not an absolute precondition for its interpretation (Weber, 1968, p. 5).

To highlight our conflict of interpretations we could invoke other concepts as well as the distinction between experience-near and experience-distant concepts, or rather pairs of concepts, such as Pike's well-known polarization between *emic* and *etic* (1967) or, more relevant here, the distinction between *illness* and *disease*[19] in medical anthropology. However, the differences between psychiatric and anthropological interpretation have been made quite clear by this stage: where some perceive symptoms as natural signs (having no original meaning) of a psychopathological reality, others observe a cultural product which refers to a world of meanings.

There are still other significant differences in our conflict of interpretations, such as the fact that for anthropology there is no need to distinguish between the normal and the pathological. For example, the ethnographic description of Elvira does not attempt to diagnose or reveal a pathological process, either in biological terms or from a psychological or psychoanalytic perspective. What is of interest to ethnographers or theoretical anthropologists is not the same as what is of interest to clinicians, whether they be psychiatrists, psychoanalysts or psychologists and whether or not they adopt a hermeneutic approach to understand illness and symptoms. If there is something that clearly separates these two forms of understanding phenomena it is precisely this presence or absence of criteria for distinguishing the normal from the pathological. In fact, this divergence of interests is not exclusive to anthropology and psychiatry. It is, as Max Weber perceptively pointed out, the distance separating the social sciences from what he called the "dogmatic sciences." Speaking of "sociological meaning," he argued that:

> In no case does it refer to an objectively "correct" meaning or one which is "true" in some metaphysical sense. It is this which distinguishes the empirical sciences of action, such as sociology and history, from the dogmatic disciplines in that area, such as jurisprudence, logic, ethics, and esthetics, which seek to ascertain the "true" and "valid" meanings associated with the objects of their investigation (Weber, 1968, p. 4).

Although this passage makes no reference to the so-called health sciences, the distinction is enlightening. The need of the "dogmatic sciences" to distinguish between what is just and what is not, between truth and falsehood, legality and illegality, beauty and ugliness is no different as far as we are concerned from the desire of psychiatry to distinguish the normal from the pathological. Furthermore, like those sciences Weber calls "empirical sciences of action," anthropology does not attempt to find a pathological meaning in phenomena such as illness or symptoms, but rather an "autochthonous" meaning which yields another sort of information: the form in which an expression of distress or a complaint reflects a shared domain of meanings.

This is why symptoms—a word whose etymological meaning is coincidence—can be studied both by contemporary psychiatry and by interpretive psychiatric anthropology. However, we are faced with fundamentally different concepts and problems. For some, the coincidence is between manifestations and pathophysiological processes, while for others it is between meanings and cultural contexts.

NOTES

1. It may be controversial to differentiate between theoreticical and applied work, since the boundary between them is ill-defined and permeable. For some authors such as Singer, Baer or Lazarus (1990), Kleinman and Good would undoubtedly belong to clinically applied anthropology. Nevertheless, I believe that the subsequent shift of these two authors towards more critical perspectives, as well as their theoretical contribution to medical anthropology, distances them from purely applied approaches.

2. Chrysanthemums and swords are a reference to Ruth Benedict's book of the same name (1974).

3. Curiously, while psychiatry has abandoned (although not totally) the phenomenological approach, medical and psychiatric anthropology has used this paradigm as a new option to counter the weakening of the interpretive position. Various contributions have been made in this area: Corin (1990) applied phenomenological principles to the field of schizophrenia; Kleinman and Kleinman (1991) reconverted illness into forms of experience and developed the theoretical basis of an "ethnography of interpersonal experience;" and Csordas (1993, 1994) outlined an "anthropology of embodiment."

4. Medicine and psychiatry also use the term "symptom" in its broad sense, which includes both signs (objective symptoms) and symptoms (subjective symptoms). Here, to prevent terminological confusion, I shall use the distinction sign/symptom and not the distinction objective symptom/subjective symptom.

5. Here I am using Peirce and Eco's distinction between "semiosis" and "semiotics": the former is the phenomenon of meaning, while the latter is the discipline which studies semiosic phenomena. See Eco (1996) and also Peirce (Collected Papers of Charles Sanders Peirce [CP], 5: 484). See also Chapter 9 in this book.

6. Even "heart" can mean different things for physicians of different national traditions, as Thomas Ots has pointed out in his article "A heart is not a heart is not a heart is not a heart" (1993).

7. This is generally true for European psychoanalysis; for example, the Lacanian school, which is closer to the humanities than to biomedicine and biomedical psychiatry. This is evident from a glance at Lacan's *Écrits* (1966).

8. Abduction is recognized to be a form of inference different from both deduction and induction. See Eco for abduction (1984). An interesting interpretation of this concept coined by Peirce can also be found in the *Diccionario de Filosofía* by Ferrater Mora (1988).

9. Obviously, this would not be valid for structuralism in which, as is well known, the signifying logic prevails over meanings. For a critique of the formalism of structuralism, see Ricoeur (1979).

10. For the analogy between symptom and signifier, see Barthes (1985). See Chapter 9 in this book for an in-depth review.

11. Ricoeur has spoken of the text as a unit which is different from the sentence or the word within a sentence (1969) and has attempted to apply the text model to analyze social action or "meaningful action" (1979). The text model has had important repercussions for interpretive anthropology not only in the work of authors such as Geertz, but in that of some medical anthropologists as well. In particular, see Good & Good (1981).

12. Geertz would not agree with this. He says: "The diagnostician doesn't predict measles; he decides that someone has them, or at the very most *anticipates* that someone is rather likely shortly to get them" (197, p. 26). This is a curious intellectual pirouette which enables him to force the analogy between biomedicine and a non-predictive discipline such as anthropology. However, clinical medicine, including psychiatry, also makes predictions, albeit only once the disease has got under way. A neoplasia which indicates a life expectancy of six months or a wound which is certainly fatal are clear cases of prediction.

13. Although Geertz does not say so, this statement is problematic, because from a point of view akin to depth psychology it could be said that a twitch encodes a message.

14. See also Ryle's example of "to knit one's brow" (1967, p.66). See also Ryle (1960).

15. For the priority that contemporary psychiatry gives the signifier over the meaning, see Young (1991).

16. The institution of *millora* or *mejora* is complex and has various forms which, for obvious reasons, are beyond the scope of this chapter. A classic analysis of this topic can be found in Lisón (1983).

17. The literature on culture-bound syndromes is very extensive. There is an interesting compilation in Simons & Hughes (1985).

18. A recent application of the concepts experience-near and experience-distant to the ethnographic and psychiatric interpretations of a case can be found in the work of Shigeyuki Eguchi on *Kitsune-Tsuki* or "fox possession" in a mountain village in Japan (1991).

19. Provisionally we can use Kleinman's definition of these two concepts: "By illness I mean the way individuals and the members of their social network perceive symptoms, categorize and label those symptoms, experience them, and articulate that illness experience through idioms of distress and pathways of help seeking." And: "By disease I mean the way the illness experience is reinterpreted by practitioners in he terms of their theoretical models and through clinical work. When I speak of disease etiology in general, such as in the social production of disease, I am referring to biomedical reformulations of disease as malfunctioning, maladaptation, or structural abnormalities in biological systems" (1986, p. 225).

Part One

On Psychiatric Observation...
Symptoms as Organic Manifestations

Disease is nothing more than an effort made by Nature who, to save the patient, works with all its might to remove the morbid material...Nature uses a method and a chain of symptoms to remove the malignant, harmful material which, should Nature not intervene, would deliver a fatal blow to the machine [my translation].

—Sydenham, *Observationes medicae circa morborum acutorum historiam et curationem*

CHAPTER 2

The Dream
of A Biomedical Psychiatry

We are in an era of remarkable, almost incredible, advances in molecular biology,
in psychiatry—in medicine, in general. And various technological advances have
allowed us to learn remarkable new things from patients that can guide our treatments. Yet these same technologies can also serve to distance us from patients.
While seeing more, we are often at risk of hearing less.

—S. Jackson
The Listening Healer in the History of Psychological Healing.
American Journal of Psychiatry

Few statements define contemporary psychiatry better than the observation that seeing has eclipsed hearing. With the development of molecular
biology and techniques such as computerized tomography (CT), magnetic
resonance imaging (MRI) or the more recent positron emission tomography (PET), new possibilities have become available for increasing our
knowledge of the biological bases of psychopathological processes. To these
advances should be added the boom in psychopharmacology (antidepressants, neuroleptics, anxiolytics, lithium, etc.) and electroconvulsive therapy
(ECT) as well as the development of hypotheses about the neurochemical,
hormonal, genetic and even viral[1] causes of various mental disorders.

In contrast to these spectacular "advances," the psychological and psychosocial tendencies that based their practice on listening attentively to the
patient, empathy, and the meaning of symptoms have been pushed into the
background (Jackson, 1992). Mental disorders are no longer perceived as

peculiar anomalies whose symptoms can be traced to psychological, experiential or biographical mechanisms. Now mental disorders are understood as physical diseases and their symptoms as more or less direct expressions of organic anomalies (Robins & Helzer 1986). "Auditory hallucinations," "paranoid ideations," "feelings of hopelessness," "antisocial behaviors," "irritability," "low self-esteem" and many other manifestations are seen as signs of an underlying biological dysfunction. No longer are they symbolic forms of expression whose meaning is embedded in biography or intrapsychic conflicts, but natural signs which, like the tip of an iceberg, imply a neuropathological reality.

In theory, the treatment of mental disorders as physical diseases has brought psychiatry closer to the model of Western medicine or biomedicine. However, this has not been a clear-cut process, but one characterized by uncertainty. Attempts to place psychiatry within the biomedical framework have come up against the following problems: a) the difficulty of defining specific pathophysiological processes leading to mental disorders; b) the obstacles to direct and specific intervention in etiological pathways; c) the problematic search for universally applicable diagnostic criteria; d) the limited capacity of existing technology to reveal the physical signs of mental disorder; and e) the elusiveness of the special link that is assumed to exist in mental disorders between the affected organ (the brain) and the patient's consciousness.

Contemporary psychiatry, then, has a problematic nature. On the one hand, it attempts to assimilate itself to biomedical theory and practice through research that seeks to locate the biological sources of mental illness, and by promoting the use of brain imaging and treatments such as electroconvulsive therapy (ECT). On the other hand, however, the acceptance of this model reveals the limitations mentioned above. Of these, the most serious is the lack of any etiological knowledge about most mental disorders.

BIOMEDICINE AND PSYCHIATRY: SOME
SILENT ASSUMPTIONS

In *Naissance de la clinique* (*The Birth of the Clinic*), Foucault brilliantly demonstrates how modern medicine arose from what he defines as a modification of the clinical gaze. The turning point which gave rise to positivist medicine is revealed in his comparison of a description by Pomme, an eighteenth-century clinician who tried to cure a case of hysteria with ten to twelve hours of baths a day for ten months, with one by Bayle, a nineteenth- century doctor who was the first to observe and describe the encephalic lesions of general paralysis of the insane (GPI) or paresis (1972, p. v). In a span of less than one hundred years, medical science underwent such a transformation that the quasi-botanical classification of disease entities was overturned by this penetration into the interior of the body. The resulting reorganization of medical knowledge replaced the old "botany of symptoms" with a new "grammar of signs,"[2] the prior emphasis on nosological classification with a study of the sequence of events which give rise to diseases, and the premodern doctor's first question—"What is the matter with you?"—with "Where does it hurt?" (p. xiv).

The features outlined by Foucault in his description of the newly-formed "positive medicine" can be found in the characteristics of contemporary biomedicine. If this emergent science was still a long way from Henle-Köch's bacteriological paradigm, which would provide Western medicine with a model for understanding and eradicating infectious diseases, and the method of clinical experimentation introduced in 1865 by Claude Bernard, it was nonetheless very close to achieving the epistemological conditions which would bring it into being through Bichat's work in pathology and Broussais' physiological approach (Laín Entralgo, 1947; Canguilhem, 1966; López Piñero, 1985). Neo-Hippocratic medicine was already being transformed into a science capable of identifying pathological processes through the penetration of the physician's gaze into the silent and natural universe of the organs.

At first, the paradigm of the clinical gaze was to be the dissection of cadavers, but subsequently there were innovations such as the introduction of radiological examination and laboratory tests at the beginning of the century (Jackson, 1992). The ability to localize abnormality would establish the preeminence of seeing over hearing and, as a result, the analysis of the signs of disease over the interpretation of symptoms. This is the hallmark of a fully-formed biomedical model from which, as we can deduce from the quotation which opened this chapter, we have not yet emerged.

The development of biomedicine has also been associated with a series of theoretical and epistemological principles traditionally regarded as scientific and objective, and therefore unquestionable. This is what Mishler, in an interesting critique of contemporary medical knowledge, calls the "silent assumptions" of the biomedical model (1981, p. 1) or what Gordon, in a subsequent study, refers to as "tenacious assumptions" of Western medicine (1988, p. 19). In fact, both Mishler and Gordon, as well as various scholars of medical anthropology and social medicine, have attempted to demonstrate that the fundamental premises of biomedical knowledge are ideological assumptions rather than objective principles. Here I would like to devote some space to a deeper analysis of three of Mishler's "silent assumptions": first, the definition of disease as a deviation from normal biological functioning; second, the doctrine of specific etiology; and third, the supposed scientific neutrality of biomedicine.

First, one of the most important assumptions of biomedicine is that disease can be distinguished using objective criteria to detect deviation from a biological norm (Mishler, 1981). In other words, the symptoms and signs of disease are expected to be the same in different historical periods and cultural contexts. Even though we cannot deny the proven value of this idea in the analysis and treatment of many diseases, we should not regard it as an unshakable premise. The reality of facts, the "reality" to which the defenders of biomedicine constantly appeal, shows us that numerous disorders, such as culture-bound syndromes, defy the supposed uniformity of both pathological manifestations and criteria of biological anomaly. There are, in fact, no criteria of normality which exist independently of the sociocultural characteristics of different populations (Mishler, 1981, p. 4). And this principle of relativity (not necessarily of relativism) is applicable not only to existing cultural diversity but also to the multiplicity of groups sharing the same cultural context. It is well known that the same physical disorder is experienced very differently by a Wall Street executive, a lumberjack, a monk, and a combat pilot. Hypotension, for example, may pass unnoticed by the monk but may be a most worrisome disorder for the pilot.

If biomedical knowledge is limited, like all knowledge, by the construction of categories and criteria which establish the reality of facts, can these criteria be totally independent of the context of cultural values, aesthetic forms, and political-economic conditions within which they have been produced? In reply to this question, let us consider a simple example: the fact that up until only twenty years ago, psychiatry understood homosexuality as a perversion, and therefore as a pathological phenomenon (Ey, Bernard & Brisset, 1978). Are we dealing with a deviation from normal biological functioning? Obviously not. Rather it is an arbitrary—and clearly moralizing—cultural construction. Faced with such notions of normality and abnormality, we should ask: normal for whom? And normal for what? (Mishler, 1981, p. 4). In short, the golden rule which the biomedical model uses to distinguish disease is not an aseptic, value-free criterion but a socially normative concept of what is biologically normal. Canguilhem sheds light on this question in *La Connaissance de la Vie*: "*Toujours le concept du 'normal', dans l'ordre humain, reste un concept normatif et de portée proprement philosophique*" [The concept of the normal, in the human order, always remains a normative concept of inherently philosophical import] [my translation] (1992, p. 169).

Second, no less interesting is the so-called "doctrine of specific etiology" of diseases (Dubos, 1959, [1952] 1992; Mishler, 1981). This notion realized its full potential when the so-called Henle-Köch paradigm, which ushered in the bacteriological era, became the dominant model in the study of the causal processes of diseases (Rosen, [1958] 1993; Trostle, 1986), pushing anti-contagionist theories into the background.

This doctrine is based on the idea that all diseases can be traced to a single biological cause. The justification for this approach is the pragmatic efficacy of germ theory in the treatment of infectious diseases, a success story that has tended to reduce history and culture to insignificant and epiphenomenal factors in disease causation. However, different knowledge traditions from within Western medicine, such as social medicine or social epidemiology, and from the social sciences, such as medical anthropology and medical sociology, treat this argument more as an ideological assumption than as an unquestionable principle. Let us consider two classic examples which have a certain illustrative value.

The first is the historico-demographic research carried out by McKeown (1976) on tuberculosis in England and Wales, where death rates from this disease decreased before there was any effective chemotherapy.[3] McKeown's explanation for this paradox is the gradual introduction over the course of the nineteenth century of fundamental changes in the nutritional status of the population as a result of advances in agriculture and an increase in the food supply. These changes probably cannot be isolated from the socioeconomic transformations that shook Britain during this period. But whether we limit our explanation to simple technological improvements or extend it to include the development of capitalism, what is important is that the cause of tuberculosis cannot be understood as an exclusively biological phenomenon, nor can effective treatment (chemotherapy and the BCG vaccination) alone account for the decrease in death rates. On the contrary, from McKeown's perspective, disease incidence, frequency, etiology, outcome, and mortality rates are the result of complex and multicausal networks involving a multiplicity of factors.[4]

The second example is that of voodoo death, a phenomenon in which the breaking of a social norm results in the almost immediate death of the transgressor. Often a medicine man or someone of certain ritual standing predicts the future death of the person concerned.[5]

From a strictly biomedical point of view, voodoo death cannot be explained. However, in the 1940s, Cannon attempted to outline a hypothesis describing a series of associated factors which form a vicious circle (1942). The social isolation caused by the loss of the kinship network, a social death that sets in motion the rituals of mourning, which sever any remaining connections to the world of the living; the victim's acceptance of inevitable death; the sense of panic; and the excessive activity of the sympathico-adrenal system would interact complexly to cause a reduction in the volume of circulating blood and a fall in blood pressure. According to this hypothesis, death would result from this special interaction of social, psychological and biological factors subjecting the victim to ever-increasing pressure.

Despite the passage of time and the sometimes ethnocentric tone of Cannon's article, his hypothesis is one of the most important predecessors of the so-called social support-stress-disease theory, a paradigm that regards disease as the consequence of a complex and multicausal process in which both social and biological factors intervene.[6] Although Cannon believed that voodoo death was "so extraordinary and so foreign to the experience of civilized people that it seems incredible" (1942, p. 169), very similar processes have been observed in Western societies for some time. For example, various prospective epidemiological studies have revealed that the loss of social networks in these societies is associated with an increase in death and morbidity rates (Berkman & Syme, 1979; House, Landis & Umberson, 1988), a clear indication that the impact of social isolation on health levels should not be interpreted as a phenomenon alien to industrialized societies. Similarly, labeling—another element of voodoo death—is known to affect the health of first-world populations. This is the case of the Bloom and Monterossa study monitoring over seventy North Americans wrongly diagnosed as having hypertension. The authors show how simple labeling involves a considerable worsening of health and the appearance of depressive symptoms (1981, p. 1228). To sum up, studies such as McKeown's and Cannon's demonstrate that, biomedical perception notwithstanding, disease is the consequence of multicausal networks in which biological processes are influenced by such exogenous and apparently epiphenomenal elements as labeling and social networks.[7]

Third, the doctrine of specific etiology and the associated notion of disease as a deviation from a biological norm have increased the pragmatic efficacy of biomedicine and consolidated its hegemony over other systems of medical knowledge. This supremacy has not only given rise to a taxonomy of disease presumed to be universal, but also to a confusion of bio-medical categories with actual pathological reality. As Mishler points out: "The biomedical model is treated as *the* representation or picture of reality rather than understood as *a* representation" (1981, p. 1) [italics in original].

This identification between representation and reality is revealed in such supposedly insignificant matters as the names used to identify medical traditions. Western biomedicine is simply "medicine," while other therapeutic systems require adjectives to qualify and identify them: Chinese medicine, Ayurvedic medicine, osteopathic medicine, homeopathic medicine and so on (Hahn & Kleinman, 1983; Rhodes, 1990).

It is even more problematic to argue that psychiatric diagnostic catego-ries are *the* representation rather than *a* representation of psychopathologi-cal reality. The difficulty here lies in the continuing absence of a "cartography" of insanity, mood disorders or personality disorders that assimilates the cat-egories to the phenomena they represent. Even so, this does not prevent contemporary psychiatry from using the notion of isomorphism between representation and reality to introduce an assumption which is just as ques-tionable: the scientific neutrality and objectivity of medical theory and prac-tice.

Of course, if biomedical categories represent reality then it is feasible to believe in the neutral, objective, rational and value-free nature of the knowl-edge system itself. In other words, both diagnosis and treatment are per-ceived as neutral processes in which the values of the professional are neither important nor relevant to clinical practice and medical research. Biomedi-cine (and biomedical psychiatry) emerges, then, as a knowledge system free from metaphors and unaffected by social, political and economic factors. The functionality of this assumption is, according to Mishler, obvious:

> Thus, the view of medicine as a science serves to justify physicians' control over technical, esoteric knowledge, and at the same time such control sup-ports claims for professional autonomy and self-regulation (1981, p. 18).

The idea of the autonomy of the professional group is one of the most frequently reiterated arguments in biomedical literature and one of the pil-lars on which the notion of scientific neutrality has been built. An interesting example is a statement by Klerman, one of the most emblematic representa-tives of contemporary psychiatry, about corporate self-regulation in psychia-try:

> In discussing the history of psychiatry, one of my premises is that professional groups, such as medical specialties, are able to determine their own destiny to a greater extent than most other occupational groups (1984, p. 539).

The force of this assertion is scarcely blunted by the final words of the quotation: "to a greater extent than most other occupational groups." In fact, it is hardly surprising that biologically oriented psychiatry should amplify the ideological features that define the biomedical model. Historically, psychiatrists have struggled to defend their territory among the medical sciences, with the added burden of knowing that successes in their field paled into insignificance beside the successes of biomedicine: their knowledge of etiology, the localization of the pathological nucleus, the effectiveness of treatment, etc. Klerman's statement reveals an ideological project which transcends the frontiers of the history of psychiatry: the history of medicine controls itself, it is in command of its own destiny.

The myth of neutrality and objectivity has also been applied with no perceptible differences to clinical practice. Again, to quote from one of the defenders of the biomedical model in psychiatry:

> Whether the diagnosis is...mania, schizophrenia, or obsessional neurosis...is more important treatment, course or outcome than whether the individual is male or female, black or white, educated or ignorant, married or divorced, well adjusted or not, religious or not, etc. (Guze, 1977, p. 25).

Here diagnosis is seen as a neutral activity which should not be affected by human diversity in any form: ethnicity, sex, age, religion or social class. What is important is the diseases, their treatment, course and outcome, not the characteristics of the patients. Nevertheless, this conclusion is contradicted by a more recent data on the hospitalization of patients in the United States according to their ethnic group:

> Blacks and Native Americans are considerably more likely than Whites to be hospitalized; Blacks are more likely than Whites to be admitted as schizophrenic and less likely to be diagnosed as having an affective disorder; Asian American/Pacific Islanders are less likely than Whites to be admitted, but remain for a lengthier stay, at least in state and county mental hospitals (Snowden & Cheung, 1990, p. 347, cit. in Good 1993, p. 431).

The differences between Guze's expectation and the results of the study by Snowden and Cheung speak for themselves. Where Guze perceives only the objectivity of science, the facts suggest the partiality of its practitioners. The differences in diagnosis, psychiatric hospitalization and length of hospitalization according to ethnic group reveal the fragility of the supposed neutrality of clinical medicine, maintained by unreflexive practices which render it impervious to social realities. It is hardly surprising that medical anthropologists have perceived biomedicine as a peculiar cultural system whose ideological nature is revealed, paradoxically, in its rejection of ideology and its aseptic self-representation in strictly scientific and technical terms.

The Argentinian anthropologist Menéndez (1981), for example, has placed Western medicine in its sociopolitical context by speaking of the "Hegemonic Medical Model" (*Modelo Médico Hegemónico*). This is a Gramscian concept similar to biomedicine and defined as a theoretical-practical model characterized by biologicism, individualism, ahistoricity and asociality, as well as such other factors as mercantilism and pragmatic efficacy. Here Western medicine seems to be defined in negative terms: asociality and ahistoricity.

Rhodes (1990), inspired by Geertz's idea that a cultural system is both a model *of* reality and a model *for* reality, defined biomedicine as a cultural system which simultaneously endows social and psychological reality with meaning and objective conceptual form, and shapes this reality to itself (Geertz, 1973). Like religion or art, biomedicine as a system structured on this double activity of expressing and shaping reality, on this relationship between the symbolic dimension and the domain of experience, creates what Geertz has characterized as an "aura of factuality" through which the images produced by the cultural system about the world come to seem unquestionably real. Thus the principle of objectivity is transformed perhaps not into an illusion, but certainly into a cultural construction.

For both Menéndez and Rhodes, biomedicine has ceased to be a knowledge system whose objectivity excludes it from anthropological analysis. The analysis to which it is subject may be termed anthropology of medicine, anthropology of biomedicine, anthropology of psychiatry or anthropology of Western medical systems. No category, premise or concept is immune to anthropological scrutiny. As Kleinman and Good have pointed out for psychiatry: "Psychiatric categories and theories are cultural, no less than other aspects of our world view" (Kleinman & Good, 1985, p. 3). Anthropological critiques of biomedical knowledge seem to have the special role of demonstrating that the scientific premise is not in fact an objective principle, but a cultural assumption.[8]

BETWEEN CLASSIFICATORY RATIONALITY AND THE ETIOLOGICAL IDEAL

One of the constants in the history of psychiatry is the tension created by its attempt to join itself to the biomedical model, and the obstacles which prevent its adherence to the ideals of this model. If, as we have seen, the assumptions of biomedicine can be regarded as cultural constructions, in psychiatry the fragility of these principles becomes even more evident, because contemporary psychiatric knowledge remains unable to make pathophysiological processes "visible," determine the etiology of most mental disorders and, consequently, establish biological norms endowed with the appearance of "unquestionable realities." If any given cultural system bases its "aura of factuality" on a set of principles, we may say that, in the case of psychiatry, these principles are excessively contradictory. For this reason, it is hardly surprising that psychiatry has drawn harsh criticisms that still retain their evocative power: mental illness is a bourgeois myth that threatens the rights of the individual (Szasz ,1970); the asylum was not a response to the need to provide care, but a strategy of social and political control (Foucault, 1964); "medical symptoms" and "mental symptoms" are radically different things (Goffman, 1969); and the hospitalization of mental patients is merely another facet of a repressively custodial policy (Basaglia, 1976).

Although the efficacy of organic therapies (mainly psychopharmacology and ECT) has deprived these arguments of some of their force, the fact remains that their critical content cannot be completely disregarded. Because the organic origins of most mental disorders have yet to be demonstrated, psychiatry is suspended uncomfortably between taxonomic rationality and the ideal of etiological knowledge.

One of the historical moments most representative of this tension is the birth of positivist medicine in the first half of the nineteenth century. While biomedicine opted for a causal view of disease at the expense of classifying pathological phenomena, in the emerging field of psychiatry a similar debate was taking place.

On the one hand, the alienist approach initiated by Pinel, which was grounded in the theory of the *moral* cause of mental illness and the possibilities of *traitement moral*,[9] had gained general acceptance. In this view, the clinical process was understood as a combination of careful observation of the patients' behavior and attentive listening to their narratives, with the aim of understanding the events triggering the natural history of the disease (Weiner, 1992). The search for an organico-cerebral location for mental illness was regarded as unfounded speculation, and the methical classification of disease symptoms was advocated (Pinel, 1800).

At the other end of the spectrum, hypotheses were beginning to emerge concerning the organic sources of this type of pathology, turning towards the interior of the body in the search for knowledge about the origins of mental illness in the diseased brain (Castel, 1980). In this case, observation transcended the field of phenomena to which the taxonomic rationality of alienism seemed to be restricted.

The alienist trend merged with the late eighteenth-century "medicine of species" model, while the organicist vision was absorbed into the domain of positivist medicine. In medical knowledge, the penetration of the clinical gaze into the universe of the organs had managed to establish its hegemony; that is to say, positivist medicine had displaced the taxonomic and almost botanical medicine of species. However, in the emerging field of psychiatry, the classificatory model championed by the alienists[10] continued to predominate, despite the fact that in 1822 Bayle had shown that paresis was associated with certain encephalic lesions. This discovery would give rise to a new model of mental illness which would eliminate several diagnostic categories, such as melancholy or monomania, leaving only the simplest range of signs and symptoms consistent with brain lesions. Even so, Bayle's approach was initially regarded with great skepticism by the emerging psychiatric profession, which at that time had adopted the name of "special medicine." The alienists had obvious professional reasons for rejecting an approach that threatened their *traitement moral* model, but these considerations were not incompatible with their defense of the moral theory of mental illness on the grounds that the organic etiology of insanity and its manifestations had not been established (Castel, 1980).

The difficulties in establishing the organic causes of mental illness throughout the nineteenth century reduced the optimism surrounding the brain lesion paradigm. In fact, the invisibility of most types of insanity in the universe of the organs forced the retention of a taxonomic approach closer to the "medicine of species" than to positivist medicine, and therefore psychiatry was dominated by a nosological rationale rather than an etiologic ideal (Castel, 1980). This meant that psychiatry acquired a distinctive character in the context of medical knowledge which has been maintained to a greater or lesser extent to the present day.

We are not dealing only with a nineteenth-century problem. The relationship that contemporary biomedicine establishes between signs, nosologies and causes cannot be extrapolated to the context of psychiatry, at least not totally. The continuing search for an organic etiology of mental disorders has not yielded such brilliant results as it has in biomedicine. For example, in an interesting collection of correspondence among North American psychiatrists between 1890 and 1940, Gerald Grob pointed out the inability of early twentieth-century psychiatry to adopt the single-cause bacteriological paradigm of biomedicine. About this period he writes: "Psychiatric nosology remained descriptive; with the exception of paresis, the etiology of mental illness remained a mystery" (Grob, 1985, p. 185).

At present, with a few exceptions such as the so-called organic mental disorders (the very name of which refers to a biological cause), possible organic etiologies are still rooted in conjecture. This is not to say that associations or statistical correlations have not been established between a series of organic processes and certain symptomatological sets or syndromes which are believed to be more or less discrete units. Different studies have now shown that there is an association between some types of schizophrenia and organic factors such as hyperactivation of the dopaminergic cerebral pathways, dilation of the ventricles of the brain, or cortical lesions (American Psychiatric Association [APA], 1994). As far as mood disorders (mainly depression) are concerned, various clinical experimental studies have opted either for a neurohumoral theory—monoamine disorder—or a hypothesis based essentially on a disorder of the serotonin receptors (Gastó & Vallejo, 1991). A genetic predisposition in most of the severe mental disorders such as psychosis and the affective disorders has also been discussed (McGue, 1989). In short, discovery of the biological bases of mental illness has begun to seem possible. However, the knowledge acquired to date is hypothetical, and hypothesis is not corroboration nor conjecture a certainty. For this reason, psychiatric classifications nowadays are clinical (based on signs and symptoms) and/or pathochronological (based on the course), but not etiopathogenic (causal) or anatomopathological (based on the location of the disorder) (Vallejo, 1991). In other words, what diagnostic classifications express is not knowledge about disease processes, but the manifestations of these processes: their signs and symptoms.

Modern taxonomies, such as DSM-III, DSM-IIIR and DSM-IV (*Diagnostical and Statistical Manual*) in North America and the ninth and tenth version of ICD (*International Classification of Diseases*) published by the World Health Organization, consist of lists of signs and symptoms which can be associated with other factors such as course, evolution, outcome and prognosis (APA, 1980, 1987, 1994; World Health Organization [WHO], 1992a). These taxonomies, with some exceptions which have been mentioned above (organic mental disorders), consist of a wide range of phenomena lacking any specific organic cause. For this reason, the adoption of the biomedical paradigm in psychiatry should be understood as a singular development which assumes an organic cause for most mental disorders, although the proof of this is still a long way off. Contrary to all reasonable expectations, psychiatry takes itself to be a biomedical and objective practice, based on observation and universal taxonomies which are impervious to the socio-historical realities in which they are embedded. What is it, then, that allows its theoretical and practical model to be defined as biomedical?

THE BIOMEDICALIZATION OF PSYCHIATRY

One of the most important factors in the biomedicalization of contemporary psychiatry has been the development of organic therapies. Between 1932 and 1940, somatic treatments such as the use of pentylenetetrazol (Metrazol), CO_2, insulin and, on a different level, electroconvulsive therapy (ECT) and lobotomies had already been developed (Freedman, 1992). Grob (1991a) has pointed out that the last two were in frequent use in most North American psychiatric hospitals. The adverse effects of ECT, notably the pain involved in its administration, were considered to be minor in comparison to its advantages: simple to apply and efficient at mitigating the symptoms of the psychosis. Lobotomies, for their part, increased dramatically after 1940.[11]

All the same, the success of ECT and psychosurgery was somewhat diminished by the appearance of two particularly significant drugs: chlorpromazine, which was effective in mitigating the symptoms of psychosis; and imipramine, which was successfully tested on depressive patients (Davis, 1992; Grob, 1991a; Freedman, 1992). Psychopharmacological treatment had advantages that ECT and psychosurgery did not: it was cheap, and its use did not require the patient to be hospitalized. Their greater effectiveness enabled psychiatry to draw progressively, though in fits and starts, nearer to the ideal of biomedicine.

Strangely enough, the development of psychopharmacology at first overlapped with the heyday of the psychosocial and psychoanalytical models after the Second World War, particularly in the United States and Great Britain. Even though these models were introduced into each country at historically different moments and in different ways,[12] we can summarize some of the principles of the psychosocial trend: a) the boundary between health and mental illness is considered to be fluid since healthy individuals can become ill if they are exposed to traumatic conditions; b) mental illness can be regarded as a continuum stretching from the least pathological extreme, for example neurosis, to the most serious extreme of psychosis; c) a harmful environment and/or intrapsychic conflict is assumed to cause mental illness; and d) pathological phenomena are affected by psychological mechanisms (the so-called principle of psychogenesis) (Wilson, 1993; Grob, 1991b).

The psychosocial model was first introduced in the English-speaking countries, and competed during the 1950s and 1960s with the less successful biological tendencies with which it had always coexisted. In the United States, for example, the psychosocial model was a synthesis of Freudian theories and environmentalist approaches. One of the most representative exponents of this trend was the Meyerian model, an etiological theory of mental illness based on the idea of the individual's reaction to biological, social and psychological factors. The hegemony of Meyer's approach in North American psychiatry can be observed in the so-called DSM-I (*Diagnostical and Statistical Manual*)[13] and, to a much lesser extent, in the DSM-II[14] published by the American Psychiatric Association in 1952 and 1968, respectively (Spitzer, 1980; Spitzer & Williams, 1992; Robins & Helzer, 1986; Grob, 1991b).

But the psychosocial model progressively declined in favor of the biological approach. Wilson, for example, pointed out that the psychosocial approach had not paid enough attention to the distinction between health and mental illness and, in the latter, between different psychopathological types. What is more, since etiology was regarded as social or psychological in nature, priority was given to analysis of the patient's narrative and interpreting the meaning of symptoms. The advent of psychopharmacology changed this emphasis, creating a need for more sharply defined clinical categories that would make somatic treatment feasible. Diagnostic consensus based on etiological classifications of a psychosocial and psychodynamic nature such as DSM-I and, to a lesser extent, DSM-II (Wilson, 1993) became more and more problematic as the development of psychoactive drugs, backed by the powerful pharmaceutical industry, began to show experimental results that were increasingly at odds with these classifications (Guimón, Mezzich & Berrios, 1987). To this was added the opposition to the psychosocial model on another front: the antipsychiatry discourses which attempted to discredit psychiatric practice by turning one of its own principles—the indeterminacy of the normal and the psychopathological—against it. If mental disorders could not be traced to pathophysiological processes, the argument went, then they did not belong in the same category as physical diseases. And if this were the case, there was no reason why they should even be considered disorders, as long as diagnostic categories referred to pathological realities and not to the clinician's moral judgment.

The influence of these factors progressively eroded the psychosocial model and prompted the resurgence of organicist tendencies based on experimental research, the use of psychopharmacology and the search for "valid," "reliable," "objective" diagnostic classifications.[15] As Grob pointed out in a historical analysis of North American psychiatry:

> After 1970 the character of American psychiatry underwent a marked transformation. As psychodynamic and psychoanalytic leaders who had dominated the speciality for nearly a quarter of a century retired, their places were taken by those more committed to biological explanations of mental disorders. Less concerned with the role of broad environmental and psychological factors in the shaping of personality, these individuals stressed the importance of integrating psychiatry and medicine and exploiting new medical technologies that might eventually illuminate the biology of mental disorders (1991a, p. 301).

By the 1980s, pharmacological therapy was the main psychiatric treatment, not only in the United States, but in most Western countries (Klerman, 1984; Kleinman, 1988b). This meant that psychiatry became more clearly integrated into the territory of biomedicine, adopting the allopathic notions of monocausality, the biological definition of disease, the universality of symptoms, the neutrality of practice and the view of symptoms as manifestations of organic pathology. These assumptions are not new to psychiatry—we have already seen that they can be traced back to some nineteenthth-century psychiatric approaches—but in psychopharmacology they find firmer grounding.

Therefore, the development of psychopharmacology shifted mental illness from a psychological and psychosocial terrain to an essentially biological domain. In this new space, clinical pictures can be defined and classified not only on the basis of their symptomatology, but also in accordance with the efficacy of the treatment. This efficacy, nevertheless, is debatable, not because the substances administered do not produce the desired effect, but because this effect is the alleviation of signs and symptoms rather than the resolution of the underlying pathology.

With organic therapies, mainly psychopharmacology, as the main point of contact, contemporary psychiatry achieves biomedical status, but the deficiencies of etiological knowledge compel it to construct its nosology on the basis of simple clinical description. The psychiatric gaze, then, fluctuates between the possibility of treating some level of biological reality and the impossibility of shedding light on the still-opaque universe of the organs.

The DSM-III, the DSM-III(R) and the DSM-IV exemplify this descriptive nosological rationality. Unlike DSM-I and DSM-II, DSM-III and its successors are based on the apparently "atheoretical" description of clinical pictures and the elimination of such psychoanalytically-oriented categories as "neurosis." Though defined as manuals integrating the various currents of psychiatric theory and practice, they represent the hegemony of the curing-centered approach over the healing-centered approach, of symptom description over symptom interpretation, of the natural-science approach over the more hermeneutic tendencies, of seeing over hearing; in short, the triumph of the view of mental illness as a physical anomaly over the view of mental illness as a psychological and psychosocial disorder.

Within psychiatry, there have been some attempts to show that the emphasis on biomedicine, despite its advantages, has led to an impoverishment of clinical psychiatry (Kessler, 1990; Jackson, 1992; Freedman, 1992; Wilson, 1993) through the marginalization of more theoretical tendencies linked to therapies now regarded as "soft" (psychoanalysis, systemic therapy or social psychiatry). This is not to say that their use has been totally eliminated, but that the role they play is now secondary to pharmacological and electroconvulsive treatment. The culture of the precise, objective diagnosis has eclipsed those models based on clinical theorizing, and as we shall see in greater detail in Chapter 4, the newer versions of DSM represent this biomedical approach. They offer little freedom to the more hermeneutic, interpretive approaches which are now regarded as "prescientific," stressing instead the possibility of a positivist approach to disorders or psychopathological manifestations. This is what in contemporary psychiatry has been termed the return of the speciality to its medical roots,[16] a return which adopts the visual metaphor as its epistemological paradigm and therefore regards symptoms as physical signs. But before we embark on an analysis of the psychiatric model which dominates contemporary practice —the psychiatric era from which we have not yet emerged—it may be useful to ask ourselves the following question. What does this return to medical roots mean?

NOTES

1. For an interesting debate on the theory of contagion in schizophrenia, see Crow & Done (1986) and the belated reply of Butler & Stieglitz (1993).
2. Foucault's approach to signs and symptoms is clearly different from the one I use in this book. For Foucault, symptoms are the physical manifestations (fever, cough, etc.), and signs the transformation of these natural signs into medical language. In Chapter 9 I will analyze this position in greater depth.
3. McKeown observes that the death rates for infectious diseases such as scarlet fever, whooping cough, bronchitis, pneumonia and influenza have similar tra-

jectories.

4. An interesting critique of the monocausal theory of disease can be found in Janes, Stall & Gifford (1985).

5. Voodoo death has also been seen as the opposite of another enigmatic phenomenon: the placebo effect. It has been associated with the production of neurochemical substances induced by the patients themselves (Csordas & Kleinman, 1990).

6. The "social support-stress-disease" model has been applied recently to a number of diseases and is the subject of several publications. Some general references are Cassel (1976), Berkman & Syme (1979), Broadhead et al. (1983), Berkman (1984) and Bloom (1990). For mental disorders, see Dean (1986) and Palinkas, Wingard & Barret-Connor (1990).

7. Of course, to these two social variables, we can add a long list of factors which are no less important; for example, social inequality, processes of acculturation, or lifestyle. Some classic studies of social factors in disease causation can be found in Marmot & Syme (1976), Marmot, Rose, Shipley & Hamilton (1978) and Karasek, Baker, Marxer, Ahlbom & Theorell (1981).

8. A similar approach can be found in three articles by Young (1993), Rhodes (1993) and Fabrega (1993), all of which make an anthropological criticism of contemporary psychiatry. See also Lock & Scheper-Hughes (1990) and Good & Good (1993).

9. As Weiner (1992) has pointed out, moral should not be confused with its connotation in English of "moralizing." *Traitement moral* means psychological rather than physical treatment.

10. Castel (1980) points out that the registration categories of Pinel and Esquirol, the creators of the great synthesis of alienism, were still being used in an 1874 report by the inspector general of asylums.

11. According to Grob, in 1940, 684 lobotomies were carried out in the United States. By 1949 the figure had risen to 5,074, and by 1951 to 18, 608 (Grob 1991a).

12. See Comelles and Martínez-Hernáez (1994) for an analysis of the situation in Spain and Catalonia.

13. DSM-I, prepared by George Raines, was a classification based on the taxonomic system devised by Meninger for the Veterans Administration. It makes frequent use of such concepts as "reaction," "psychoneurotic reaction" and "schizophrenic reaction," which reveal the influence of Meyerian theories on the development of this nosology. On the other hand, it is also quite clear that the psychoanalytical schools influenced the use of the notion of defense mechanisms to explain neuroses and personality disorders. DSM-I is obviously a psychodynamically oriented diagnostic manual (Grob, 1991b).

14. DSM-II, published in the 1960s (the study committee began work in 1965), is not very different from its predecessor. It was devised under the auspices of the American Psychiatric Association and attempted to adapt the ICD in use at the time (ICD-8) to the North American context. This manual is perhaps most sig-

nificant for its rejection of the concept of reaction, the possibility of multiple diagnoses—alcoholism in a case of depression, for example—and the use of wide-ranging diagnostic terms unsupported by a well-defined theoretical structure. Although DSM-II is less explicit about its theoretical approach, some authors have defined it as an extension of DSM-I (APA, 1994; Robins & Helzer, 1986).

15. At first, the most emblematic group representing the biological approach was the Department of Psychiatry at Washington University, St. Louis, and in Europe, the departments of some universities in Great Britain and the Scandinavian countries (Robins & Helzer, 1986).

16. For a critical vision of this return to the biomedical roots of psychiatry, see Kleinman (1988b).

CHAPTER 3

Kraepelin Versus Freud: A Retrospective

The main precursor of contemporary psychiatry is Emil Kraepelin, a German psychiatrist who at the end of the nineteenth and the beginning of the twentieth century advocated a biomedical view of mental disorders in opposition to the rising importance of psychoanalysis. In fact, Freud (1856-1939) and Kraepelin (1856-1926), undoubtedly the two most influential psychiatrists by 1920 (Beer, 1992, p. 507), also represent two clearly rival and conflicting positions.[1]

The first great bone of contention emerges from their respective methodologies. Freud's more hermeneutic tendencies stand in contrast to Kraepelin's biomedical positivism, which was also openly critical of the methodological principles of psychoanalysis:

> Intuition is indispensable in the fields of human relations and poetic creativity, but it can lead to gross self-deception if used in research. As intuition is greatly influenced by one's own prejudices and needs it lends an air of deceptive yet powerful plausibility. This is especially worrying as we have no objective yardstick for this confidence...It is dangerous to construct an edifice of learning which cannot be validated against another. This is the mistake made by the psychoanalysts (Kraepelin, 1992a [1920], p. 512).

In terms of research interests, the opposition is revealing. Freud's interests center on deep motivational structures, while Kraepelin's focus is on the clinical description of the symptoms, course, evolution and prognosis of mental illnesses. For Freud, symptoms are part of a structure of meaning; for Kraepelin, symptoms are manifestations of biologically-based processes. In classical psychoanalysis, the biography of the subject is fundamental, while for Kraepelin, in spite of his careful clinical histories, the first priority is the correct classification of psychopathological species: what is generic rather than specific in mental illness. But let us go step by step.

SAXA LOQUUNTUR²

> It is a pity that one cannot make a living, for example, by interpreting dreams.
> —S. Freud
> Letter to Fliess of 21 September 1897

There seems to be a certain consensus in defining psychoanalysis as a theory positioned between the natural and the human sciences, between the search for causal explanations (*Erklärung*) and the search for meaning (*Verstehen*). Ricoeur has spoken of the indeterminacy of the distinction between a *herméneutique* (hermeneutics) and an *énergétique* (energetics), of the dual character of psychoanalysis, which is an attempt to achieve both a comprehensive investigation of meaning, and an economic, dynamic and even hydraulic explanation of instincts (1965). For Ricoeur, one of the most important issues raised by this indeterminacy lies in the centrality of affective life to psychoanalytic theory and, in particular, the role of desire as an ambiguous and enigmatic place where "there is, at the same time, the possibility of *passing* from force to language, but also the impossibility of completely *recovering* force within language" (1965, p. 77) [italics in original].

Habermas, for his part, defined classical psychoanalysis as a new science which linked hermeneutics to practices seemingly reserved for the natural sciences (1989), as knowledge which cannot be understood as an interpretation of meaning in the sense of merely linguistic translation, but rather as a process through which the analyst teaches patients how to read "their own languages." The notion of a linguistically-oriented hermeneutic approach is thus modified by the introduction of self-reflection as one of the ultimate objectives of understanding (*Verstehen*) (1989, p. 228).

In the field of anthropology, Obeyesekere, whose own interpretation of Freudian writings is of the most hermeneutic sort, has nonetheless argued recently for a multidimensional view of Freud himself, a "multiple Freud" not silenced by simplistic and hasty categorization in terms of some sort of essentialism, whether empiricist or hermeneutic (1990, p. xxiii).

As is already evident, Freud's writings prompt divergent responses, and can only be situated definitively within either hermeneutics or the natural sciences with great difficulty. Freud is both a decipherer of dreams and symptoms, and the would-be founder of a psychology grounded in physiology. The hermeneutist Freud who strives to uncover the meaning of parapraxes also predicts the future substitution of psychotherapy by psychopharmacology. This ambiguity should also be seen in the context of the evolution of Freudian thought over time. If the Freudian project began as an attempt to construct a physiologically-based psychology, it gradually developed into a more hermeneutic approach, although it was never totally free of the energetic or natural-science elements inherent in psychoanalytic discourse (Standard Edition [SE], XIII, p. 165).

In Freud's first works, the energetic approach is explicitly linked to the project of constructing a physiologically-based psychology. The emblematic work of this period is undoubtedly *Project for a Scientific Psychology* which, although published posthumously[3] (1950), dates from 1895. Shortly before this, Freud and Breuer had published *Studies on Hysteria*, a work that foreshadowed Freud's belief that the universe of biography was the strategic domain of analysis. However, it is in his *Project* that Freud attempts to ground psychological theory in the premises of the natural sciences:

> The intention is to furnish a psychology that shall be a natural science: that is, to represent psychical processes as quantitatively determinate states of specifiable material particles, thus making those processes perspicuous and free from contradiction (SE, I, p. 295).

Toward this end, he introduces such categories as "nervous system," "permeable neurons," and "impermeable neurons," as well as a whole range of complex explanations about the articulation of these systems with various quantitative laws (SE, I, p. 300). In *Project* we also find a number of mechanical and energetic concepts—discharge, excitation, inhibition, neuronal inertia, contact-barriers, current, apparatus, paths of conduction, connection, Q (quantity), Q-screens, replacement—in addition to the better-known concepts of resistance and cathexis[4] (SE, I, p. 295). The psychology that Freud was aiming for, then, was decidedly physical in nature. In this work, even his definition of *Ego*, a concept that would not acquire any real relevance in his writings until after 1920, is that of "a network of cathected neurons well facilitated in relation to one another" (SE, I, p. 323). *Project* is in fact a physical and physiological theory of psychological functions, an attempt to join quantitative concepts to a neurological theory using as a model the principles of energy conservation which Mayer had developed in 1842 and Brücke subsequently transferred to physiology.[5]

However, the subsequent development of his work reflects a slight distancing from this physicalist image of normal and abnormal psychology. Only a year later, in an article on the etiology of neurosis, the complex rhetoric of *Project* gives way to a more clinical discursive style. In this article, Freud criticizes the theories of Charcot and his followers (Guilles de la Tourette, Guinon and Janet)[6] who regarded heredity as a cause of neurosis (SE, III, p. 147). Freud points out that heredity is a "precondition" but not a "specific" or "concurrent cause" in the etiology of neuroses.[7] Its effect is comparable "to that of a multiplier in an electric circuit which exaggerates the visible deviation of the needle, but which cannot determine its direction" (SE, III, p. 147).

Using the metaphor of the electric circuit, Freud questions both hereditary and degenerationist theories. As far as he is concerned, everything can be represented as a combination of conditioning factors. A slight hereditary tendency would require a greater degree of specific cause and vice versa: causes of lesser importance could be added to greater hereditary conditioning. Heredity and specific causes can be substituted for each other in the quantitative dimension and achieve, through an additive process, the same pathological result. But the important thing is not so much this compensatory mechanism, in which we can detect an energetics very close to that of *Project*, but what he considers to be the most fundamental of all the specific causes of neurosis: the patient's sexual life, whether present or past (SE, III, p. 149). This idea had been outlined in *Project*, but appears here stripped of its physical and physiological rhetoric.

Freud formulates a clinical classification based on situating sexual problems within biographical space. For neurasthenia and anxiety neurosis, symptoms are linked to disorders in the patient's present sex life. On the other hand, for hysteria and obsessive neurosis, the causal relation must be traced back to a "precocious sexual event" prior to puberty, consisting of sexual seduction by an adult. In fact, in hysteria and obsessive neurosis, the search for an etiology opens up clinical knowledge to the domain of biography and experience: a first approach to hermeneutics. For Freud, heredity may aggravate the condition, but the definitive cause of neuroses must be sought in biography, in the experience of a historical subject inhabiting a body. Etiologies, then, must be sought within this space: a space of memory which Freud evokes through the metaphor of archaeological ruins. The analyst must excavate this site in order to make the invisible visible:[8]

Imagine that an explorer arrives in a little-known region where his interest is aroused by an expanse of ruins, with remains of walls, fragments of columns, and tablets with half-effaced and unreadable inscriptions...If his work is crowned with success, the discoveries are self-explanatory: the ruined walls are part of the ramparts of a palace or a treasure-house; the fragments of columns can be filled out into a temple; the numerous inscriptions which, by good luck, may be bilingual, reveal an alphabet and a language, and, when they have been deciphered and translated, yield undreamed-of information about the events of the remote past, to commemorate which the monuments were built. *Saxa loquuntur!* ["Stones talk!"] (SE, II, p. 192) [italics in original].

It is no coincidence that the paragraph finishes with an allusion to "stones talk." The symptoms derive, fundamentally, from establishing traumatic events as mnemic symbols, as commemorative inscriptions of a historical or, in this case, a biographical moment.[9] In this view, the meaning of symptoms is intimately linked with the patient's experience (SE, XVI, p. 269).

Contrary to common belief, in Freud's work symptoms have not one meaning but several, since meaning is a consequence of a) a sexual representation or fantasy which is necessary, though not sufficient in itself, for the symptom to be produced; and b) an apparent polysemy, which is an expression of unconscious mental processes. In fact, as Freud showed in *Fragments of an Analysis of a Case of Hysteria*, a symptom may acquire contradictory meanings through the interplay of desire and censorship. In addition, hysterical symptoms such as coughing or loss of speech may change their meaning in the course of the illness. In these cases, as Freud points out, the symptom is "in the words of Gospel, like new wine into an old bottle" (SE, VII, p. 54). In short, symptoms are symbols whose meaning can change over time.

According to Freud, symptoms may also be individual or typical: individual when they are mainly idiosyncratic and, therefore, strongly linked to the subject's life history; and typical when they show no individual variation but are directly to a specific disease, such as the case of "topophobia" or fear of spaces (SE, XVI, p. 270). The symptoms most amenable to psychoanalytic interpretation are the individual ones, for the obvious reason that the more idiosysncratic the symptom, the easier it is to reconstruct its meaning in relation to the patient's life history. For typical symptoms, the possibilities of psychoanalysis are more reduced:

So we are now faced by the depressing discovery that, though we can give a satisfactory explanation of the individual neurotic symptoms by their connection with experiences, our skills leave us in the lurch when we come to the far more frequent typical symptoms (SE, XVI, p. 271).

However, this is not regarded as a limitation of psychoanalytic theory, but rather a consequence of its youth. For Freud, there is no basic ontological difference between individual and typical symptoms. In fact, if the former guide us to a knowledge of what is personal, since their origins are biographical, the latter may open the doors to a knowledge of what is typical, an understanding of events and processes common to the whole of humanity.

In assigning meaning to symptoms, the analytical task is characteristically an interpretive one, carried out through symbolic decoding, deciphering the hidden meaning of these phenomena. But this interpretive approach was consolidated through the study of a phenomenon not of the pathological order: dreams.

If the paradigm example of Freud's physicalist approach was, as mentioned above, the *Project for a Scientific Psychology*, one of the leading works of the hermeneutic approach is *The Interpretation of Dreams*. Strangely enough, both of these works include principles and hypotheses for analyzing the production of dreams. But whereas in *Project* dreams are defined in terms of their lack of "motor discharge" and "the absence of spinal precathexis owing to the cessation of discharge" (SE, I, p. 338), in *Interpretation* the underlying model is quite different: "In short, we have treated as Holy Writ what previous writers have regarded as an arbitrary improvisation, hurriedly patched together in the embarrassment of the moment" (SE, V, p. 514).

Freud uses the paradigm of textual analysis as a model for the interpretation of dreams—and not just any text, but "Holy Writ": the original object of study in hermeneutics. In chapter VII of *Interpretation*, one of the most complex passages in Freudian literature, Freud replaces the anatomic location of psychological mechanisms with a more abstract concept:

> What is presented to us in these words is the idea of *psychical locality*. I shall
> entirely disregard the fact that the mental apparatus with which we are here
> concerned is also known to us in the form of anatomical preparation, and I
> shall carefully avoid the temptation to determine psychical locality in any
> anatomical fashion (SE, V, p. 536) [italics in original].

The neuronal mechanisms described in *Project* have given way to a "psychical locality" that requires no anatomical point of anchorage. Here the energetic dimension of psychoanalysis has been detached from its basis in physiology, and the result is a series of energetic concepts such as libido[10] which will gradually lose their organic referent. This change of approach makes *The Interpretation of Dreams* a turning point in psychoanalytic theory.[11] The textual model of dreams marks the progressive shift of psychoanalysis towards the hermeneutic approach. Nevertheless, the work of the psycho-analyst is not quite identical to that of the interpreter of texts.

Freud begins by defining the interpretation of dreams as the process of translating the "language of dreams" into another known language. The former is the language of the manifest, confusing and apparently meaningless. The latter is the language of the latent which, once learned, allows the dream to be correctly deciphered. The image which Freud evokes to explain the rela-tionship between these two languages is that of the hieroglyph. The analysis of the dream is likened to cracking a hieroglyphic code which at first seems to be absurd and nonsensical: a boat is on top of a house, to the right of which there is a letter and then a human figure (SE, IV, p. 277). All of this makes up a disjointed universe which can be identified as the manifest lan-guage of dreams. Nevertheless, it ceases to be incomprehensible once the latent code of dreams is discovered. The initial appearance of incoherence is only the result of superficial observation; that is to say, a perspective charac-teristic of previous interpretive efforts, in which the analytic model for the analysis of dreams was based on visual analogies such as pictorial composi-tion. For Freud, however, the pictorial analogy did not yield a sufficiently accurate interpretation of dreams, particularly when compared to the textual or hieroglyphic model in which dreams were not senseless or incoherent, but vehicles of meaning that can be reconstructed in translation (SE, XIII, p. 169).

Hieroglyphics and dreams share several features. In both there are ele-ments that are meaningful as well as elements that are merely determinative, whose sole function is to facilitate comprehension. Likewise, the multiple meanings of some elements and the omission of others means that, in both, meaning must be deduced from context.[12] Up to this point, then, interpreting a dream resembles solving a crossword puzzle or translating an inscription partly effaced by centuries of wear and tear. However, the next step will be to introduce some nuances into this identification of text and dream, exege-sis and psychoanalysis.

In principle, dreams are not objective and stable products against which different interpretations or readings may be tested. Dreams are one of the expressive forms of unconcious psychic activity and are, therefore, subject to censorship by the dreamer himself. In this way, dreams pass into the realm of consciousness to form part of a universe in which the author's intention-ality is more complex, split between the conscious and the unconscious world. Furthermore, what the patient or informant describes is not the dream itself, but the narrative of the dream. Freud himself tested subjects by asking them to recount the same dream on multiple occasions, but the narrative never proceeded the same way twice (SE, V, p. 515). The problems created by the idiosyncratic nature of dreams do not, then, seem to be so very different from the difficulties and enigmas involved in the interpretation of a damaged inscription. For the philologist the important thing is the conscious intent behind the inscription; for Freud, however, this is not the ultimate aim. Damaged or missing elements, whether in inscriptions or dreams, obscure meaning for the philologist, but not for the psychoanalyst, who finds in them the most primordial of meanings. The alteration of dreams by censorship in the conscious realm, the forgetting of specific items or the substitution of some dream images by others, are processes that Freud regards as being far from arbitrary. In fact, these missing or distorted phenomena are as important as the actual content of the narrative. Their very resistance to conscious expression is of great analytic importance:

> My request to the patient to repeat his account of the dream has warned him that I was proposing to take special pains in solving it; under pressure of the resistance, therefore, he hastily covers the weak spots in the dream's disguise by replacing any expressions that threaten to betray its meaning by other less revealing ones. In this way he draws my attention to the expression which he has dropped out. The trouble taken by the dreamer in preventing the solution of the dream gives me a basis for estimating the care with which its cloak has been woven (SE, V, p. 515).

The fact is that what interests psychoanalysis is not only "the meaning of a text," but also "the meaning of the distortion of a text" (Habermas, 1989, p. 221). It is the search for this second kind of meaning which obliges the analyst of dreams to proceed in reverse, working backwards through the process in which the dream was produced, formed, deformed and mutilated. To use Freud's own metaphor, the cloak which has been woven with such care by the patient must be unwoven[13] in order to find in its construction process the keys to the production of dreams or "dreamwork," the set of rules according to which latent ideas and deep motivational content are transformed into dream images.[14] It is this interpretive effort that characterizes hermeneutic psychoanalysis, by contrast with forms of interpretation based on organicist approaches in psychiatry and neurology, for which dreams are "a purely somatic phenomenon without meaning or significance" (SE, XIII, p. 169)—that is to say, a phenomenon hardly worth scientific attention. As Freud remarked in another of his works, *On Dreams*, "Serious-minded people smile at these efforts: 'Träume sind Schäume'—'dreams are froth'" (SE, V, p. 634).

The hermeneutic nature of psychoanalytic interpretation and the consequent rejection of an exclusively organic explanation for dreams extended to other areas of psychic life. Freud's textual model for analyzing dreams also became his model for analyzing symptoms. But dreams cannot be treated as symptoms, and symptoms as dreams, unless these two phenomena are of the same nature. On the surface, they are both products of "unconscious psychic activity," but a deeper analysis reveals the weaknesses of the analogy.

Earlier in this chapter, I noted that in one of Freud's first articles, symptoms are regarded as symbolic representations of trauma, and thus clearly not of the same nature as dreams. Symptoms are the consequence of real events; for example, seduction in early childhood by an adult. However, dreams are not necessarily the result of a real biographical event, but a fantasy fed both by desires and by censorship. The theory of symptoms, then, cannot be transferred wholesale and without alteration to the fantasy life of dreams.

In *On the History of the Psycho-Analytic Movement*, Freud explains the nature of this transformation. If at first Freud had understood symptoms as being mnemic and repressed symbolizations of a traumatic event, the observation of clinical cases gradually convinced him that seduction was not always a factor; sometimes it was merely a part of the patient's explanatory repertoire. Having come this far, Freud had two options: to discard his entire body of work to date; or to adapt his theoretical model to an object that did not seem to be grounded in objective reality. In choosing to adapt rather than reject his previous approach, he came to understand hysterical "fantasy" as a "psychical reality," of a different order than objective reality, but nonetheless real:

> If hysterical subjects trace back their symptoms to traumas that are fictitious, then the new fact which emerges is precisely that they create such scenes in phantasy, and this psychical reality requires to be taken into account alongside practical reality (SE, XIV, p. 17).

The falsity of the seduction trauma—of which Freud is already aware in his letter to Fliess of September 21, 1897—was to develop into an argument that both placed symptoms and dreams within related fields of reality, and led to an understanding of sexuality as a set of psychic structures already in existence from the very first moments of life. As Freud wrote later in his autobiography, the step from the image of the seduced child to the hypothesis of the child's desire to be seduced was to be his first contact with the Oedipus complex (SE, XX, p. 34).[15]

But Freud was unable to avoid a certain awkwardness. It is more difficult to corroborate the existence of a psychic reality than it is to demonstrate a material and objective reality. In fact, it is by no means unreasonable to think that his subsequent foray into anthropology with the publication of *Totem and Taboo* is, in the final analysis, an attempt to ground a psychic structure in a supposedly real event that may lead back to the origin of culture. Freud himself said that of all his books, this one had given him the greatest intellectual satisfaction, because in writing it he resolved his anxiety as a neurologist trying to come to grips with the slipperiness of a psychic reality lacking a demonstrable organic basis.

In the final pages of *Totem and Taboo*, Freud reveals his deepest theoretical interests. Having analyzed the anthropological literature of the period on the suject of totemism and its relationship to exogamy and the prohibition of incest, Freud sets out to state his hypothesis. In general terms, the Oedipus complex can be regarded as the origin point of morality, religion, society and art—in short, of culture. After a complex description of clinical data, the most fundamental of which is infantile zoophobia (a rejection of contact with animals which he regards as a displacement of the father figure onto the figure of an animal), and anthropological data taken from Frazer, Robinson Smith, Atkinson and Lang, among others, Freud speculates on the possibility of an original moment in human history: the murder of the patriarch of the horde by his sons, motivated by their lack of sexual access to the females. The jealousy of the father generated feelings of ambivalence in the sons towards their progenitor. This ambivalence was resolved through parricide because the males, unable to gain access to the females, resorted to homosexual practices which gave rise to a conspiracy. But the story does not end here. The murder itself would lead to cannibalism, motivated by the desire to absorb the properties of the victim. Once the victim had been totally consumed, the murderers would experience feelings of guilt and repentance induced by their ambivalent relationship with the patriarch. Their repentance for this act would lead them to renounce any possible subsequent benefits, and prevent it from ever happening again. As a result, guilt is represented in the norms and prohibitions inherent in the totem: the prohibition on eating the animal (the father) except on specific ritual occasions; identification with the totem (the victim); and the law of exogamy, which would prevent further conflict between the young males of the horde (SE, XIII, p.141).

Apart from the highly speculative nature of this work, which was criticized at the time of its publication by Alfred Kroeber (1952 [1920]) from the anthropological point of view, *Totem and Taboo* is a representative example of the conflict in Freudian literature between the hermeneutic approach and the natural-science approach. Since the evidence did not support the theory of seduction trauma as the possible origin of neurosis, the natural-science aspects of Freudian thought required drastic action to resolve what was, from Freud's point of view, the precariousness of the theoretical model. As the author himself argues:

> The analogy between primitive men and neurotics will therefore be far more fully established if we suppose that in the former instance, too, psychical reality—as to the form taken by which we are in no doubt—coincided at the beginning with factual reality: that primitive men actually did what all the evidence shows that they intended to do (SE, XIII, p. 161).

The end of *Totem and Taboo* removes any remaining doubt concerning the author's objectives:

> But neurotics are above all inhibited in their actions: with them the thought is a complete substitute for the deed. Primitive men, on the other hand, are uninhibited: thought passes directly into action..."in the beginning was the Deed" (SE, XIII, p. 161).

Despite Freud's attempts to trace this "psychic reality" back to an original moment in human history, in the domain of clinical medicine he had to resign himself to the absence of any proof—which seduction trauma might have provided—that such a moment ever existed. However, this vacuum was productive because it brought together two apparently disparate objects— symptoms and dreams—and placed them both within the order of psychic reality. It was of little importance that one could be regarded as an outcome of normal processes, and the other as the result of pathological processes, because psychoanalysis observes "an unexpected amount of affective disturbance and blinding of the intellect in normal no less than in sick people" (SE, XIII, p. 175).[16] The process of symptom-work is, then, very similar to that of dream-work:

> Alongside the indication of distortion in the symptom, we can trace in it the remains of some kind of indirect resemblance to the idea that was originally repressed. The paths along which the substitution was effected can be traced in the course of the patient's psycho-analytic treatment; and in order to bring about recovery, the symptom must be led back along the same paths and once more turned into the repressed idea (SE, XI, p. 27).

The path analogy can be found both in symptom formation and in the dream-work process: it is the substitution of latent by manifest content. In both cases the task of interpretation consists of working backwards: passing from the manifest to the latent. It is this identification of symptoms with dreams that gives psychoanalysis its double identity as both therapy and theory. At this point, the barrier between normal and pathological psychology also breaks down—not, however, at the cost of rejecting the idea that organic factors (mechanical, toxic, or infectious) may have considerable influence on the genesis and development of mental disorders, but by restricting its field of activity to the psychic domain and the analysis of the formation and deformation of meaning.

This becomes more explicit when Freud touches on the analysis of psychosis. Freud has no doubt about the organic etiology of *dementia praecox*, the term used by Kraepelin, as we shall see below, which refers to the disorder currently known as schizophrenia (SE, XIII, p. 174). Although psychoanalytic treatment may not be feasible in these cases, the organic hypothesis does not prevent an analytic interpretation from also being relevant. The "stereotypies" (monotonously repeated movements and gestures) and delusions characteristic of schizophrenia, those manifestations regarded by clinical psychiatrists as incoherent, absurd and meaningless, are perceived by psychoanalysts as objects to be deciphered. The procedure is the same as that for the analysis of dreams, and it is this which distances the use of analytic methodology from the normal procedures of psychiatry. In a classic study of a case of paranoia, the Schreber case, Freud writes:

> The interest felt by the practical psychiatrist in such delusional formations as these is, as a rule, exhausted when he has ascertained the character of the products of the delusion and has formed an estimate of their influence on the patient's general behavior: in his case marvelling is not the beginning of understanding. The psycho-analyst, in the light of his knowledge of the psychoneuroses, approaches the subject with a suspicion that even thought-structures so extraordinary as these and so remote from our common modes of thinking are nevertheless derived from the most general and comprehensible impulses of the human mind; and he would be glad to discover the motives of such a transformation as well as the manner in which it has been accomplished. With this aim in view, he will wish to go more deeply into the details of the delusion and into the history of its development (SE, XII, p. 17).

In this passage, Freud not only stresses the interest of analytic interpretation in processes of symbolic transformation—in this case, in delusional disorders —but clearly articulates the difference between psychiatry and psychoanalysis. The former rejects the possibility of understanding and, therefore, discovers in incomprehensible speech the principle according to which pathology is defined. The latter, by contrast, analyzes apparently incomprehensible speech in such fine detail that understanding becomes possible and, perhaps for this reason, also establishes a close theoretical relationship between normal and pathological processes. Where arbitrariness seemed to reign supreme, the psychoanalytic interpretation finds order and coherence by regarding these manifestations as meaningful forms of expression.

When this archeology of meaning (latent meaning) is given priority over the search for a biological explanation of psychopathological disorders, relationships begin to appear among apparently different symptoms. Take, for example, three cases: a hysterical woman with repeated vomiting; an obsessive neurotic who takes painstaking measures to prevent infection; and a paraphrenic who accuses someone of trying to poison her. Despite surface differences, in all these cases the latent content remains the same: the repressed and unconscious desire to have a child; or, alternatively, the patient's defense mechanism against such a desire.

As can be seen from this last argument, what Freud seeks in the study of psychoses is not so very different from what he is looking for in the case of hysteria or obsessional neuroses, or even in the phenomena of normal psychic life. Dreams and parapraxes are closely related despite their outward differences, which diminish in importance under analytic scrutiny. Psychoanalysis is not subject to astonishment in the same way as psychiatry. Both are born of surprise, but where the latter reacts by distancing itself from the object of study, the former uses its own perplexity as a means for understanding and reflecting on the analyst's own psychic processes.

NATURA LOQUINTUR

Unlike Freud, Kraepelin limits his analysis of psychopathology to an interpretation of mental disorders. Restricting himself to the realm of the objective, to what can be discerned by the senses, Kraepelin is best known for his effort to create an orderly psychiatric nosology from an empirical, descriptive and biologicist perspective. This approach, as we shall see in the next chapter, is still largely in use today.

Kraepelin carefully dissects the various psychopathological species, placing particular emphasis on psychoses and organic mental disorders represented with the greatest frequency in asylum environments of the sort in which he practiced. Therefore, whereas the paradigm examples of psychoanalysis are hysteria and neuroses, Kraepelin's theoretical model emphasizes psychoses, in particular manic-depressive insanity and *dementia prae-cox* (now known as schizophrenia). In fact, the precise definition of schizo-phrenia is widely recognized as one of the greatest taxonomic achievements in the history of psychiatry.[17] Kraepelin defines this disorder not only by its phenomenological appearance but also in terms of its course and prognosis, characterized by progressive deterioration and incurability (1988 [1904], p. 29). Though he concedes the possibility of slight improvements in *dementia praecox*, this will generally be episodic and brief, and the inevitable relapses will lead to progressive and irreversible feeble-mindedness.

In this context, the symptoms of dementia praecox ("flattening of af-fect," "loss of drive," destruction of will," "automatic obedience," "stereo-typies," "negativism," "auditory hallucinations," etc. are regarded as reflections of cerebral abnormality, although at present its nature remains unknown. For Kraepelin, there is no ontological difference between *demen-tia praecox* and diseases of known etiology, such as progressive paralysis in syphilitics or dementia produced by severe infections. Comparing *dementia praecox* with general paralysis (paresis), he writes:

> The foremost place among these is held by the widely-diffused varieties of *dementia praecox*. Obvious as may be the clinical resemblance of this disease to general paralysis in many respects, it is yet improbable that it is produced by any external injurious influence (1988 [1904], p. 34).

Thus, the Kraepelinian vision of *dementia praecox* is clearly organicist. In other words, what is at issue here is not moral causes, psychosocial fac-tors or seduction traumas, but brain injuries and toxins:

> We can hardly doubt that we have to deal with toxins in such cases, and these experiences suggest the conjecture that ordinary *dementia praecox* may also have poisoning of the cerebral cortex for its immediate cause, although we are not yet in a position to discover their more remote origin (1988 [1904], p. 342).

Kraepelin's fundamental problem, then, is to define correctly the etio-logical agents responsible for the production of different types of insanity.

At first, this knowledge seems to be a long way off, but this is no reason not to assume that mental disorders are the result of pathophysiological pro-cess. On the contrary, Kraepelin believes that this knowledge will gradually form the solid basis of a "scientific psychiatry" in which "the physical foun-dation of mental life...should occupy most of our attention" (1988 [1904], p. 1).

Faced with this lack of etiological knowledge, the Kraepelinian project strives for a precise definition of insanity, no small task considering the varied and imprecise nature of the symptomatology of different forms of madness: *dementia praecox*, manic-depressive psychosis (*manisch-depressive Irresein*), epileptic insanity (*epileptische Irresein*), infectious insanity (*infektiöse Irresein*), paresis (*Dementia paralytica*), and senile and presenile dementia (*senile und präsenile Irresein*), among others. But sorting out this universe which, seen from some angles seems to be extraordinarily diverse while from others exceptionally homogeneous, is not a task Kraepelin regards as impossible:

> It can still only too well remember the perplexity with which I faced throughout very many years, the vast number of states of mental weakness harboured by every large asylum. Their manifold manifestations were to a certain extent grouped together, but, in spite of all variety in outward form, definite characteristic features recurred with surprising uniformity (1988 [1904], p. 204).

The possibility of discerning and defining disease entities, therefore, lies in noting down and dissecting "recurrent" and "characteristic" features; that is to say, in careful observation of disease manifestations. Kraepelin's whole taxonomic project is based on this observation for two different but related reasons. First, Kraepelin is a faithful representative of biomedical positivism and empiricism and, therefore, of approaches which concentrate more on the observation of patients' behavior than on listening to their accounts. Second, it should be noted that when he began to outline the most fundamental principles of his nosology, between 1886 and 1892, he was living and working in the city of Dorpat (now Tartu in Estonia), an environment that was linguistically and culturally foreign to him. While there, he worked among non-German speakers and had to rely on an interpreter for his clinical interviews (Berrios & Hauser, 1988; Beer, 1992). These linguistic limitations caused his observation of insanity to assume even greater importance, and he was to maintain this priority throughout his work. But what exactly did Kraepelin observe?

Some of the most representative features of Kraepelinian psychiatry are the concepts of course, evolution, outcome and prognosis. In fact, the analysis of course replaces knowledge of the etiological bases of mental disorders, while the link between cerebral lesion and the clinical picture remains hypothetical in the absence of any corroborating evidence. This emphasis on the course of the disease gives rise to a new concept of mental illness: whereas the old model of psychiatry was fundamentally "symptomatological," the new model was to be eminently "clinical" and included prognosis as a fundamental criterion. Observation through time was the means by which those symptoms which are simply episodic manifestations could be differentiated from those which are more stable and thus more accurately classifiable (Kraepelin, 1992a [1920]).

Kraepelin's diachronic approach to mental illness—course, evolution and prognosis—is not at all like Freud's. The temporality contained in these concepts is restricted to directly observable phenomena, not to the mnemic imprints of biographic history. This type of temporality no longer requires the expertise of an archaeologist or the skill of a hermeneutist, because what is revealed is not the psyche but the very nature of the pathology itself, understood as a biological aberration. In his analysis of the concept of schizophrenia as it was conceived by Bleuler, Schneider and Kraepelin, Hoenig wrote:

> What was felt to be lacking in Kraepelin's description of the clinical picture was the psyche. The symptoms were symptoms of the underlying disease process. The patient's life history, his premorbid personality, even his own experience of the illness had no assigned place in the scheme of things. They were an irrelevancy (1983, p. 549).

Kraepelin's interpretation of clinical pictures, therefore, undervalues what the clinical gaze discerns to be biographically individual and specific. What importance can the idiosyncratic and biographical meaning of the disturbed person's forms of expression have in comparison with the general tendencies of organic processes? Clinical histories are important for Kraepelin to the extent that they transmit universal information, in the sense that they are manifestations of a generic and classifiable disease process which results, like physical disease, from an organic cause. In this view, symptoms are expressions of organic pathology. In other words, the "language of stones" is replaced by the amorphous and asemiotic sound of the organs. Nevertheless, this reading of Kraepelin is polemical.

In their analysis of Kraepelin's works, Berrios and Hauser (1988) have questioned this vision of a profoundly organicist Kraepelin little concerned with individual clinical histories. They believe that the problem lies in the selective interpretation of Kraepelin's writings. Although they agree that his first works were indeed organicist, descriptive and classificatory in nature, part of a project to constitute clinical psychiatry within the framework of positivist medicine, they believe that his point of view underwent certain transformations in his subsequent writings.

What Berrios and Hauser are referring to is that Kraepelin, after the publication of the eighth edition of his *Lehrbuch der Psychiatrie* (*Textbook of Psychiatry*) in 1909, seems to criticize his own initial assumptions, particularly with respect to the undervaluation of life histories and the biographical significance of symptoms. In order to demonstrate this change in perspective, they point to one of Kraepelin's later articles, entitled *Die Erscheinungsformen des Irreseins* ("The manifestations of insanity"):

> ...it seems absurd to propose that syphilis causes patients to believe that they are the proud possessors of cars...rather the general desires of such people are reflected in these delusions... (Kraepelin, 1920, p.2, cited in Berrios & Hauser, 1988, p. 814).

This quotation seems to support their claim.[18] Here, Kraepelin does not appear to be a staunch organicist. Delusional symptoms are not approached as the direct result of a cerebral abnormality. However, what Berrios and Hauser do not say is the importance that Kraepelin attaches to the expressive content of symptoms. Even though it is true that "The Manifestations of Insanity" introduces some variations with respect to his initial positions, such as the possible mediation of psychobiological factors in the pathological process, it hardly represents a significant transformation of his biomedical, positivist approach. Let us examine it in the context of his other writings.

Works prior to "The Manifestations of Insanity" also raise questions about the extent of Kraepelin's interest in symptoms and the biography of the patient. His writing, which is of great descriptive richness, is full of painstaking observations of his patients. Generally, he introduces the cases with sketches of the following type:

> The stately gentleman, aged sixty-two, who presents himself before us with a certain courtly dignity, with his carefully-tended moustaches, his eye-glasses, and his well-fitting if perhaps somewhat shabby attire, gives quite the impression of a man of the world (1988 [1904], p. 142).

> The merchant, aged twenty-five, whom you see before you to-day, has made himself conspicous by putting leaves and ferns into his buttonhole. He takes a seat with a certain amount of ceremony, and gives positive, concise, and generally relevant answers to our questions (1988 [1904], p. 153).

The account is not limited to superficial descriptions of the patients who are the subjects of the clinical session. He usually describes the content of the symptoms as well: if the patient feels that he is being persecuted, Kraepelin records by whom and in what way; if the patient is delusional, then the content of the delusion is specified (German emperor, high-ranking executive in German colonial politics, well-known artist, etc.). Where, then, is the biomedical Kraepelin for whom the biography of the patient is irrelevant? Life history and the specific content of symptoms seem to be of some importance here.

A deeper analysis of his expository style allows us to see that his interest in content pales by comparison to the urgency with which he pursues other, more important realities: the invariable forms of the symptoms, their purest and most universal identity as natural signifiers. It is not a question of whether Kraepelin links the meaning of a symptom directly to an organic dysfunction, but whether this particular meaning is considered relevant within his nosological edifice. As Kraepelin himself points out in the introduction to his lecture on paranoia:

> The different forms of delusions—the delusions of greatness and insignificance, the delusion of sin, the physical delusion of persecution, and so on—have often been considered as characteristics of distinct forms of diseases. According to our present experience, conclusions as to the clinical *meaning* of a picture of a disease from the existence and purport of the delusions are only permissible to a very limited extent (1988 [1904], p. 142) [italics in orginal].

This passage makes it quite clear that what interests Kraepelin is not the specific content of the symptoms—whether the patient is experiencing delusions of guilt, persecution or grandeur—but the fact that the delusion can be related, as a physical sign or natural signifier, to other signs and symptoms and to the course of the illness.[19] The content of symptoms, then, is reduced to a superficial element, because what is at stake in his methodology of knowledge is not the understanding (*Verstehen*) of meaning, but the explanation and naturalist classification of disease entities. If the signifier takes precedence over the signified, there is no point in trying to trace the specific content of symptoms to a supposed cerebral dysfunction. On the other hand, the same cannot be said about formalizations such as "delusion," "hallucination," "flattening of affect" or "slurred speech," since here the psychopathological order reveals their real relationships to an underlying biological reality. It is no coincidence that, in Kraepelin, the invariable classificatory features are almost always limited to this formal dimension of symptoms. However, this is problematic for the construction of a universally applicable set of disease categories.

It is likely that among the most decisive experiences of Kraepelin's scientific career are his ethnopsychiatric excursions.[20] His trips to Java, Cuba, Mexico and the United States allowed him to observe crosscultural differences in the frequency of mental illnesses and in the way the symptoms are manifested. One interesting example is furnished by the results of his comparative study of 100 European and 100 South Asian patients. Although similar frequencies of *dementia praecox* are found in both groups, there is significant variability for the categories of epilepsy (*Epilepsie*), imbecility

(*Imbecillität*) and manic-depressive psychosis (*Manisch-depressive Irresein*). The most important results, however, are not the slight variations in the ratios of these types of illnesses, but the absence of alcoholism (*Alkoholismus*) and paresis (*Paralyse*) among the South Asian patients. These two disorders were very common in Europe at the beginning of the twentiethth century.[21]

Not only does the frequency of mental disorders vary by ethnic group; so does their phenomenology and symptomatology. *Dementia praecox* among native Americans does not manifest itself in delusions or hallucinations, nor does it seem to be associated with such symptoms as "negativist stupor" or "auditory hallucinations" among indigenous Javanese. This was subsequently to be attributed to the insignificant role of discourse in the thought of Javanese patients (Kraepelin, 1992a [1920], p. 516). Observations of this type prompted Kraepelin to change his organicist model of *dementia praecox* slightly, making room in it for what he somewhat vaguely called "culture" and "living conditions".[22]

But where the psychopathological landscape changes most dramatically is in the most culturally idiosyncratic phenomena: *amok, latah* and *koro*.[23] Faced with these three culture-bound syndromes of Southeast Asia, he had essentially two options: either to include these "exotic" forms in the nosology by introducing new categories or to force them into the existing categories. Kraepelin chooses the latter course, and identifies these phenomena as ethnic manifestations of epilepsy, hysteria and depression, respectively. As he writes in the eighth edition of his *Lehrbuch*:

> The Latah of the Malayans is expressed in attacks of automatism or coprolalia, triggered by fear and closely related to hysteria.... Most of the cases of Amok that I studied in Java were undoubtedly epileptics.... Recently I observed in a European suffering from circular depression what Van Brero described as "the Koro obsession," in which the penis retracts into the abdomen (1909, p. 157-8) [my translation].

This strategy overcomes an important obstacle to the development of a universal classification of mental disorders, but at the same time it makes it necessary to introduce an explanatory model *ad hoc* in order to account for this symptomatological variability. A certain indeterminacy thus creeps into the project of constituting a stable classification based on the assumption that symptoms are the reflection of a specific organic pathology. Griesinger's well-known aphorism,[24] to which Kraepelin also subscribed—diseases of the mind are diseases of the brain—must be modified to allow for the inclusion of psychological, biographical and cultural variables. Nevertheless, the result is not a great transformation of Kraepelin's original principles. He remained very much within the epistemological field of biomedical positivism, and this continuity is still evident in "The manifestations of insanity."

Without abandoning his belief in the existence of specific cerebral pathologies, Kraepelin introduces in "The manifestations of insanity" the idea that between the underlying disease process (*Kranskheitsvorgänge*) and the clinical symptomatology there are biological and psychological preconditions which may account for the extraordinary clinical variability he observed. This would explain why the same pathology can give rise to symptoms of widely differing form and content.

This idea is not new in psychiatry. In fact, Kraepelin makes use of two already existing and quite similar models. The first is the distinction between the essence and the presentation of a disease, first discussed by Kahlbaum (1828-1899), whose intellectual influence Kraepelin acknowledged. The second is the model that differentiates between pathogenicity and pathoplasticity, introduced by Birnbaum (1878-1958), which Kraepelin takes up again in order to distinguish between the physical cause of disease (pathogenicity), and the circumstantial factors of ethnic origin, lifestyle and the patient's clinical history (pathoplasticity). The same example used by Berrios and Hauser can be used again here: the organic cause (syphilis) is one thing and the particular meaning of symptoms (the patient's emotional volatility) is quite another (Kraepelin, 1992a [1920], p. 513). But of what importance is the meaning of a delusion in comparison with the basic and invariable organic cause of the disease?

Pathoplasticity, from the Kraepelinian perspective, seems to be less an object of interest in its own right than a smokescreen to be penetrated. The analysis of pathoplastic factors, therefore, is clearly subordinate to the study of causal processes at the organic level:

> We shall look at diseases different in form but with the same cause. We shall try to elucidate how the above mentioned factors (pathoplasty: age, social class, profession, climate, living conditions, etc.) modulate the clinical picture even when the cause is indeed the same (Kraepelin, 1992a [1920], p. 513).

At this point, the clinical task is to transcend the order of symptomatological variability in order to arrive at correct definitions of natural disease entities. This task is made easier by the existence of invariable symptoms and features:

> We therefore cannot help but expect that in any given disease a substantial part of the clinical picture will remain constant, because it represents the natural response of the 'human machine' to a morbid insult (1992a [1920], p. 517).

In the context of this mechanical and natural-science model, the meaning of symptoms and the biographical evolution of the patient become irrelevant. What interests Kraepelin are not the Javanese, German, native American or Russian patients, but mental disorders in their most generic sense; and this theoretical approach cancels out his capacity for astonishment at the individual nature of the phenomena. Where Freud was captivated by the symbolic meaning of dreams, the supposed keys to symptoms hidden within the psychic and experiential structures of his patients, Kraepelin's perplexity gives way to the positivist meanings imposed by a strictly biomedical tradition of clinical practice:

> With the help of the ideas you have derived from general pathology, you will usually be able to find your way in a new department of medicine without any serious difficulty. But here you will be utterly perplexed at first by the essentially peculiar phenomena of disease with which you will meet, until you have gradually learned to a certain extent to master the special symptomatology of mental disturbances (1988 [1904], p. 1).

The mastery of which Kraepelin speaks in this passage involves a familiarity with diseases and their manifestations, not with the patient. Mental disorders occupy a place in what Hoenig defined above as "the order of things" and, in this sense, they are independent of individuals and their biographies. Manic-depressive insanity evolves in a circular fashion. Manic crises are characterized by their violence and suddenness. *Dementia praecox* involves progressive loss of reason and is characterized by incomprehensible and preposterous manifestations. Mental disorders, therefore, have distinctive characteristics that allow them to be dissected and classified. The fact that Kraepelin had a brother who was a botanist may account at least in part for his classificatory bent.[25]

Kraepelin's psychiatric project, on this point, resembles the general medicine that Sydenham had outlined over two hundred years earlier:

> In the first place, all diseases should be reduced to specific, defined species, with the same care and precision as the botanists took in their Treatise on Plants (Sydenham, 1816 [1666], p. XXJ) [my translation].

The most representative feature of Kraepelin's work is precisely his classificatory intent, his definition of psychopathological manifestations as the "precise and determined species" of which Sydenham spoke. Here also psychiatry seems to absorb many of the principles of the medicine of species so characteristic of the eighteenth century. As Foucault points out:

In the epistemic or epistemological system of the eighteenth century, the great
model for comprehending diseases is Linnaeus' botanical classification. It requires diseases to be considered as a natural phenomenon. As in plants, in
diseases there will be species, observable characteristics, courses of evolution
(1990, p. 166) [my translation].

The similarity of the principles defined by Foucault for the medicine of
species (observable characteristics, courses of evolution) with those of
Kraepelin's taxonomic project seem to be quite clear: recall the emphasis on
prognosis and invariable characteristics. But if the medicine of species, as
well as alienist psychiatry, had limited itself to rational classification,
Kraepelin's more ambitious botany of psychopathologies is not without etiological hypotheses. In fact, the impossibility of transcending the domain of
mere classification generates a mixed theoretical formulation in which classification and etiological explanation emerge as two interdependent exer-
cises: the former can lead to the latter and vice versa (Young, 1991).

What is most important here, however, is that the Kraepelinian project
does not particularly recognize mental illness and its symptoms as experiences and expressions of meaning inscribed in the patient's biography. In
light of this, Berrios and Hauser's claim that Kraepelin is more sensitive to
individual clinical histories and to the meaning of symptoms loses some of
its force. If there is a profound difference between Freud and Kraepelin, it is
precisely the fact that the former gives importance to the symbolic content
of symptoms, while the latter is interested in what he supposes to be the
essentially organic nature of mental disorders.

For Freud, symptoms have a meaning, even though this meaning, in the
final analysis, may be subject to mechanisms of supposed universality. In
psychiatric terms, a delusion of jealousy, for example, is in no sense imma-
terial, arbitrary or inexplicable (SE, XVI, p. 251), because the symptom has
a value in its own right despite the fact that it may initially present itself
illogically and incoherently.

For Kraepelin, on the other hand, the patient's symptoms are only important insofar as they are associated with the course of the disease and with
other symptoms, in the composition of a clinical picture which can be classified in a taxonomy of species. Symptoms are, then, natural signifiers and
what is signified is their classificatory position. Meaning is bestowed only
through clinical inference. As a result, the patient's symptoms are treated as
physical signs rather than as symptoms. Even the patient's narrative, in this
context, emerges as an erroneous and false interpretation:

If we want to study such patients we cannot afford to pay much attention to
the patient's own account of his experiences...We must be all the more careful

because the self-perception, memory and judgement of our patients is clouded by mistakes (Kraepelin, 1992a [1920], p. 512).

This passage makes it clear that in the Kraepelinian approach there is no room for attending to the patient's narrative, because the clinician can do no more than interpret what is erroneous by nature. And error cannot lead the clinician to an exegesis of the formation and deformation of meaning.

NOTES

1. This professional rivalry also had repercussions on a personal level. Freud agreed to treat the patient who proved to be one of his most famous cases, the "Wolf-man," only after he had been told that both Kraepelin and Ziehen, two of the most prestigious psychiatrists of the time, had failed to treat him successfully. See Gay (1988:326) for an account of this episode.

2. The works of Freud cited here are from the *Standard Edition of The Complete Psychological Works of Sigmund Freud* (hereafter SE) and the Spanish version by López-Ballesteros (*Obras Completas de Sigmund Freud*, hereafter OC), which was characterized by Freud himself as a "most correct interpretation" of his thought. Quotations are identified with a reference to the *Standard Edition* (SE) or the *Obras Completas* (OC), followed by the volume and page numbers.

3. Almost simultaneously, Freud had published with Breuer *Studies on Hysteria* (1893-5), a work that introduces the energetic approaches which were to appear later, fully formed, in *Project*. *Studies* is characterized by a hermeneutic and biographical approach that was problematic for him. In the "Discussion" of the Elizabeth von R. case, for example, he attempts to warn readers that his clinical histories may seem more like "short stories," but that this appearance is justified by the very nature of his hypotheses, which are concerned with the biographical and experiential universe of his patients (SE, II, p. 160).

4. The term "cathexis" is problematic, since it is not one of Freud's own words but an error in the first English translation, which used the quasi-esoteric "cathexis" as a rendering of the original *Besetzung*. See Gay (1988, p. 514) and Freud (OC, II, p. 211).

5. In short, the principle of energy conservation can be defined as the hypothesis that, in an isolated system, the sum of motor and potential forces tends to remain constant (see Ricoeur, 1965, p. 82).

6. A subsequent critique of Janet's organicist and degenerationist theory of hysteria can be found in his *Second Lecture on Psycho-Analysis* at Clark University (SE, XI, p. 21).

7. Freud defines "preconditions" as being indispensable to the production of the disorder, but of a sufficiently general nature to contribute to the etiology of many

other disorders as well. "Concurrent causes" are similar to preconditions in their general causal involvement, but they are not necessary for the development of a disorder. Finally, "specific causes" are as indispensable as the preconditions, but are of a limited nature and appear only in the etiology of the disorder to which they are specific (SE, III, p. 147).

8. The archaeological analogy is repeated in other Freudian writings. See particularly the introduction to *Fragments of an Analysis of a Case of Hysteria* (OC, I, p. 936).

9. The mnemic symbol is, simultaneously, the means by which the trauma is prolonged in the symptom. See Freud (SE, III, p. 193) and Ricoeur (1965, p. 104).

10. An interesting analysis of the progressive shift towards non-localizationalist standpoints can be found in Ricoeur (1965). I will not discuss Freud's metapsychological works here; I would only point out that they also deal with the distinctively hermeneutic dimension of psychoanalysis. Ricoeur has perceptively observed that in these works the unconscious is incorporated into the terrain of meaning. A clear example is the idea that instinct (*Trieb*) cannot be present in the unconscious without a representation or a presentation (*Vorstellung*). See Ricoeur (1965, p. 41).

11. Freud himself, in the *Preface to the Second Edition* (1908), writes: "During the long years in which I have been working on the problems of neuroses I have often been in doubt and sometimes been shaken in my convictions. At such times it has always been the *Interpretation of Dreams* that has given me back my certainty." (SE, IV, p. xxvi).

12. For Freud, interpreting a dream means deciphering the symbolic representations present in it, and here Freud's understanding of the relationship between context and symbol is ambiguous and problematic. On the other hand, he notes that symbols often have multiple meanings and that their exact meaning depends in each case on context: "as with Chinese script, the correct interpretation can only be arrived at on each occasion from the context" (SE, V, p. 353); that is to say, the polysemy of the symbol is qualified and refined by the context, even when the polysemy is excessively conventional as in the case of hieroglyphics or similar writing systems. However, he immediately goes on to make an inventory of the meanings of such symbols as "the king," "the queen," "elongated objects," etc., which in his approach are universals without polysemy. See especially section E of Chapter VI in *Interpretation of Dreams*.

13. Interestingly, Crapanzano has identified the Freudian idea of "text" with the etymological meaning of the Latin word *textus*, the past participle of *tegere*, which means "something woven" (1992, p. 119).

14. See Chapter VI, "The dream-work," in *The Interpretation of Dreams* (SE, IV). See also Ricoeur (1965) and Obeyesekere (1990).

15. Kriss has shown that Freud's self-analysis was instrumental in the development of this idea. This act of self-reflection distanced him from organic explanations of psychic life, and found its biographical counterpoint in the break-up of his

friendship with Fliess. While Fliess continued to speculate on the organic etiology of neurosis, Freud became less and less interested in these hypotheses and
attempted to formulate a fundamentally psychological theory of sexuality. See
Kriss (1985, p. 3467).

16. In fact, Freud places the so-called "parapraxes" in the category of symptoms,
because in both cases they function by repressing unconscious desires and substituting them with others (SE, XI, p. 27).

17. The term *dementia praecox* did not originate with Kraepelin. Benedict morel
had already spoken of *démence précoce* in 1857. However, Kraepelin was the
first to use it as a concept embracing catatonia, hebephrenia and paranoid dementia. Shortly afterwards, Bleuler coined the term schizophrenia to refer to this
nosological set. See Beer (1992).

18. If we continue reading where Berrios and Hauser leave off, we can see that the
importance Kraepelin assigns to the patient's story is subsequently qualified:
> It seems absurd to propose that neurosyphilis causes patients to believe
> that they are the proud possessors of cars, mansions or millions of pounds
> and that cocaine causes visual hallucinations of mites and lice. Rather, the
> general desires of such people are reflected in these delusions of grandeur.

Kraepelin continues:
> The hallucinations receive their individual stamp after the mind has worked
> through the perceptual and visual disburbances induced by cocaine. where
> external insults are concerned—destruction, injury, excitation and inhibi-
> tion affect the brain either extensively or in a locally circumscribed way...The
> kaleidoscopic nature of the picture corresponds to the antecedent condi-
> tions encountered by the morbid agent in the patient's personality
> (Kraepelin, 1992a[1920], p. 510).

19. Note the similarity between this undervaluing of content in Kraepelin, and that
which is reflected in the psychiatric report included in Chapter 1.

20. Kraepelin is also know as the founder of comparative psychiatry, a precursor of
the modern subdiscipline of transcultural psychiatry. See Kraepelin (1992a[1920])
and Jilek (1995).

21. Kraepelin was actively engaged in the struggle agains alcohol. In 1895 he became a teetotaller to set an example for his fellow citizens. In fact, he regarded
alcoholism and syphilis as two fronts that were just as important for Germany as
those that had threatened the survival of Germanism in World War I. In one of
his most explicityl political articles, he wrote of syphilis and alcoholism: "A
great people is not destroyed by an external enemy; it succumbs only to inner
distress, regardless of external pressures" (1992b, p. 269). An interesting analysis of the implications of his nationalist and conservative ideology for his clinical practice can be found in Engstrom (1991).

22. Kraepelin's concept of culture is clearly evolutionist and positivist, and he uses
it in an attempt to justify connections between what he considers to be intellec-
tually underdeveloped life forms: "primitives", children and the insane. With

respect to this comparison, Kraepelin writes: "We are helped somewhat by the comparison of these clinical signs with phenomena we have witnessed in children, in primitive races and in animals. This reveals that mental illnesses resemble conditions found in creatures representing lower forms of intellectual development" (1992a [1920], p. 519).

23. The literature on these three culture-bound syndromes is very extensive. Hughes (1985a), in his Glossary of Culture-Bound or Psychiatric Syndromes defines these disorders as follows:

> Amok: dissociative episode(s); outburst(s) of violent and aggressive or homicidal
>   behavior directed at people and objects; persecutory ideas; automatism;
>   amnesia; exhaustion and return of consciousness following the episode
>   (for amok runners who are not killed during the episode).
>
> Latah: hypersensitivity to sudden fright or startle; hyper-suggestibility; echopraxis;
>   echolalia; dissociative or trance-like behavior.
>
> Koro: intense and sudden anxiety that the penis (or, for females, the vulva and
>   breasts) will recede into the body; the penis is held by the victim or some-
>   one else, or devices are attached to prevent its receding (Hughes, 1985a, p.
>   469-505).

24. Griesinger's influence on Kraepelin, particularly on his early writings, is notorious. The first edition of his *Lehrbuch* (*Compendium of Psychiatry*), written in 1883 at the suggestion of Wilhelm Wundt when Kraepelin was 27, is in fact very similar to Griesinger's classic textbook *Pathologie und Therapie der psychischen Krankheiten* (*Mental Pathology and Therapeutics*), published in 1876. See Beer (1992).

25. Karl Kracpelin, Emile Kraepelin's elder brother, was a well-known botanist and naturalist who was director of the Natural History Museum in Hamburg between 1889 and 1914, as well as his brother's faithful companion on his various ethnopsychiatric excursions. See Boroffka (1988).

CHAPTER 4

Neo-Kraepelinism I: Nosologies

Psychiatry still lives in a Kraepelinian world and its practitioners cannot escape the blinding embrace of its episteme.

—G. Berrios & R. Hauser
The early development of Kraepelin's ideas on classification:
a conceptual history.
Psychological Medicine

In the previous chapter we saw how the Kraepelinian project attempted to describe and classify mental disorders by assuming that, one day, a particular organic dysfunction could be found underlying each specific manifestation. Avoiding any speculative etiological explanation, Kraepelin encouraged plain description of the behavior and manifestations involved in clinical cases, and differentiated between those symptoms of an episodic nature and those of longer duration which enabled the formulation of a universal and stable classification. His naturalist nosology gave greater importance to diseases than to patients' narratives and led to the hegemony of seeing over hearing, of the apparent over the implicit, of the signifier over the signified, of signs over symptoms, of form over content, of the universal over the individual, of explanation (*Erklärung*) over understanding (*Verstehen*). Although the ideal of a specific etiology could not be reached for the time being, psychiatric practice was moving closer to the biomedical model.

Given Kraepelin's interest in achieving a scientific psychiatry, it is not surprising that in the history of psychiatry he is identified as the precursor of modern clinical medicine (Comptom & Guze, 1995, p. 196). This may seem to be a mere anecdote, a product of the positivist history which Canguilhem has criticized as "anecdotal history." This is the sort of history which a discipline writes about itself in which "strokes of genius" light the way towards definitive knowledge (Canguilhem, 1989, p. 235). There are, however, some similarities between the principles of contemporary psychiatry and those of Kraepelin, particularly the early Kraepelin, which can be traced back, not in a superficial and anecdotal way, but through an epistemological-conceptual analysis of a type advocated by authors such as Canguilhem (1955).

One of the most important resemblances is the assumption that the separation of mood/affect from cognitive processes of judgment, memory, and attention could yield an exclusively phenomenological description of different disorders.This idea had already been outlined by Kraepelin who, on the basis of Wundt's psychological model, differentiated between affective disturbances and cognitive or thought disorders. These notions have acquired taxonomic currency in various diagnostic manuals in use at present because they distinguish between disorders such as schizophrenia (the manifestations of which are delusions and hallucinations), and mood disorders, such as major depression (Young, 1991, p. 175).

The idea that symptoms provide information about the course, evolution and outcome of the disease, is also an old principle that has now been revitalized in psychiatric studies. For example, modern research speaks of positive and negative symptoms in schizophrenia. The former are those florid and striking expressions of psychosis: hallucinations (auditory, visual, kinesthetic), the so-called "disturbances in the form of thought" (neologisms, loosening of associations) and the "disturbances in the content of thought" (persecutory delusions, delusions of reference, delusions of being controlled, etc.). The negative symptoms refer to such manifestations as "flat affect," "apathy," "anhedonia," "social isolation and social withdrawal," or "marked impairment in role functioning." What is important for my purposes here is less the possibility of establishing a typology in these terms, than the persistence of the notion that some symptoms are indicative of a good outcome (the positive symptoms) while others (the negative symptoms) are related to a deteriorating course (Andreasen, 1985; Andreasen & Grove, 1986; Andreasen & Carpenter, 1993; Deister & Marneros, 1993).

The similarities also affect the currency of diagnostic categories which sometimes persist under superficial differences in nomenclature (we no longer speak of *dementia praecox* but of schizophrenia, and manic-depressive insanity or psychosis is now bipolar disorder) while others are clearly revealed by the use of identical terminology, as in the case of the diagnostic category of erotomania (Segal, 1989).

Erotomania has been defined as a disorder which primarily, but not exclusively, affects women from modest social strata. It is characterized by the persistent delusional idea that the woman concerned is loved passionately by a man, generally one of higher economic and social status and prestige than her own. The fact that such a suitor is unattainable does not prevent the patient from explaining most convincingly how the supposed admirer has declared his love, or from providing details about the telepathic messages and attentions of which she has been the recipient. These ideas may last for some time, despite their obvious lack of foundation, and the patient's attitude fluctuates between indignation at her admirer's proposals and recognition that she also shares his supposed affection. In any case, the category of erotomania, skillfully analyzed by Kraepelin and absent for some time from diagnostic manuals, has reappeared in the more recent taxonomies such as DSM-III-R and DSM-IV in which it has resumed a position very similar to its original space in the nosographical map. Thus, whereas Kraepelin considered erotomania to be a subcategory of delusions of grandeur, which was in turn a subcategory of paranoia, it is now regarded as a type of delusional disorder alongside those characterized as "grandiose," "jealous," "persecutory" or "somatic" (APA, 1987, p. 200).

As we can see, the extent of these similarities goes beyond mere appearances to reveal important genealogies of knowledge. It is no coincidence that the hegemonic paradigm in contemporary psychiatry is known as neo-Kraepelinism, both by its defenders (Compton & Guze, 1995; Robins & Helzer, 1986) and its critics (Good, 1993; Young, 1991).

THE TAXONOMIES OF NEO-KRAEPELINISM

Neo-Kraepelinism has been defined as a movement which classifies and describes psychopathological pictures and opposes the psychoanalytical viewpoint. Likewise it takes an interest in clinical and epidemiological research and desires "the return of psychiatry to its medical roots" (Guimon, Mezzich & Berrios, 1987, p. 5). It is the outcome of the hegemony of the biomedical viewpoint in the professional sectors of North American psychiatry, which currently dominates.

The emblematic taxonomies of this paradigm are DSM-III, DSM-IIIR and the more up-to-date DSM-IV.[1] The relation between the three is not only one of continuity but also of continuism, because, apart from the timid introduction in DSM-IV of the cultural dimension of mental disorders, the reader notices immediately that they are practically identical. But let us begin from the beginning.

The first of them, DSM-III, is a diagnostic manual coordinated by Spitzer and published in 1980. Previously, other taxonomies of a similar nature had been published, notably the Feighner criteria and Research Diagnostic Criteria (RDC). However, none of these diagnostic criteria had an impact on contemporary psychiatry equal to that of DSM-III. This is made quite clear by the fact that, even though it was originally produced only for use in the North American context, it has subsequently been published in twenty different languages and in numerous countries, and has even had more editions than the WHO International Classification of Diseases. For example, the latest version of the ICD (ICD-10) (WHO 1992a) has incorporated many semantic and nosological criteria from the DSM-III(R), thus reflecting the worldwide hegemony of North American psychiatry.

DSM-III was produced in the context of the biomedicalization of contemporary psychiatry as discussed above. This process would force demand for a classification that departed from the more psychosocial and psychoanalytical approaches of its predecessors, DSM-I and DSM-II. In this psychiatric context, the aim of DSM-III was to create a useful classification "for making treatment and management decisions" based on reliable diagnostic categories resulting from dialogue between the varying theoretical orientations of importance at the time (including, at least in theory, both psychosocial and psychoanalytical approaches). The new diagnostic criteria would also have to be compatible with the WHO International Classification of Diseases, enable a consensus about the meaning of psychiatric categories, and permit the elimination of categories (for example, neurosis) that had lost their usefulness (Spitzer, 1980). These objectives were to give rise to much debate and many questions not only in psychiatry, but also in anthropological critiques.

One of the principles that came in for the harshest criticism was the effort to produce a classification integrating the various theoretical tendencies. This criticism was based on two related questions.

First, an attempt was made to show the clear hegemony of those who defended the neo-Kraepelinian orientation in the advisory committees and in the task force. Here we should recall that one of the defining characteristics of neo-Kraepelinism is its opposition to psychoanalytic theory. Because of this, despite the involvement of professionals representing different theoretical traditions, DSM-III reflected the supremacy of one theoretical tendency over all others and was not the result of a neutral and integrating process. As Michels has pointed out:

> The task force that forged DSM-III was not representative of the interests, the values, or the theoretical diversity of the profession. It was composed of an invisible college that is only one college in the university of American psychiatry (1984; p. 549).

The "invisible college" to which Michels refers is, undoubtedly, the neo-Kraepelinian orientation which had been developing since the 1960s in the Department of Psychiatry of the University of Washington, St Louis (Robins & Helzer, 1986). Its hegemony in the forging of DSM-III has also been pointed out by Allan Young. In principle, the forging of DSM-III was defined by its principal architects as an open and plural process. Nevertheless, Young believes that

> It is hard to believe that so many people representing so many different points of view would simultaneously want to replace the established psychiatric language with a new one...the spirit of pluralism was, without exception, limited to shaping DSM-III's content, i.e. mainly the texts making up the individual entries. On the other hand, the structure of DSM-III was the product of a relatively small and homogeneous circle of people, known among themselves and to their critics as "neo-Kraepelinians." (Young, 1991, p. 176).

Young seems to be right in this respect. DSM-III is a classification whose structure is reminiscent of the Kraepelin taxonomies, which are based on objectivizing the distinctive features of different clinical pictures. The elimination of the concept of neurosis and the attenuation of the heuristic value of the concept of psychosis are evidence of the scant attention accorded to psychoanalytic theories in DSM-III. The fact that the diagnostic categories allow for the use of some terms that are closer to the psychodynamic model is of little value because, while the structure as a whole tends towards neo-Kraepelinism, the logic of DSM-III would prevent the formulation of a theory in contradiction with the model which gave rise to it.

Second, criticism has been directed at the procedure for establishing the validity and reliability of diagnostic categories. In epidemiology, the validity of a category is understood as its ability to represent reality; that is to say, its potential for defining what it is meant to define.[2] Reliability is regarded as the extent of professional agreement on a series of cases; in other words, the extent to which some cases or species are systematically differentiated from others. It is defined more precisely by the epidemiological manuals in the following way:

> *Validity* is the extent to which the results of a measure correspond to the true nature of the phenomena they are measuring. Another word for validity is *accuracy*.

And also:

> *Reliability* is the degree to which repeated measurements of a relatively stable phenomenon fall close together. *Reproducibility* and *precision* are other words for this property (Fletcher, Fletcher & Wagner, 1988, p. 22) [italics in original].

Because of the difficulties involved in establishing the validity of categories and diagnostic criteria in psychiatry, the DSM-III criteria were developed on the basis of diagnostic reliability. Thus, prior to the completion of the final draft, the reliability of diagnosis was assessed by having pairs of clinicians diagnose hundreds of patients (Spitzer, 1980). The reliability proved to be greater in DSM-III than in previous classifications, such as DSM-II. Nevertheless, reliability is only an index of agreement between diagnostic judgments, not a measure of validity. Thus, although validity always requires some measure of reliability, the categories agreed upon by the majority emerged as the most reliable. In an interesting critique of DSM-III, Faust and Miner emphasize that:

> There is no empirical basis from which to argue that a system on which people agree has greater inherent scientific validity. In fact, many great scientific discoveries were initially rejected by the majority (1986, p. 963).

In the final analysis, the only thing which demonstrates reliability is that the group of professionals who have to make clinical judgments is sufficiently homogeneous to agree on certain assumptions. In this context, the diagnostic categories and criteria supported by the majority become the most reliable nosologies. No less important is the problem of validity, of whether the representations in use really correspond to the phenomena they are intended to define, which still remains a mystery. In short, both the hegemony of neo-Kraepelinism and the demonstration of its superiority using the artifact of category reliability, make DSM-III a clear example of how declarations of unifying intent can combine with obviously partisan purposes.

However, this North American nosology is deliberately and self-consciously atheoretical and descriptive. Apart from particular cases of known etiology, as in "organic mental syndromes and disorders," DSM-III makes no attempt to introduce causal hypotheses or to propose treatments, but simply describes the set of symptoms and characteristics associated with each disorder. As Spitzer points out in the introduction:

> Because DSM-III is generally atheoretical with regard to etiology, it attempts to describe comprehensively what the manifestations of the mental disorders are, and only rarely attempts to account for how the disturbances come about, unless the mechanism is included in the definition of disorder. This approach can be said to be 'descriptive' in that the definitions of the disorders generally consist of descriptions of the clinical features of the disorder (1980, p. 7).

The revised version of DSM-III (DSM-III[R]) reiterates the atheoretical and descriptive nature of the taxonomy (Spitzer & Williams, 1987). Even in DSM-IV, despite its less positivist tone, its clearly empiricist orientation can be detected from the very first lines (APA, 1994).

The atheoretical nature of DSM-III is justified by the difficulty of integrating the various theoretical tendencies around particular etiological hypotheses. The example of phobic disorders is used as a paradigm of possible conflicts. Those who favor the psychodynamic approach may believe that these disorders represent "a displacement of anxiety resulting from the breakdown of defensive operations for keeping internal conflict out of consciousness." The behaviorists, on the other hand, understand phobic symptoms in terms of "learned avoidance responses to conditioned anxiety." Finally, those who support an organic hypothesis associate phobic disorders with a "dysregulation of basic biological systems mediating separation anxiety" (Spitzer, 1980, p. 7). Given this diversity of hypotheses and theoretical approaches, DSM-III was apparently designed to make diagnosis based on clinical manifestations acceptable to different schools of thought despite widely divergent explanations of the origins of the symptomatology.

The rationale behind DSM-III is revealed, therefore, as fundamentally classificatory: it is an attempt to define disease manifestations—"easily identifiable behavioral signs or symptoms" such as "mood disturbance," "disorientation" or "psychomotor agitation"—as accurately as possible to reduce the need for clinical inference. In fact, signs and symptoms are classified according to supposed similarities which are made up of various umbrella categories such as anxiety symptoms, mood/affect disturbances, personality traits or physical signs and symptoms, among many others (APA, 1987). This classification of symptomatic species combines with the taxonomy of diagnostic types and subtypes to produce a complete map of the psychopathologic universe. Each syndrome is assumed to be characterized, despite individual variation, by a more or less stable set of symptoms which, as in

Kraepelin's project, enables certain phenomenological patterns to be identified.

In this complex description of clinical pictures, priority is given to those factors which correspond to biological dimensions, although rhetorically psychological and behavioral dimensions are also considered important. Social factors, however, are excluded as determinants of the severity of a particular disorder:

> In DSM-III each of the mental disorders is conceptualized as a clinically significant behavioral or psychological syndrome or pattern that occurs in an individual and that is typically associated with either a painful symptom (distress) or impairment in one or more important areas of functioning (disability). In addition, there is an inference that there is a behavioral, psychological, or biological dysfunction, and that the disturbance is not only in the relationship between the individual and society. (When the disturbance is limited to a conflict between an individual and society, this may represent social deviance, which may or may not be commendable, but is not by itself a mental disorder.) (Spitzer, 1980, p. 6).

DSM-IIIR and DSM-IV reiterate this point:

> Neither deviant behavior (eg. political, religious or sexual) nor conflicts that are primarily between the individual and society are mental disorders unless the deviance or conflict is a symptom of a dysfunction in the individual (APA, 1994, p. xxii).

In the new DSMs, then, there seems to be a clear divide between what is social and what is psychological and biological. Social criteria are not regarded as principles from which psychopathological phenomena can be analyzed. Emphasis is placed on the apparently atheoretical nature of these taxonomies, as well as on their objectivity and scientific neutrality. The new psychiatry is impervious to moral judgments and cultural values. However, in practice, this aseptic and individualizing approach makes it difficult to distinguish between what is behaviorally pathological and what is socially normative; between the psychological and biological background of the symptoms and the cultural universe in which they are produced; between clinical work and the bias introduced by the moral judgments of the professional; and between objective classification and a sort of corporate "common sense."

Perhaps the most representative example of disagreement on such matters is the so-called "antisocial personality disorder" (APA, 1980, p. 320; APA, 1987, p. 344; APA, 1994, p. 645; Widiger & Corbitt, 1995, p. 103). DSM-IIIR stipulates for this diagnosis a pattern of irresponsible and antisocial behavior since the age of 15. Here, "antisocial" refers to such behaviors and attitudes as: "is unable to sustain consistent work behavior;" "fails to conform to social norms with respect to lawful behavior;" "is irritable and aggressive;" "repeatedly fails to honor financial obligations;" "fails to plan ahead, or is impulsive;" "has no regard for the truth;" "is reckless regarding his or her own or others' personal safety;" "if a parent or guardian, lacks ability to function as a responsible parent;" "has never sustained a totally monogamous relationship for more than one year;" and "lacks remorse" (APA, 1987, p. 345). Surprisingly, only four of these ten criteria are needed to diagnose antisocial personality disorder.

DSM-IV has removed two items (irresponsible parenting and failure to sustain a monogamous relationship), added two others to the general criterion of consistent irresponsibility, and reduced the number of criteria for making a diagnosis from four to three. Even so, these changes are not intended as a corrective for the moralizing tone of some of the criteria. The one about monogamous relationships is still included as an example in the text discussion which accompanies the diagnostic criteria for this disorder. But let us look more closely at possible combinations of three criteria, as in the following example: "failure to conform to social norms with respect to lawful behaviors," "deceitfulness, as indicated by repeated lying, use of aliases," and "lack of remorse." Is this combination not applicable to any clandestine political activist? Even the general diagnostic criteria introduced into DSM-IV to prevent confusion between "personality traits" and "personality disorders"—for example, "an enduring pattern of inner experience and behavior that deviates markedly from the expectations of the individual's culture" or "the pattern is stable and of long duration" (1994, p. 633)—are so vague that they can easily be applied to any number of individuals and behavior patterns. Therefore, it is hardly surprising that studies of prison populations have revealed percentages of antisocial personality disorder as high as 80% (Widiger & Corbitt, 1995, p. 106). On the contrary, the surprising thing would be to find lower percentages using these criteria.

However, what should be highlighted here is the odd way in which the definition of mental disorder is separated from its social context when the behaviors and attitudes which make up the diagnostic criteria are related to a particular ethic, acquiring their pathological meaning from a clear pattern of social abnormality. In fact, antisocial personality disorder is a clear example of this obvious contradiction between a biomedical ideal of asociality and the impossibility in practice of adhering to this model.

The biomedical inspiration of DSM-III(R) and DSM-IV is also evident in another no less important point: the definition of "mental disorder." In various diagnostic manuals the concept of "mental disorder" does not have precise boundaries, but is as ambiguous as such notions as "mental and physical health" or "physical disorder" (APA, 1994, p. xxi). It is also stressed that a classification of disorders such as this does not attempt to classify individuals: diseases are one thing, and the individuals who suffer them quite another:

> A common misconception is that a classification of mental disorders classifies people, when actually what are being classified are disorders that people have. For this reason, the text of DSM-IV (as did the text of DSM-III-R) avoids the use of such expressions as "a schizophrenic" or "an alcoholic" and instead uses the more accurate, but admittedly more cumbersome, "a person with Schizophrenia" or "a person with Alcohol Dependence" (APA, 1994, p. xxii).

This principle was an attempt to discredit a traditional assumption which marginalized psychiatry because of its object of knowledge; namely, the idea that if most physical diseases reflect *suffering* or *having* ("J suffers from coronary heart disease"), mental disorders are mainly associated with *being* rather than *having* ("J is a schizophrenic"). Breaking with this assumption brings about an ontological and epistemiological reconciliation between physical diseases and mental disorders, in effect marginalizing the psychoanalytic model in favor of the biomedical model (recall that in classical psychoanalysis, psychopathology is closely linked to the patient's life, personality and family history). For a scientific psychiatry this association between being and pathology, between biography and mental disorder, is at best inaccurate and at worst simply wrong (recall Kraepelin's prioritizing of diseases over patients).

By locating diseases outside being, the new DSMs bring into play two assumptions which, although closely interrelated, are analytically separable. In the first instance, those individuals who suffer from a mental disorder are not further burdened by stigma. However, in the second instance, this understanding of pathological phenomena enables psychiatry to counter any attempt at marginalization with respect to the biomedical model, because *having* seems to be more relevant to the domain of the body (*soma*) than to the domain of the mind (*psyche*). Here, there is a need to differentiate between the disease and the patient in order to justify the objectivity, rationality and neutrality of psychiatric knowledge. This assertion, however, is not unproblematic. As Fabrega has pointed out,

> Whereas disease accounting in general medicine and surgery is a commentary *about* the physical body and indirectly *about the self*, disease accounting in

psychiatry is a direct commentary *on* the self and *of* the self. (1993, p. 167)
[italics in original]

What constitutes being, and what suffering? Taking as a reference some symptoms which are used as diagnostic criteria in the most recent DSMs, we can see how the symptomatological definition itself introduces considerable ambiguity: "is reluctant to confide in others;" "is critical, blaming, and derogatory toward self;" "flattening of affect;" "is pessimistic;" "feelings of hopelessness;" "irritability and aggressiveness;" "disorganized behavior;" and "is overconscientious, scrupulous and inflexible about matters of morality, ethics or values," among many others. Even in disorders with a more clearly organic etiology, such as schizophrenia, it is hard to differentiate between the effects of a neurochemical or cerebral abnormality (eg. hallucinations, delusions or catatonic stupor) and individual idiosyncracy. Where, for example, can we place symptoms such as flattening of affect or social isolation? What is the exact criterion for differentiating between a foreign entity that upsets bodily equilibrium, and an aspect of the patient's self? This way of separating the mind from the body reflects a model, prototype or pattern, rather than a discovery or a scientific finding. Mind/body dualism is deeply rooted in Cartesian doctrine, but this is not to say that it is an invariable feature; it is simply an ideological and cultural assumption.

Another of the characteristics of the neo-Kraepelinian taxonomies is their ambiguity about whether the diagnostic categories reflect discrete diseases. The introduction to all the manuals states that the categories should not be regarded as separate entities, with strict limits which differentiate them from other mental or physical disorders. For example, DSM-IV states:

In DSM-IV, there is no assumption that each category of mental disorder is a completely discrete entity with absolute boundaries dividing it from other mental disorders or from no mental disorder (APA, 1994, p. xxii).

This is an attempt to sidestep the old polemic about whether the different disorders simply reflect quantitative differences or clear qualitative discrepancies. This had been a question of the utmost significance, not only in the confrontation with the psychosocial theories—recall that the psychosocial model regarded mental illness as a continuum going from mental health to psychosis, passing through neurosis[3]—but also at the heart of the more biomedical tendencies which debated the utility of psychosis or depression as a unitary diagnosis. In this context, the new DSMs seem to take a neutral position: they neither affirm nor deny similarities among psychopathological species. In the final analysis, however, different disorders are constructed as discrete entities. Diagnostic practice always involves delimiting the clinical picture. The orientation of the neo-Kraepelinian taxonomies is clearly pro-diagnostic and not anti-diagnostic, as some theoretical positions within the psychosocial model had maintained;[4] in addition, the analogy of mental disorders as discrete disease entities can be inferred from the internal structure of the manual, since it is essentially classificatory, and its logic demands bounded psychiatric categories.

The intent of the new DSMs, however, is not merely classificatory. Their structure not only makes it difficult to infer connections between its main types and subtypes (anxiety disorders, schizophrenia and other psychotic disorders, personality disorders, etc.) but also contradicts the theory that mental illness may be appproached processually. Here there are no concepts like Freud's "unconscious processes" or Meyer's idea of "reaction," which allow for connections between different pathological processes. In fact, the very need to describe the different disorders with clear, observable, accurate features reinforces the appearance of each species as a discrete entity similar to any physical pathology. For example, if we were to analyze the category "delusional disorder," we would observe that one of the essential criteria for its diagnosis is that "Criterion A for Schizophrenia has never been met" (APA, 1994, p. 301). One of the three requisites for diagnosing major depressive disorder is also that "There has never been a Manic Episode, a Mixed Episode or a Hypomanic Episode" (p. 345). Most of the disorders require a differential diagnosis, a contrast, if they are to be correctly recognized. In other words, the priority of the new DSMs is to define the boundaries separating different disorders, not to trace their similarities.

Both DSM-III(R) and DSM-IV introduce a multiaxial system which makes it possible to diagnose a varied repertoire of disorders in the same patient (co-morbidity). In DSM-IV, the first axis is for the so-called "clinical disorders and other conditions that may be a focus of clinical attention;" the second is for "personality disorders and mental retardation;" the third for "general medical conditions;" the fourth for "psychosocial and environmental problems;" and finally, the fifth for "global assessment of functioning." The following is a case example given by the authors:

> Axis I: 296.23 Major Depressive Disorder. Single Episode, Severe Without Psychotic Features.
> 305.00 Alcohol Abuse
> Axis II: 301.60 Dependent Personality Disorder. Frequent use of denial
> Axis III: None
> Axis IV: Threat of job loss
> Axis V: GAF=35 (current) (1994; p.33).

Of these five axes, the first three are the ones that are normally included in clinical reports, while the last two are of an anecdotal nature because they are often used only in specific studies. Strangely enough, these two axes provide not only qualitative but also quantitative information. For instance, the result of Axis V is found by using a scale (GAF scale) which consists, paradoxically, of a continuum numbered from 0 to 100 in which the clinician assesses the patient's "psychological, social and occupational functioning" (APA, 1994, p. 30). Fortunately, in DSM-IV Axis IV is not measured quantitatively. It should be pointed out, however, that in DSM-IIIR this axis is subject to quantification. On a scale from 1 to 6 for measuring psychosocial stressors, "broke up with boyfriend or girlfriend" had a value of 2, "marital separation" 3 and a "divorce" 4 (APA, 1987, p. 11).

In the first three axes, the different diseases are clearly defined and there are no references to their possible origins. Even the individual who gives form to this wealth of categories, diseases and circumstances appears to be practically annulled as a referent, because the various disorders are expressed in a logic of their own which needs no biographical shape. As in Kraepelin's project, the emphasis is on diseases and not on patients, reinforcing the idea that an individual "suffers from a disorder" rather than "is disturbed." The cataloguing of the disorders inhabiting the patient's body ("major depression," "alcohol abuse," "dependent personality disorder") reasserts the model of "suffering from," and weakens the links between the disease and the patient's "being." The patient is thus converted into a mute space in which different pathological species coincide. It is of little importance that an appendix included in DSM-IV provides a glossary of culture-bound syndromes and appears to stress the importance of cultural and social factors in the etiology, course and outcome of mental disorders.[5] The patients' voices have no place in the multiaxial system of neo-Kraepelinism. This naturalist approach denies us access to large or small worlds of meaning, to the cultural categories and political-economic relations that a complaint may contain. Like Kraepelin's taxonomies, the new DSMs disregard the possible understanding of the patient's narrative in favor of a botany of mental illnesses.

Taking the relationship between the new nosologies and the Kraepelinian project much farther than most, Michels, one of the fiercest critics of DSM-III, feels that the analogy between mental disorders and physical diseases was not the result of neo-Kraepelinism but rather of a "hyper-Kraepelinism" which would have made Kraepelin himself uncomfortable (Michel, 1984, p. 549). While the Kraepelinian project attached a certain importance (albeit limited) to psychological variables,[6] Michels argues, the psychic order in DSM-III is conspicuous only by its absence.

The question of whether DSM-III and its successors give any real importance to psychological and social variables has been a highly controversial topic. For those who represent the neo-Kraepelinian and biomedical approach, the new classifications constitute one of the most important advances in modern psychiatry. Its unexpected success, they argue, is proof of its usefulness, noting that nowhere does it discount the possibility of a psychological and psychosocial approach to mental disorders. In fact, they normally characterize the orientation of the DSMs as biopsychosocial, pointing to its atheoretical nature and the multiaxial structures which allow for the inclusion of different types of data. The DSMs are held up as an example of possible collaboration between different theoretical viewpoints, as simple collections of species which permit the naming of psychopathological phenomena.

Nevertheless, this aseptic and objective image has been challenged by those sectors of the profession whose concerns are not reflected in these nosologies and see in their application the dangers of a biomedicalized, static, descriptive, falsely objective and reductionistic practice (Faust & Miner, 1987; Michels, 1984; Pascalis, Perceau, Théret, Jarraya & Achich, 1988). The problem is that, even though the DSMs are defined as integrative nosologies, if their diverse but practically clonal multiaxial structures are observed closely, it can be seen that they have two axes for diagnosing mental disorders and a third for physical diseases. As in Kraepelin's early work, in these axes there seems to be no room for the psychic, whether this is understood in terms of a defense mechanism model, an intrapsychic conflict model, or existentialist model. Strangely, this closing off of the psychic domain cannot be blamed on to the lack of an appropriate axis, because the second one is particularly appropriate for personality disorders. It is an outcome of the restrictive and purely diagnostic logic used in these manuals.

A similar situation emerges from the last two axes (IV and V), which provide supposedly psychosocial information, but because they are not indispensable for diagnostic purposes, they often go practically unnoticed. What is more, as we have seen above, the structuring of information on psychosocial and environmental problems and on psychological, social and occupational functioning is inappropriate for a sociocultural contextualization of the case, since a biomedical model is being applied to complex data of a non-biomedical nature. Scotch had already warned against this danger in a programmatic article on medical anthropology: "To be sure, medical research which has encompassed sociocultural variables has not always been particularly sophisticated. Physicians tend to use such variables in crude and unsystematic ways" (1963, p. 31).

In the case of the new DSMs we may speak, perhaps, of greater sophistication—though in fact this often comes down to technical and quantitative pseudo-sophistication—but under no circumstances can we speak of psychosocial variables being treated in an appropriately contextualized way. The model for understanding physiopathological phenomena is systematically transferred to the domain of social and behavioral phenomena, with the result that a culturally relative condition such as "threat of job loss" ends up reified in terms that are not so different from evidence of "major depressive disorder."

These taxonomies reveal a clearly biomedical point of view in spite of the fact that the reader may initially notice a slight terminological discrepancy: namely, that even though the biomedical approach often appears to be a reductionistic one in which social aspects can be subsumed in psychological terms (which, in the final analysis, can be included in a biological order), the DSMs are explicitly presented as biopsychosocial models which seek to integrate explanatory variables from different dimensions of reality. However, if the structure of these manuals is examined in greater depth, we observe that these dimensions are not given equal weight, but are ranked in the same order as the terms bio-psycho-social.[7] This order of priorities reveals the extent to which the DSMs are grounded in reaction against psychological and psychiatric theories that locate the origins of psychopathological processes in nonbiological spaces. This reaction was particularly virulent in the United States (probably as a result of the considerable impact that psychosocial and psychodynamic theories had after the Second World War) but it was soon to become the hegemonic model of the psychiatric profession the world over. For the defenders of the model, this internationalization is "not entirely the result of psychiatric imperialism, but rather springs from a correspondence between these categories and phenomena in the real world that have parallels to physical diseases" (Robins & Helzer, 1986, p. 410).

Here there is an interesting identification between categories and real phenomena which enables psychiatric nosologies to be presented as neutral entities, and therefore independent of cultural and historical context. Such a correspondence between words and things reveals a positivist and empiricist bias.

THE COPY OF FACTS

Neo-Kraepelinism, like biomedicine in general, is closely related to philosophical-empiricist approaches to language. Such diverse authors as Laín

Entralgo (1961), Givner (1962) and Good (1977) have attempted to demonstrate that Locke's theory of human understanding and its constitutive processes developed out of the medical research of his friend Sydenham, particularly with respect to the concepts of designation and classification.[8] Although we should point out that Locke is more a rational empiricist than a crude empiricist, the fact remains that these authors are correct in establishing a link between empiricism and Western medicine. In medical discourse since Sydenham, naming and classifying have become activities necessary for the development of knowledge. Neither speculative nor conscious of the distance which separates words from things, this kind of knowledge joins names to objects in an isomorphic relation. In this way any distinction between biomedical categories (ideational) and pathological processes (real) is eliminated. A diagnostic category is not perceived as a more or less arbitrary social construction characterized by its embeddedness in a particular cultural and historical context which is the product of historical forms of treatment. Biomedical psychiatry regards categories as real, universally valid units which are simply the consequence of the evolution of medical knowledge, experimental research and epidemiological analysis. In other words, they are the consequence of an internal logic which, by approximating itself to the real world, rejects the erroneous categories and concentrates on the true ones (Robins & Helzer, 1986).

Undoubtedly, the DSM's aforementioned claim to represent an atheoretical and purely descriptive taxonomy is one of the clearest indicators that it subscribes to this ideology of knowledge. An epistemological assumption is being made here. The process of knowledge is seen as directional; that is to say, it moves from fact to theory, not from theoretical hypothesis to fact. If DSM is a simple presentation of disorders, syndromes, symptoms and manifestations, the pathway to theory is the unfinished task which every clinician must undertake, armed with the knowledge at his disposal. But this is a problematic quest. Is a nosological description possible in the absence of some sort of theory? Do not even simple taxonomies rest on an underlying theory?

Faust and Miner, in an article cited above on the connections between empiricism and DSM-III, have attempted to demonstrate the impossibility of an atheoretical approach such as the one advanced in this nosography:

> We will argue that DSM-III's appearance of objectivity is largely illusory. Theory and inference have perhaps been reduced somewhat but eliminated nowhere—the document is replete with presuppositions and theoretical assumptions (1986, p. 963).

From this point of view, the DSM-III is by no means free of theoretical assumptions. In fact, it is precisely the denial of theory that allows us to situate this manual in the terrain of empiricist ideology. For Faust and Miner, DSM-III's attempt to impose limits on inference and theory represents the application of the Baconian principle that nature reveals itself through directly observable facts and objective phenomena. Indeed, precise description reflects in its categories an order of irreducible reality which is discovered rather than constructed. According to Faust and Miner, this goal is unattainable, not only for psychiatry, but for any scientific discipline.

Similarly, Fabrega (1987) has attempted to place the taxonomic model of DSM-III within the framework of a naturalist epistemiology of mental disorders. In a fitting comparison between North American nosology and botanical classifications, he suggests that achieving an exact reproduction of phenomena is much more difficult in a classification of psychiatric disorders than in other types of facts and/or phenomena, because botanical taxonomies differ ontologically from classifications of psychiatric disorders. In the former, according to Fabrega, an object and a category are in closer contact. However, in psychiatric classifications the situation is much more complex because the manifestations of mental disorders are essentially behavioral realities, and hence more abstract. To clarify this distinction, he uses the example of co-morbidity discussed above: when various diagnostic categories are present in the same case, it is difficult to determine what is related to what. Why is the patient behaving aggressively? Is his behavior the product of a schizophrenic disorder, a personality disorder or a substance-related disorder?[9]

Fabrega's appraisal coincides with that of Faust and Miner, observing that the list of symptoms, courses, complications and diagnoses which comprises DSM-III is anything but atheoretical. It is undergirded by an empiricist theory of language, a doctrine which places categories and phenomena in an isomorphic relation. In the neo-Kraepelinian taxonomies, diagnosis becomes the simple exercise of applying predetermined names to things. This maneuver is an attempt to limit theoretical inference, just as the positivist tradition attempted to restrict its theoretical scope to being "a copy of the facts" (Habermas, 1989, p. 93). Categories emerge as representations adapted to a psychopathological reality, just as classical positivism believed that thought adapted itself to facts. The DSMs are not, therefore, atheoretical taxonomies; rather, theory (again, as in positivist schools of thought) is restricted to the justification for suppressing reflection concerning the relationship between the subject and object of knowledge, between representations and facts (or other representations), and between diagnostic categories and psychopathological manifestations.

The empiricist bias would not assume such importance if it were a question of classifying species of trees, fossils or even skin diseases. However, as Fabrega points out, more is at stake in the case of mental disorders because of the degree of abstraction involved. Here we are dealing not only with facts, but also with human behavior, experience, and emotions.

In clinical practice, psychiatrists encounter not signs but symptoms: linguistic, cultural and semiotic realities which cannot be understood without considerable inference. Abdominal swelling means nothing in itself. "My heart aches" or "I feel depressed," on the other hand, are messages that imply a sender, a context and a code of meanings. However, the DSMs quickly and superficially circumvent the problem of meaning by reifying the symptoms, transforming them into objective realities on the same level as eczema or abdominal swelling. Let us take a look at some illustrative examples.

An individual has schizophrenia if, in its active phase (for at least a month), he exhibits symptoms such as "delusions" and "disorganized speech" accompanied by social and occupational dysfunction, and his "continuous signs of the disturbance persist for at least six months" (APA, 1994, p. 285). Another individual suffers from a "dysthymic disorder" if, for at least two years, he experiences depressed mood and at least two symptoms from a possible list of six (e.g., "feelings of hopelessness" and "low self-esteem"). This diagnosis is excluded in cases of major depressive episodes, manic episodes, disturbances that take place during a chronic psychotic disorder or when the symptoms are the direct physiological effects of medication or other substances. A third individual suffers from "psychoactive substance abuse" if, for instance, he makes "recurrent use [of the substance in question] in situations in which use is physically hazardous (e.g., driving while intoxicated)" for at least a month (APA, 1987, p. 169). A fourth patient suffers from a "paranoid personality disorder" if he exhibits four of seven possible manifestations; for example,

1. "suspects, without sufficient basis, that others are exploiting, harming or deceiving him or her;"
2. "is preoccupied with unjustified doubts about the loyalty or trustworthiness of friends or associates;"
3. "reads hidden demeaning or threatening meanings into benign remarks or events" (for example, he believes that a neighbor puts his rubbish out early with the sole intention of annoying him);
4. "persistently bears grudges," i.e., is unforgiving of insults, injuries or slights (APA, 1994, p. 637).

What is striking here is not only the fragility of the criteria, but also the way in which they are deployed. On the one hand, it is clear that "bears grudges," "is unforgiving of insults" or "suspects that others are exploiting her or him" are not directly observable phenomena. On the contrary, they require not only close reading, but multiple and contrasting interpretations: those of the spouse, relatives and friends of the supposed victim of a "paranoid personality disorder" as well as that of the patient himself. But, on the other hand, the list of diagnostic criteria treats these manifestations as stable elements which can, for diagnostic purposes, be disengaged from their cultural and historical context. While it is true that DSM-IV places special and unprecedented emphasis on the analysis of the patient's social and cultural environment, it is difficult to take cultural contextualization very far when the point of departure is a set of biomedicalized diagnostic criteria. In fact, although most of the criteria refer to symptoms in the strict sense, they are treated as objective and individualized physical signs reflecting a universal and recognizable order of reality. The clinician's task is to identify the criteria corresponding to a psychopathological species of the same order as diseases of known physical etiology, and to arrange these manifestations in a logical sequence and temporal frame that yields a diagnosis. However, the groupings introduced by the new DSMs are not representations which account for observed phenomena, but representations of other representations. The manuals do not place sufficient emphasis on the need to understand symptoms as messages endowed with local, original and polysemous meaning; instead, diagnostic criteria are presented as facts or natural signifiers not subject to cultural variability. "Auditory hallucinations," "suspects that others are exploiting her or him," "feelings of hopelessness" or "low self-esteem" are considered to be factual phenomena rather than the inevitable results of cultural interpretation and contextualization. In this way the categories and criteria are reified and converted into objective, natural and directly recognizable facts. Here some obvious questions emerge. What are "feelings of hopelessness," and from whose point of view? How is low self-esteem determined? Why should low self-esteem be considered pathological? What is a "sufficient basis" for feeling exploited? Not to mention such questions as: Is it true or false that a neighbor puts his rubbish out early with the sole intention of annoying the patient?

Apart from the need to differentiate between truth and deceit, a task which is not only the clinician's but also the ethnographer's, clearly these questions can only be answered through an analysis of the social and cultural context in which low self-esteem or feelings of hopelessness and exploitation acquire meaning. The bizarre and inappropriate nature of some types of behavior is revealed in the play of contrasts between the socially normative and the socially abnormal. However, we already know that the DSMs, albeit in a somewhat contradictory fashion, deny the diagnostic value of social criteria in identifying psychopathology. How, then, do they work?

The immediate answer is that, despite the introduction of cultural dimensions of mental illness in DSM-IV, the understanding of symptoms seems to be highly ethnocentric. The neo-Kraepelinists, however, would disagree, very likely arguing that the diagnostic criteria reflect manifestations which, stripped of their cultural context, reflect universal pathological processes. That is to say, their answer would not be so very different from the way in which Kraepelin used the distinction between pathoplasticity and pathogenicity to explain away variety in the expression of insanity: epiphenomenal manifestations are one thing, while underlying pathology is another.

However, to what extent do the symptoms adopted as criteria in the modern taxonomies refer to universal pathological processes? Is this not a transformation of the patients' expressions (symptoms), which are individual, into natural phenomena (physical signs), which are supposedly universal? It is only possible to speak of "low self-esteem," "feelings of hopelessness" or "auditory hallucinations" in a general and universal sense because they have been reified. To the extent that "I hear voices" is transformed into "auditory hallucinations," the experience loses its original meaning, which is a product of its social and cultural embedment. The symptom has been converted into a natural signifier, a physical sign whose only meaning is determined by clinical practice.

The difficulties of the neo-Kraepelinian nosologies generally arise out of these two problems: deploying categories as a copy of the facts, and reifying symptoms as physical signs. Of course, the distance separating categories (ideal) from phenomena (real) is not an issue limited to psychiatry, but one shared by all forms of knowledge. However, it is more problematic in psychiatry than for other biomedical disciplines in which pathophysiological processes can be observed, because the symptomalogical criteria deployed in DSM-III(R) or DSM-IV do not normally reflect a mute and asemiotic reality discoverable through clinical observation as physical signs, but belong to the domain of the patient's experience and forms of expression as symptoms. Here the contradiction involved in reifying the patient's symptoms as objective and isolated facts becomes evident. A case of eczema or an X-ray showing a malignancy have little to do with low self-esteem. But those symptoms which constitute syndromes cannot be diagnosed without understanding that the object of knowledge is a human being whose behavior is located in a context of meaning and experience. Any other approach risks confining the meaning of symptoms within the boundaries of a sort of professional common sense, or to a notion of diagnostic reliability in which there is no room for cultural variation. By this I do not mean that the reliability of diagnostic criteria is unimportant or unnecessary for the development of a valid classification of mental illnesses, nor that it is impossible to validate diagnostic categories to some extent. The problem is rather that the validity of a category in psychiatry requires interpretation of the context in which symptoms acquire their meaning, and a degree of reflexivity concerning the usefulness of the categories themselves. As Kleinman rightly points out:

> Validation of psychiatric diagnoses is not simply verification of the concepts used to explain observations. It is also verification of the meaning of observations in a given social system (a village, an urban clinic, a research laboratory). That is to say, observation is inseparable from interpretation. Psychiatric diagnoses are not things...Categories are the outcomes of historical development, cultural influence and political negotiation. Psychiatric categories are no exception (Kleinman, 1988b, p. 12).

True, the new DSMs point out that it is not the manual that interprets symptoms and mental disorders but the clinician, once the diagnosis is established. Nevertheless, the descriptive structure of a given set of diagnostic criteria seriously limits interpretation of the patient's narrative. Symptoms reconstructed as physical signs block both understanding (*Verstehen*) and interpretation (*Auslegung*). And all this in the interest of diagnostic categories which, in the final analysis, are not stable but adrift, unmoored to any knowledge of illness etiology.

In short, the most crucial problem of the neo-Kraepelinian taxonomies is the way their descriptive structure, grounded in the model of representations as a copy of facts, forecloses the interpretation of symptoms. But in this case the facts themselves are representations: meaningful behaviors and forms of expression. Of course, this positivist exercise in objectification eliminates certain inconveniences. In the domain of clinical practice, for example, the idea of isomorphism between categories and facts eliminates the risk of inaction; we should not forget that psychiatry is also a therapeutic technique that requires quick response on the part of the clinician. In the domain of psychiatric theory, however, something else is achieved: the elimination of reflexivity and a certain critical distance from one's own diagnostic categories. This danger was pointed out by Breuer, in a passage in *Studies on Hys-*

teria , a work co-authored with Freud and published at the end of the nine-teenth century (1893-5). Having developed his argument on hysteria, Breuer then called the reader's attention to the gulf separating reality, which always remains just out of reach, from the representations of it that he and Freud had constructed. Of these representations, Breuer concluded, "we must always say ...what Theseus in *A Midsummer Night's Dream* says of tragedy: 'The best in this kind are but shadows'" (SE, II, p. 250).

NOTES

1. Here I will not analyze the taxonomies of the World Health Organization: International Classification of Diseases, versions nine and ten. Even so, much of this chapter will also be applicable to them.
2. Spitzer and Williams (1992), two authors belonging to the neo-Kraepelinian group, have suggested the possibility of different types of validity not necessarily linked to the strict sense of the term. Some of these are: "apparent validity" (agreement at first sight between category and real phenomenon), "descriptive validity" (the singularity of the features which make up a category in comparison with their presence or absence in other categories), "predictive validity" (the relation between diagnostic category and the expected effect of the treatment and/or the prognosis of the disease), and "construct validity" (consistency of the category with an etiological hypothesis). In all these cases the validity of the categories is apparent and hypothetical, not corroborated.
3. It should be pointed out here that not all psychosocial and psychoanalytical tendencies have maintained the idea of a continuum of mental illness. The Lacanian school, represented at present by the European School of Psychoanalysis, considers that there are three main groups of clearly defined psychopathology: neurosis, psychosis and perversion.
4. See Robins and Helzer (1986) for an analysis of debates prior to DSM-III between pro-diagnostic (neo-Kraepelinian) and anti-diagnostic positions.
5. For a discussion on the place of culture in psychiatric nosologies, see Mezzich, Fabrega and Kleinman (1992) and Fabrega (1992). These works reflect the critiques and commentary directed to the task force in charge of developing DSM-IV by leading cultural experts during a conference in Pittsburgh in 1991. Thanks to contributions of this sort, as well as consultants on transcultural issues in DSM-IV, the task force made relative improvements in the assessment of the relations between culture and mental disorders. Nevertheless, these improvements were, in the final analysis, too timid to make a difference. DSM-IV attempts to combine a naturalist approach, which is clearly hegemonic and was already present

in DSM-IIIR, with a culturalist orientation which is clearly subordinate. The final result is that cultural and social factors are treated as biomedical variables.

6. This statement is more relevant to the later Kraepelin than to the earlier; that is to say, to the reflective Kraepelin who thought deeply about his excursions into ethnopsychiatry; the Kraepelin who wrote the eighth edition of his *Lerhbuch* and "The manifestations of Insanity."

7. The term bio-psycho-social condenses a professional hierarchy in which the psychiatrist controls the principal content (biological), the psychologist the secondary content (psychological), and the social worker the third-order content (social). Within this hierarchy there are routes which lead downward (bio-psycho-social), but not upward (socio-psycho-biological).

8. Locke himself refers to his friend Sydenham in his "The Epistle to the Reader" which opens *An Essay Concerning Human Understanding*. See Locke (1975, p. 9).

9. For an interesting review of the phenomenon of co-morbidity, see Manser and Dinges (1992). Although their approach is fundamentally neo Kraepelinian, it also makes use of anthropological literature to account for this phenomenon among Native Americans in Alaska.

CHAPTER 5

Neo-Kraepelinism II: Epidemiologies

The epidemiologist views the etnographer's task as "impressionistic", "uncontrolled," "messy," "soft," "unrigorous," "anecdotical," "unscientific;" the etnographer, in near perfect counterpoint, regards the epidemiologist's work as "superficial," "biased," "pseudoscientific," "invalid," "unscholarly."
— Arthur Kleinman & Byron Good
Culture and Depression

In recent decades, psychiatry has found in large-scale epidemiological research a source of reliable and generalizable knowledge about mental disorders, measuring their prevalence and incidence,[1] analyzing their courses of evolution, and studying their signs and symptoms. However, this interest in epidemiological studies should not be regarded as a new phenomenon. As we have seen above, Kraepelin had already outlined the principles of a comparative psychiatry in later editions of his *Lehrbuch* and in "The Manifestations of Insanity." It should also be pointed out that ambitious studies were undertaken during the psychosocial period: for instance, the Midtown Manhattan Study (Srole et al., 1962), the New Haven study of prevalence (Hollingshead & Redlich, 1958), and the early sociological research on the prevalence of schizophrenia in the city of Chicago (Faris & Dunham, 1939).[2]

Contemporary epidemiology, therefore, belongs to an already existing tradition, although it is no coincidence that it shares more similarities with Kraepelin's comparative project than with the studies of the psychosocial era. In fact, we can be detect a fundamental difference between the aims of neo-Kraepelinism and the psychosocial tendencies which made the so-called "golden era of social epidemiology" possible in the United States (Klerman, 1986, p. 159). Whereas the Midtown Manhattan and New Haven studies stressed such psychosocial variables as urban anomie, social isolation, the changes caused by industrialization, and individual psychodynamics, the present emphasis has shifted to the prevalence, symptoms, signs, course and prognosis of mental disorders. This is due to an epistemiological change of considerable significance: psychiatry has replaced an epidemiology of mental health with an epidemiology of mental disorders (Klerman, 1986). The most cursory glance at the existing literature shows that the psychosocial perspective, grounded in the idea of a continuum between health and mental illness (also understood as a continuum running from neurosis to psychosis) has given way to an approach based on discrete nosological categories: schizophrenia, depression, anxiety, etc. This is what Klerman has called the beginning of a "new era in psychiatric epidemiology" (1986, p. 165).

In this new approach to mental illness, clinical psychiatry and epidemiology are unusually interdependent. First of all, contemporary epidemiological research requires precise definition of disease processes based on diagnostic criteria such as the DSM-III(R), DSM-IV or the various ICDs (eighth, ninth or tenth editions). Second, epidemiological findings are intended to adjust the diagnostic criteria for the various psychopathologies; to deepen understanding of their courses and outcomes; and to reveal, or at least suggest, possible etiological factors. Even so, we should keep in mind that psychiatric epidemiology, especially cross-sectional or longitudinal research, is considered more useful for improving clinical practice than for discovering etiological processes. The reason for this is that neo-Kraepelinism, unlike the psychosocial model, deemphasizes the sociocultural context of mental illness etiology, which includes processes of anomie, social mobility or economic inequalities. The emphasis on biological processes in contemporary psychiatry limits the development of causal knowledge almost exclusively to the area of experimental design studies, that laboratory epidemiology in which variables are controlled from the outset by the researcher, new drugs are tested, and the presence or absence of symptoms— evidence of changes in an underlying physical reality—are observed.

In the context of this new epidemiology, any dialogue between psychiatry and anthropology would seem irrelevant and anecdotal, at least if we compare the biological interests of neo-Kraepelinism with those of the psychosocial model. However, this is not in fact the case. The results of epidemiological research have opened up new areas of interest and debate about the possible relation between psychopathological processes and certain sociocultural variables. The epidemiological interest in defining the universal signs and symptoms of each psychopathological diagnosis has come up, as it did in Kraepelin's work, against cultural realities not easily be contained by a homogeneous framework. For example, the symptoms which constitute psychiatric categories have shown a wide phenomenological range cross-culturally. Similarly, the courses and outcomes of mental diseases bear the imprint of social and cultural factors. These observations have given rise to debates between psychiatry and anthropology reminiscent of the classical confrontations between the two disciplines: a) the conflict between universalist (epidemiological) and particularist (ethnographic) positions; b) the opposition between biomedical positivism and the often antipositivist tone of ethnographic work; c) the contrast between quantitative techniques and the qualitative or mixed techniques which medical and psychiatric anthropology employs; and d) the problem of relativity in clinical psychiatry, particularly in the case of culture-bound syndromes.

One of the most striking features of the new dialogue is the increasingly technical nature of the debates, owing to the more biomedical nature of contemporary psychiatry: greater emphasis is given to the reliability of measurement instruments (eg. scales, tests, diagnostic schedules) and to the use of sophisticated mathematical methods and computer technology. These innovations have brought about a change, a rhetorical one at least, in this interdisciplinary dialogue. Discussions about whether a particular item of a particular diagnostic instrument can accurately identify a psychopathological state, symptom or process within a specific cultural context are now more common in the literature than debates on Oedipus complexes and psychological defenses. This does not mean that the dialogue between anthropology and psychoanalysis has been exhausted: a review of the literature suggests that this is not so (Kurtz, 1991; Spiro, 1992; Kurtz, 1993). It simply means that the main topics of discussion in a psychiatry that marginalizes psychoanalysis must logically be of a different nature.

Generally speaking, the new debates can be divided into two main areas: a) those factors that research findings have been unable to account for; and b) the debates that have arisen about the validity of measurement instruments. I shall call the former "findings" and the latter "instruments."

FINDINGS

The decade of the sixties was undoubtedly an important moment for psychiatric epidemiology, at least if we give credence to the accounts of veteran researchers (Sartorius, 1993). During these years, both the Division of Mental Health of the World Health Organization and the various centers in the United States and Great Britain decided to give fresh impetus to epidemiological research on an international level. From this impetus several studies emerged.

The first was the US:UK Project, which highlighted the lack of international agreement on diagnostic criteria. A series of cases both in the United Kingdom and the USA were analyzed using the Present State Examination or PSE, a semistructured clinical interview, and the results were somewhat surprising: the North American psychiatrists used a wider-ranging schizophrenia category than their British colleagues who, unlike them, diagnosed more cases of depressive psychosis and mania (Cooper et al., 1972; Leff, 1988; Sartorius, 1993). The significance of this investigation, apart from the fact that individuals could change their diagnosis simply by crossing the Atlantic, was that it revealed a lack of consensus, and therefore suggested that clinical judgments were not reliable. As a consequence, the criteria used by professionals in different countries would have to be reviewed and more reliable ones prepared which could serve both for international communication and for research purposes. This prompted the World Health Organization to initiate one of the most important research projects in the history of psychiatric epidemiology: the so-called International Pilot Study of Schizophrenia (IPSS). The first phase of the project took place between 1966 and 1975, but the follow-up is still underway (Sartorius, 1992).

The IPSS is a multicentric epidemiological study comprising a total sample of 1202 patients in nine different countries: Colombia, China, Denmark, USA, India, Nigeria, United Kingdom and the former Czechoslovakia and USSR. The study had two aims: to respond to various questions about the cross-cultural frequency and symptomatology of schizophrenia; and to initiate international contact among professionals as a basis for future studies and, of course, as a way of developing standardized research instruments and reliable diagnostic criteria. The US:UK Project continues to cast a long shadow.

The choice of schizophrenia was not fortuitous, and was motivated by several considerations. The 1973 report states that schizophrenia (a) is a disease of "evident universality," (b) affects a considerable proportion of the world population, and (c) had already been subject to extensive epidemiological study (WHO, 1973, 1976). However, one of the main reasons was also the phenomenology of schizophrenia, a disorder which has more obvious manifestations than such psychopathologies as anxiety or depression. If consensus could not be reached about schizophrenia, what hope was there of acquiring epidemiological and transcultural knowledge of other disorders?

The IPSS sample was selected using the following inclusion criteria: a) a minimum residence time of at least six months in the participating institution; and b) subjects had to be between 15 and 44 years of age. The first criterion made the process of monitoring the sample easier, while the second restricted the age range to that in which, according to the literature, the onset of schizophrenia takes place. Some clinical exclusion criteria were also included: a) no history of alcohol or drug abuse and b) no present or past history of gross organic cerebral disorder. The information was collected, as in the US:UK Project, with the PSE among other instruments and the results were analyzed with computer software (CATEGO) prepared specially for the purposes of the project.

Although the IPSS research subjects were drawn from hospital populations, the WHO attempted to make the most of the effort by subjecting the patients to a follow-up (WHO, 1973, 1976, 1979; Left, Sartorius, Jablensky, Korten & Ernberg, 1992). The information generated about the course and outcome of schizophrenia is thus not merely descriptive and symptomatological, but also processual.

Generally speaking, the IPSS results confirmed expectations. However, there were also some unexpected results which have been the subject of interesting controversy and subsequent epidemiological and ethnographic research. The most significant conclusions were the following:

1. The patients in the developing countries enjoy a better clinical and social outcomes than the patients in the developed countries (Jablensky et al., 1992; Sartorius, Gulbinat, Harrison, Laska & Siegel, 1996).

2. Although the clinical uniformity of schizophrenia is emphasized, it is also recognized that the patients' symptomatology may vary according to the ethnic category to which they belong. For example, in Agra (India) there is a greater frequency of catatonic symptoms than in the other centers (WHO, 1976, p. 164; Leff et al. 1992, p.131).

The most surprising finding was undoubtedly the difference in the outcome of schizophrenia, because, as in Kraepelin's comparative psychiatry, the symptomatological variation may be a consequence of the plasticity of the disease itself. Nevertheless, these results had to be treated with a certain caution. Although the IPSS was a highly significant epidemiological study, the sample was, after all, hospital-based. As Sartorius et al point out:

> The IPSS was not an epidemiological study in the strict sense (patients meeting specified inclusion and exclusion criteria were recruited from consecutive admissions to the psychiatric facilities of the centers), and inferences from the study sample to the wider universe of schizophrenic and related conditions that might exist in the relevant populations were open to uncertainty (1986, p. 910).

This uncertainty suggested that the better outcome of the patients from the developing countries was less a product of different sociocultural contexts than of sampling bias, because individuals who present with a more acute schizophrenic episode generally have a better outcome than those who experience an insidious onset accompanied by essentially negative symptoms (anhedonia, alogia, apathy, asociality, etc.). Additionally, in industrialized societies (IS) individuals with schizophrenia are typically treated by the mental health services, but the same cannot necessarily be said of non-industrialized societies (NIS). Might it not be that the euphemistically-called developing countries were mainly treating the most acute cases and, therefore, the cases with the best outcome, while the developed countries were treating both acute-onset and insidious-onset cases? To dispel this doubt, and also to shed light on some possible associated variables , the WHO carried out a second great epidemiological project on schizophrenia: the Collaborative Study on Determinants of Outcome of Severe Mental Disorders (DOSMD or DOSMeD) (Sartorius et al., 1986; Jablensky et al., 1992).

The DOSMD is also a transcultural study comprising ten countries (half of which were the same as in the EPIE) and thirteen centers (Aarhus, Agra, Cali, Chandigarh/rural, Chandigarh/urban, Dublin, Honolulu, Ibadan, Moscow, Nagasaki, Nottingham, Prague and Rochester). The criteria of the International Classification of Diseases ninth edition (ICD-9) were used and the total sample was 1,379 individuals. The most striking innovation was that the DOSMD had adopted the more rigorous design format of the incidence-based sample studies. That is to say, unlike the IPSS, which was a prevalence-based sample study, the DOSMD recruited patients from among those who had already suffered an initial episode of schizophrenia. To this end, the researchers turned to such helping agencies as psychiatric hospitals, general polyclinics, psychiatric outpatient facilities or social work agencies as well as traditional healers and religious healers or shrines (Sartorius et al.,

1986). Specific studies were also designed within the DOSMD to assess how the outcome of schizophrenia might be influenced by variables such as "life events" (Day et al., 1987), the perception of psychotic symptoms by the patient's family (Katz et al., 1988) or the family atmosphere (expressed emotion) (Leff et al., 1990).

The DOSMD and IPSS results are similar. Generally speaking, they show an annual incidence of schizophrenia per 100,000 of the population at risk (age 15-54) ranging from 1.5 for Aarhus (Denmark) to 4.2 for Chandighar (India) when the broad sample is used. When the sample is reduced to the clearest cases of schizophrenia it ranges between 0.7 for Aarhus and 1.4 for Nottingham. This was not the cause of any great controversy since several previous studies yielded similar results (Jablensky et al., 1992). This is not to say, however, that this information was completely accepted. On the one hand, WHO considers the incidence of schizophrenia to be approximately the same in different countries. But on the other, it has been observed that simply reducing the sample to the clearest cases seems to bring the rates closer. The relevant question here is: By reducing the sample, are we not artificially biasing the results? Is the research design prioritizing the homogeneity of clinical pictures over phenomenological variation across cultures? I will not go into the debate about incidence here since it is tangential to my purposes. I would only point out that the very design of the DOSMD reflects the interests of a psychiatry concerned more with universality than with the diversity of phenomena. This tendency can be seen both in the design of the project and in the interpretation of the results (see Kleinman, 1988b).

Even so brief a discussion of the data on the incidence of schizophrenia raises interesting questions concerning the evidence for considerable variation in outcomes, confirmed by the DOSMD study, and the problem of the symptomatological diversity of schizophrenia.

Outcomes

For a discipline such as psychiatry, elucidating the typical prognosis of a disease involves forecasting its turning points, its advances and reverses, the variation in its signs and symptoms and the evolution of its underlying disease processes. This is the context in which the IPSS and DOSMD results concerning the variability of the prognosis in schizophrenia and the questions they raise should be understood. What is the temporal basis for the nosology of schizophrenia? How should the relation between symptoms and course be interpreted? What is the source of cross-cultural variation in the outcome of schizophrenia?

Many different hypotheses have been developed about this difference in prognosis. In the IPSS report, the WHO suggested a number of possible avenues for subsequent studies: a) elements inherent in different cultural contexts (e.g., family structure, economic factors) might be involved; b) the variability in prognosis might be traceable to differences in treatment; or c) the symptoms observed might correspond to different diseases (WHO, 1979).

The cultural hypothesis gains strength in the last DOSMD report. It states: "It is clear that 'culture' is confirmed as an important determinant of outcome" (Jablensky et al., 1992, p. 2). Likewise, although only incidentally, the report provides some results having to do with the treatment hypothesis; for example, in IS anti-psychotic drugs are prescribed more and over longer periods of time than in NIS (p. 93). This interesting fact is only briefly mentioned in the report, probably because it is highly controversial since it casts doubt on the psychopharmacological treatment currently given to millions of patients. But first let us go back a few years.

An analysis of the outcome of schizophrenia can be found in an article by Cooper and Sartorius entitled "Cultural and Temporal Variations in Schizophrenia: A Speculation on the Importance of Industrialization" (1977). After a discussion pointing out that the high rates of infant and perinatal mortality in the Third World may mean that fewer of those who are most vulnerable to chronic schizophrenia will survive, the authors put forward a sociocultural hypothesis. Not only may the industrialization process enable more of the genetically vulnerable individuals to survive, but also—and this is the most significant idea in the study—the social structure and family size (extended families) of the NIS may have a beneficial effect on the outcome of schizophrenia because of such factors as less stigmatization, community and family solidarity, and the patient's easier access to a directly-productive role. In contrast, the "nuclear families" typical of the IS may contribute to making the schizophrenia chronic (1977). Several studies seem to reinforce this position.

In 1974 Waxler published an ethnographic study on the course of schizophrenia in Ceylon (1974). Using labeling theory, the author suggests that the fundamental issue in the variability of outcome lies in the difference in the societal response. First, she observes that the behavior of Sinhalese families faced with a case of schizophrenia has certain characteristic features. The patient's relatives do not accept a diagnosis of incurable or chronic illness. Instead they negotiate the diagnosis with the professional, who may be either a Western psychiatrist or folk healer, reasoning that the individual is not responsible for his disease, but his body or soul may be possessed, so that sooner or later he will be his old self again. This attitude removes potential stigma and reduces any difficulties the patient may have subsequently in moving from the sick role back to that of a fully functioning and socially integrated individual. In contrast, Waxler hypothesizes, in the IS the process is just the opposite, characterized by stigmatizing what is believed to be a long-lasting disease. The social construction of the sickness thus works on two levels: a) on the level of the community's expectations about the case, and b) on the level of the patient's assumption of a particular role. These two elements would have a considerable effect on the outcome of schizophrenia.

Waxler argues along the same lines in a subsequent article (1979) in which she presents the results of a follow-up study of 44 schizophrenic patients in Ceylon. All the patients were Sinhalese Buddhists from rural areas. After a five-year study, the results indicate that 45% of the patients have no symptoms of psychosis and that the prognosis of the Sinhalese is good in comparison with data obtained from the IPSS follow-up after two years. Waxler mentions three possible factors which may affect this good prognosis: 1) a kind of treatment that does not involve labeling processes which prolong the disease; 2) a belief system which locates disease etiology outside the patient and is therefore less stigmatizing; and 3) a more tolerant social response, favored by the existence of extended families.

Although controversial (Cohen, 1992; Edgerton & Cohen, 1994), Waxler's contributions reveal connections that can hardly be fortuitous. Just as a group of individuals mistakenly diagnosed as hypertensive undergo a general worsening of their health (see Chapter 2), schizophrenics may also show a worse outcome within an adverse setting of family pressure, stigmatization and assumptions of incurability. Predictably, the variables may be linked in the same complex and multifactorial fashion as Cannon understood the causal process of voodoo death. Perhaps for this reason the stigmatization argument is not the only one used currently in the interdisciplinary field that has come to be called the "new cross-cultural psychiatry" (Kleinman, 1977; Littlewood, 1990; Hopper, 1991). More variables have to be taken into account in explaining the enigma of schizophrenia outcome. Below I shall organize into four main groups the most important ethnographic and epidemiological arguments currently being investigated: 1) the possibility that the results are caused by a sampling bias; 2) the role of work and political-economic variables; 3) the possible involvement of family structure and social networks; 4) the importance of cultural beliefs. It will become evident that, with the exception of the first, the rest are not mutually exclusive but can be regarded as interdependent arguments.

First, Alex Cohen has recently taken up the hypothesis of the sampling bias once again: Is it not the case that while everybody with schizophrenia is hospitalized in the IS, only the most acute cases are treated in the NIS (1992, p. 64)? This argument could certainly be applied to the IPSS since it was a hospital-based sample study, but it falls a little short of the mark after the results of the DOSMD, as several critics have observed (Sartorius, 1992; Hopper, 1992; Warner, 1992, Waxler, 1992). The DOSMD results are quite clear on this point:

> The difference in outcome between developing and developed countries re-
> mained significant when patients with acute onset of disease and those with
> insidious onset were studied separately (Jablensky et al., 1992, p. 2).

Nevertheless, in a recent article, Cohen, this time together with Edgerton (1994), seems to insist that accepting a difference between IS and NIS in schizophrenia prognosis is still premature. In a somewhat disorderly fashion, as if they were attempting to attack from all possible sides, they criticize the concepts of "developed" and "developing" countries accepted by WHO, analyze the possible biases of the DOSMD (problems of diagnosis, sample losses, gender differences, etc.) and, just in case the biases do not completely account for the differences in prognosis, argue that the more benign course of schizophrenia in NIS is not necessarily the consequence of cultural differences, but may be affected by malaria, trypanosomiasis, drug use, diet and so on (p. 230).

Why not? Well, let us take it step by step. We may agree with the criticism of the asystematic use that the WHO makes of the concepts "developing" and "developed" countries. It is probably more appropriate to speak of "industrialized" and "non-industrialized societies" or even to use the dichotomy of "rich countries" and "poor countries," which is as materialist as it is true. We may also agree with Edgerton and Cohen that cultural factors are not necessarily the cause of the difference in prognosis. Although they do not suggest it, there is the possibility that the greater perinatal and infant mortality rates in NIS constitute a selection process in which the cases with subsequent worst outcome are not among the survivors. This argument can account for some of the differences in diagnosis without recourse to socio-cultural arguments. On another level, we could even refer to the aforementioned evidence that patients in NIS receive fewer anti-psychotic drugs and for shorter periods than patients in IS. Therefore, paradoxically, the difference in outcome would be the result of the greater or lesser chronicity as a consequence of psychiatric treatments. Of course, all these ideas are viable as hypotheses. However, why should cultural variables be epiphenomenal in the course of schizophrenia, particularly when the data point us precisely in this direction? Cohen and Edgerton simply do not address this question.

Second, Warner is undoubtedly the most interesting author who has expounded the second hypothesis. Although he was an anthropologist who initially followed in the theoretical wake of Waxler (Warner, 1983), he was subsequently to develop some political-economic ideas of considerable interest (1985). I believe that two parallel and deeply interconnected arguments of Warner's are worth mentioning here. First, Warner points out that whereas in IS it is difficult for the patient to gain access to a productive role because of the competition inherent in the capitalist system, in NIS it is easier, meaning that more individuals with schizophrenia return to work and, consequently, enjoy a better prognosis (1983). Second, Warner attempts to show that there is a close relation between unemployment and recovery rates for schizophrenia, arguing that in societies where unemployment is high, the hospital and treatment conditions for psychotic patients tend to be worse and not conducive to recovery. When unemployment is low, however, "human hospital conditions" are better and there are more rehabilitation programs (1985, p. 99).

In favor of Warner's arguments it can be said that they agree with some of the observations that Waxler had made about her Ceylonese sample: almost all individuals with schizophrenia took on some kind of occupation, and competition was diluted by the network of kinship which redistributed the work as a gesture of solidarity to mitigate the lower productive capacity of the patient (Waxler, 1979, p. 144).

Some epidemiological data about industrialized societies also seem to fit in with these arguments:

1. The course of schizophrenia in women is better. This has been linked not only to delayed onset but also to the fact that social pressure is not as great for them to have a productive role beyond the domestic sphere (Goldstein & Kreisman, 1988).

2. Although the relation between low socio-economic status and bad outcome can be interpreted causally in both directions, it may be an index of the effect of unstable working conditions on the course of schizophrenia (Link, Dohrenwend & Skodol, 1986).

3. There is a strong association between poverty and schizophrenia (Susser & Struening, 1990).

Warner's hypothesis is suggestive because it joins several pieces of the puzzle, despite the fact that, as Estroff points out, the inverse relation between unemployment and recovery rates may have an alternative explanation: "Recovery rates may also be influenced by the number and type of mental health professionals who are employed, and who want to keep those jobs because others are not available or pay less" (1993, p. 270). This lucid and ironic remark only serves to reaffirm the multiple connections which may exist between employment and the outcome of schizophrenia, as well as the effect of economy and politics on mental illnesses. However, as Hopper (1991, p. 316) points out, we know very little of the processes involved in this interaction of variables; for example, the lower threshold of productivity ability required in agricultural contexts, and the better prognosis of schizophrenia in non-industrialized societies. What is more, the relation between work and prognosis can be interpreted at least in two different ways:

a) Individuals with working roles may have better outcomes. This situation, however, is not wholly applicable in Western contexts in which the lack of importance given to some productive tasks may have the opposite effect on the patient's self-image (see Estroff, 1981, 1982).

b) Alternatively, however, individuals may develop a working role because their disease has a better outcome.

As yet we do not know which of these propositions takes precedence over the other.

Third, the role of the family is a variable which has traditionally been used to account for the origin and development of schizophrenia. Two examples may be helpful here: Bateson's double-bind theory which understood schizophrenia to be the result of contradictory messages in the family (1972) and Laing's criticism of the bourgeois family from an antipsychiatric standpoint (Laing & Sterson, 1965). However, current discussion on the relation between family and schizophrenia is generally restricted to less political and conflictive topics, such as variation in outcome, number of relapses and continuity of symptoms.

In this context, the idea that the extended family has a beneficial effect seems to have become a coherent, empirically-based dogma. El-Islam (1979) has shown, for example, that patients with extended families had a better outcome than those with nuclear families. Cooper and Sartorius (1977), as mentioned above, have also echoed the possible relation between family size and the course of schizophrenia. At present, research is also being carried out in another no less important area: the effect of the family atmosphere and, particularly, so-called expressed emotion (EE), which is not only a concept but a technique for measuring relatives' emotional attitudes towards patients using criteria such as critical comments, degree of hostility and family overinvolvement (overprotection, intrusiveness).

High EE has been associated with worse outcome in schizophrenia and to a greater number of hospitalizations. For this reason it has been used to analyze cross-cultural variability in prognosis and, generally speaking, the results obtained were to be expected. Karno et al. (1987) have shown that there are differences in EE between Mexican-American and Anglo-American families with the fewest relapses occurring in the former. In a DOSMD substudy comparing a cohort from India with one from Denmark, Leff et al. (1987; see also Leff, 1988) have also shown that there is an association between lower EE (particularly fewer critical and affective responses from the family), and discussed its implications for the course of schizophrenia. EE seems, therefore, to be a predictor of the outcome of schizophrenia. However, the application of standard measurements to the communication of emotions may not be very reliable if the cultural codes which patients use to express their affection and feelings are not taken into account. An illustrative example of this is that of India—the context for the research by Leff et al. (1990)—where the Camberwell Family Interview (CFI), an instrument produced in England and based on verbal comments, did not record the emotions expressed by posture, facial movements, indirect verbal expressions, etiquette, offers of food, styles of dress and other subtle forms of expression (see Kleinman, 1988b). Considering that these difficulties derive from the measurement instruments themselves, the findings about EE should be interpreted with particular caution.

The extended-family hypothesis has suffered a similar fate. Initially, the relation between extended family and a better course for schizophrenics in NIS led to the belief that "the more relations there are, the better the outcome." However, this hypothesis begins to show its limitations when it is assumed to be universal. In the so-called University of British Columbia Markers and Predictors of Psychosis Study, for example, Erickson, Beiser, Iacono, Fleming and Lin (1989) use a social network analysis to show us that in a Canadian cohort, those patients with the most relatives in their social network have a worse outcome, while those whose social network is made up of fewer relatives and more friendship relations have a better course. This interesting study shows that, in the context of a Western society such as Canada, social networks with high family involvement may have an adverse effect—via expressed emotion, for instance—on the course of schizophrenia. It calls our attention to the risks of using sociocultural variables in a totalizing fashion.

Fourth, cultural beliefs or, alternatively, folk medical knowledge about sickness seem to have an important role in the enigma of schizophrenia outcome. Both Estroff and Fabrega have focused on the use in crosscultural epidemiological studies of an ethnocentric concept of person, and they consider that the dichotomy between thinking that one is schizophrenic and that one has (suffers from) schizophrenia is fundamental (Estroff, 1989; Fabrega, 1989). Waxler had stressed this point in 1974 when she suggested that the Ceylonese belief that schizophrenic patients were still the same persons despite their strange behavior, was of considerable importance for expectations of a cure. Similar evidence can be found in a recent study comparing concepts of mental illness among Hispanic, African-American and Euro-American families in the United States. Whereas 65% of the first group believed that the disease was curable, only 19% of the Euro-American families agreed. Likewise, whereas only 31% of the Hispanic families considered mental illness to be incurable, 81% of the Euro-Americans believed that severe mental disorders were incurable (Guarnaccia, Parra, Deschamps, Milstein & Arguiles, 1992). This interesting result may account, in part, for the better outcome of schizophrenia in some Hispanic groups.

Despite its explanatory potential, the adverse role which cultural beliefs can play in the context of IS groups has only recently been explored from an ethnographic standpoint and the results are far from clear. Two ethnographic studies published in the early 1990s have stressed: a) the relation between self-labeling, illness accounts and such sociocultural factors as social race or gender (Estroff, Lachicotte, Illingworth & Johnston, 1991); and b) the analysis of daily isolation routines (wandering around shopping centers, railway stations, etc.) as a strategy for preventing relapses (Corin, 1990). These two studies show how certain cultural categories, values, expectations, economic limitations, concepts of personhood and forms of "being-in-the-world" influence the experience of illness. However, the cross-cultural comparison of the effect of cultural beliefs on prognosis is a task of great complexity which raises a fundamental problem: the commensurability or incommensurability of cultural features and, particularly, cultural beliefs, concepts of personhood and disease concepts. It is no coincidence that this problem has generated endemic controversies in anthropology.

Symptoms

The subject of the symptomatological diversity not only of schizophrenia, but also of other mental disorders, is a reality ignored by biomedically-oriented psychiatric approaches, because the variability of disease manifestations limits the possibilities for a nosology based on the existence of central, invariable and universal manifestations for each disorder. But the cross-cultural diversity of symptoms is very similar to the outcome of schizophrenia: reality defies the expectations of the neo-Kraepelinians.

In the IPSS study, the resulting variability of symptoms was surprising taking into account the homogenization biases of the project. As mentioned above, different symptoms were recorded in a semistructured clinical interview, the PSE, which initially had close to 360 points of reference. However, to facilitate data analysis, this number of features was subsequently reduced to 27 clusters or "units of analysis" ("auditory hallucinations," "incongruity," "derealization," "lack of insight," "experience of control," "qualitative psychomotor disorder," "quantitative disorder form thinking," "flatness of affect," "disregard for social norms" or "delusions," among others (WHO 1976, p. 138). Thus, for statistical processing, the symptoms were reduced to fewer than thirty items which had to record the whole range of symptoms exhibited by the individuals in the sample.

In the DOSMD study, the situation is practically identical. Here, a more modern version of the PSE was used and, through various sophisticated procedures, 44 PSE symptoms were selected to construct a psychopathology profile for each of the various subgroups of the study population. Some of these symptoms are: "depressed mood," "morning depression," "grandiose ideas and actions," "thought insertion," "visual hallucinations," "delusions of control" or "guilt delusions" (Jablensky et al., 1992, p. 35).

The homogenization of symptoms in the IPSS and DOSMD studies can be seen as a necessity for cross-cultural comparison and epidemiological analysis. However, from the ethnographic point of view, it would be interesting to question the validity of the WHO translation, since the original expressions of the patients are not natural physical signs which can be grouped into clusters, but culturally coded symbols that resist homogenization. But, neither the IPSS nor the DOSMD approaches symptoms according to their context of meaning. They use a criterion which, at this writing, remains hypothetical: symptoms are treated as parts of an underlying and self-evident pathological reality, belonging to a medical nosology in which they find their "true" meaning.

The surprising thing is that, after these expressions of illness have been reduced to a homogenized list of categories, there is still considerable diversity. The IPSS indicates that there are more hebephrenic symptoms in NIS (Cali and Taipei) than in IS, that there are more paranoid schizophrenics in the United Kingdom than in other centers, that symptoms of derealization are much less frequent in Agra (3) than in Washington (45), that mania is most common in the Aarhus series and that in Agra, by contrast, there is a surprisingly high rate of catatonic schizophrenia and of the non-specified subtype (WHO, 1973, 1976). Although this data reflect some degree of diversity, the IPSS study concludes that the clinical pictures of the different patients were largely similar (WHO 1976, p. 83).

The DOSMD study arrives at a similar conclusion (Sartorius et al., 1986; Jablensky et al., 1992). It is first pointed out that there are double the number of cases of acute schizophrenia (40%) in NIS than in IS, and that whereas cases of catatonic schizophrenia can be as high as 10%, in IS they are practically nonexistent. Although the rate of the hebephrenic subtype has been diagnosed in 13% of cases in IS, in NIS it is as low as 4%. As is to be expected, the differences not only affect the subtypes but also specific symptoms. Thus, a greater frequency of affective symptoms, delusional mood and thought insertion has been registered in IS patients. In contrast, NIS patients show a greater frequency of "voices speaking to subject" and "visual hallucinations." Despite these differences, the 1986 report concludes that there is a clear similarity in the manifestations of schizophrenia throughout the different centers (p. 926).

In the few studies in which the different expression of schizophrenic symptoms has been the object of epidemiological research, the diversity of phenomena has also emerged as a constant. A good example is the DOSMD substudy carried out by Katz et al. (1988) comparing the symptomatological expressions of two cohorts: a 93-subject sample from Agra (India) and a 135-subject sample from Ibadan (Nigeria). The relatives were interviewed instead of the patients, so this study was innovative in that it analyzed relatives' descriptions of the patient. The investigation concluded that whereas Indian patients appear more affective and absorbed, the Nigerians have more paranoid symptoms. The result again focuses attention on symptomatological variability which, however, is not thoroughly analyzed but subjected to standard instruments such as the PSE and the more innovative Relative's Ratings of Symptoms. As a mitigating circumstance we should understand the difficulty involved in crosscultural comparison. Nevertheless, this study shows a marked tendency, as in Kraepelin's work, to reduce local meaning to an epiphenomenon.

Studies of other mental disorders have not been very different. Although research on schizophrenia has been the star of WHO's multinational projects, there are also studies of other disorders from a crosscultural perspective. This is the case of the WHO Collaborative Study on the Assessment of Depressive Disorders, a project carried out in five countries (Canada, India, Iran, Japan and Switzerland) with a total sample of 573 patients (Jablensky et al., 1981; Thornicroft & Sartorius, 1993). As in the research on schizophrenia, information was collected using a standard interview format, in this case the WHO Schedule for Standardized Assesment of Depressive Disorders (SADD). The results show "unequivocal evidence that the characteristic syndrome of depression, described since Hippocratic times, exists in different cultural settings and includes symptoms which can be assessed clinically in a very similar manner in such diverse settings" (Jablensky et al., 1981, p. 382). However, they also show cultural variation in the frequencies of symptoms when the different samples are compared. This is an interesting contradiction. More specifically, the report records that:

1. Feelings of guilt and self-reproach appear in 68% of the Swiss sample, but in only 32% of the Iranian sample.

2. Suicidal ideas have quite a varied frequency: 70% in Canada against 46% in Iran.

3. Psychomotor agitation had an average frequency of 42% but in Teheran it was 64%.

4. Likewise, somatization is greater in Iran (57%) than in the samples from Canada (27%) or Switzerland (32%) (Jablensky et al., 1981; Marsella, Sartorius, Jablensky & Fenton, 1985).

Some of the principal investigators have pointed out that Western and Westernized samples were over-represented and that it was precisely in India and Iran (the least Westernized samples) that significant differences were found in symptomatological variability (Jablensky et al. 1981).

Other studies of the manifestations of depression have also shown that, in non-Western contexts, symptoms such as "feelings of guilt," "suicidal ideas," "feelings of despair" or "self-deprecation" are rare, whereas somatic and quasi-somatic symptoms such as disturbances of sleep, appetite, energy, body sensation and motor functioning (Marsella et al., 1985, p. 306) are quite common. The idea that Westerners psychologize and that non-Westerners somatize is, in fact, a notion widely shared by epidemiologists. However, this hypothesis does not account for the symptomatological diversity to be found in the different cultural contexts which comprise the macrocategories of "Western" and "non-Western." Some studies also point out that Western patients transform their suffering into a somatic language. For instance, in an epidemiological-ethnographic study involving a small sample and intense qualitative analysis, Parsons and Wakeley were able to show that Australians of European origin evidenced a considerable number of somatic complaints associated with distress in everyday life (Parsons & Wakeley, 1991). Here, as in most of the cases cited, the ethnographic material contradicts the totalizing assertions of crosscultural psychiatric epidemiology. Somatization is not exclusive to exotic peoples. And there is a further problem: the assumption that depression can manifest itself as a series of somatic complaints is a hypothesis rather than a certainty. In the absence of knowledge about the pathophysiological basis of depression, to what extent can we claim to be observing different symptoms which reflect the same underlying process? What enables us to understand disparate phenomena as part of the same psychiatric nosology?

The contemporary model for apprehending symptomatological variability is similar to the one outlined by Kraepelin in "The Manifestations of Insanity": the idea, introduced by Birnbaum, that pathogenicity and pathoplasticity are two very different things. In contemporary psychiatric epidemiology, the first represents the form of a symptom, while the second represents it content.[3] In this way an equilibrium—albeit precarious—is achieved between two contradictory terms: the universality of psychopathology and the diversity of symptoms. This model has produced numerous publications in transcultural psychiatry, notably the classic work by Kiev (1972) and the transcultural studies undertaken by WHO. But it has also been used by some medical anthropologists to account for culture-bound syndromes or the symptomatological variations of Western nosologies (Hughes, 1985b). Leff, a psychiatrist who is known precisely for his anthropological sensibility, also adopts this model in his *Psychiatry Around the Globe*:

> In defining a symptom, it is necessary to make a distinction between form and content. Symptoms in psychiatric conditions are what patients tell you about

their abnormal experiences. The form of a symptom comprises those essential characteristics that distinguish it from other, different symptoms. The content may be common to a variety of symptoms and is derived from the patient's cultural milieu. Thus severely depressed patients may hear voices telling them they are either criminals or sinners. The religious patient is more likely to hear the latter, and the non-religious, the former. What they both experience in common are auditory hallucinations of a derogatory nature, and it is this that gives the symptom its distinctive character (Leff, 1988, p. 3).

This eclectic formula seems to vitiate the challenge to clinical psychiatry posed by the diversity of symptomatological manifestations. Evident variability is reduced to continuity of form: that significant dimension which allows symptoms to be distinguished and placed within a nosological framework in which they acquire their pathological meaning. However, a closer look at this formula reveals its many limitations. Let us first consider the example of auditory hallucination introduced by Leff.

Leff suggests that it is possible to identify a hallucination as such despite the variability with which it presents, because its content is epiphenomenal rather than overdetermined. However, it is not unreasonable to point out that if we wish to know whether a hallucination is pathological in nature, it is important to interpret its content in terms of its own cultural frame of reference (unless we want to treat winks as twitches). In other words, we must know if this experience is congruent with the patient's own cultural environment. Now we are no longer dealing simply with variation in content, but with content itself (the voice of the deceased spouse, for example, among Native Americans) as the main indicator of whether the hallucination is a pathological process or a culturally normal kind of auditory experience. The content of the symptom is not, then, an epiphenomenal reality which can be easily passed over in favor of its form. For example, in the Judeo-Christian historical tradition it is not difficult to imagine a mystic such as Saint John of the Cross or Saint Teresa of Avila hearing voices reminding them of their sins, and in these cases the understanding of content will also be decisive in determining the difference between a pathological symptom and a religious experience.

But the interplay of form and content is even more complex than this. A simple question can illustrate the problem: Is the difference between somatization and psychologization in depression a difference of form or content? This raises a different set of issues than the case of auditory hallucinations. Somatization and psychologization are clearly different ways of expressing distress. We might even think in terms of two types of language—verbal and embodied—capable of expressing similar content. An individual can verbalize a feeling of sadness or simply cry, have backache or "feel down." Here we are faced with the inverse of Leff's approach to auditory hallucination: the content (sadness or, more technically, depressive mood) will be invariable, and instead the form in which this content is expressed will vary. What, in this case, is the criterion for defining pathogenicity: form or content?

The curious thing about this theoretical model is that it proves to be fragile in both directions. If we focus on the form, the varied expressions of depression seems to suggest that there are in fact two disorders and not one. This being so, and from a clinical point of view, there is an incongruence, since the different forms reflect the same content. If we believe the content to be of prime importance, then the same model is not applicable to the example of the hallucinations in which it is the form that is invariable. Here the model of pathogenicity versus pathoplasticity (form versus content) shows important contradictions. Why, then, is such emphasis placed on establishing the pathogenic primacy of form? What is the conceptual model underlying the pathogenicity-pathoplasticity dichotomy?

Leff's text outlines a process of generalization which is characteristic of the diagnostic process: a set of diverse experiences (voices speaking of sins, crimes and other issues) are converted into pathological signs (hallucination as the sign of a biological disorder). The symptom is thus stripped of its original meaning and is modeled as a universal signifier whose content is established not by the patient, but by the professional or the observer. Here, the apprehension of the symptom is reminiscent of the way in which physical signs are diagnosed. However, a sign is not a symptom; recall that a sign is objective evidence of a disease which is not semiotically constructed. Its meaning depends on the observer. For this reason, one of the first requisites of psychiatric diagnosis is to convert the symptoms into natural signifiers so that they are "observable" as signs. Only if symptoms can be handled as mere forms is it possible to establish an analogy with the "visible" traces of physical signs which are not initially semiotic in nature. The content of symptoms such as "auditory hallucination," "delusions" or "depressive mood" will no longer reflect their link with the sender of the message but become dependent on the receiver. Thus, in the same way that doctors deduce measles from spots on the skin, or cirrhosis from abdominal swelling, psychiatrists can deduce depression, brief psychotic disorder or schizophrenia from auditory hallucinations. In other words, it is not the distinction between form and content that characterizes contemporary psychiatry, but the methodological conversion of symptoms into physical signs, of cultural realities into natural signifiers.

Epidemiological research design replicates this procedure: an established diagnostic instrument reduces expressions to types so that symptoms can be found in the same way that physical signs can be observed. In fact, symptoms are regarded as manifestations of an organic dysfunction, as expressions whose meaning is fixed by the nosological criteria of the investigator. The problem here is that symptoms, unlike signs, are always already semiotically constituted. Whereas the marks of smallpox are indicative of disease, "hearing voices" may be a conventional form of mourning, a religious experience or a pathological experience. It may be either a wink or a twitch, and this—not supposed hierarchies of form and content—is the source of the problem of the variability of symptoms.

As we shall see below, anthropology—with the exception those analytic approaches closest to the biomedical model—understands symptoms in a different way. To the extent that ethnography focuses not on disease as a pathophysiological process, but illness as a cultural construction, it is unnecessary to apply the totalizing model of physical signs to symptoms. This is not to say that anthropology denies the possible role of biological processes, neurochemical disorders or hormonal imbalances in mental disorders; it is simply points out the mixed nature of psychopathological processes.

Unfortunately, neither the epidemiological research carried out to date (IPSS, DOSMD, CSD) nor projects currently in the planning stage (International Study of Schizophrenia, ISoS) take into account this significant dimension of symptoms. As in Kraepelin's work, the positivist and quasi-botanical approach of this research constitutes an obstacle to understanding the illness narrative of the sufferer, because the patients appear in these studies as passive, mute objects. Searching the research reports for the voices of the patients themselves is fruitless.

INSTRUMENTS

Another point of controversy between psychiatric epidemiology and psychiatric anthropology is, undoubtedly, the question of measurement instruments. Although there are different types of instruments, the most frequently used are those created to distinguish psychiatric from nonpsychiatric cases such as the PSE (Present State Examination), which uses the diagnostic criteria of the ICD, the DIS (Diagnostic Interview Schedule), which is compatible with the DSM-III, the Feighner Criteria and the RDC (Research Diagnostic Criteria). Because these instruments were developed on the basis of diagnostic criteria, they are vulnerable to the same criticisms detailed in the previous chapter with reference to the new DSMs: they reify symptoms, treat symptoms as signs, adopt an empiricist and supposedly atheoretical approach, assume the existence of discrete mental disorders, etc. Here, however, we shall focus briefly on a crucial question: the problem of adapting instruments of measurement to different cultural contexts.

From the psychometric point of view, the translation of a questionnaire such as DIS or PSE is a technically complex process for which standardized procedures exist. Generally, the first step is to form a bilingual group of experts who belong both to the culture in which the instrument was originally created and the new context in which it is to be implemented. Then, the conceptual structure of the instrument is examined, the items are translated into the target language and they are tested on a monolingual group which does not know the original language of the instrument. Subsequently, the text is back-translated, this back-translation is examined and items are adjusted in accordance with their semantic and lexical meaning. There still remains, however, the question of the reliability of the instrument. This can be tested by comparing the instrument with others that have already been validated in the same social context and by different investigators judging the same cases (test, r-test). If the reliability is high, the translation is considered successful (Sartorius & Janca, 1996; Kleinman, 1988b).

Despite this technical effort, the question of the reliability and validity of instruments has aroused enormous suspicion among ethnographers (Nations, 1986; Corin, 1990). One of the reasons for this is that epidemiology tends to believe that a simple linguistic translation will suffice. Since symptoms are conceptualized as physical signs, manifestations are assumed to be uniform, and therefore easily observable once the language barrier has been overcome. But the problem is that every culture has different patterns of expression for affliction and suffering. Furthermore, the circumstances producing distress also vary among different societies. As a result, epidemiological claims become precarious, because the instruments must grapple with local realities largely incompatible with the technical categories which enable symptom recognition. Let us analyze some examples.

Manson, Shore and Bloom (1985) carried out an ethnographic-epidemiological study of Hopi Indian categories of disease. They began by attempting to translate the Diagnostic Interview Schedule into the Hopi language, but this proved to be a difficult task since Hopi is an unwritten language for which five different orthographic systems have been produced. As expected, they encountered enormous difficulties, even though Manson is a Native American anthropologist. For example, it proved impossible to retain in the Hopi version three concepts that appeared in the same item in the English version: guilt, shame and sinfulness. A team of 23 health care professionals and paraprofessionals pointed out the inappropriateness of including all three in the same item because in Hopi cosmology they had contradictory meanings. Questions about sexual behavior had to be removed in many cases because some of the participants in the survey refused to answer them.

Bravo, Canino, Rubio-Stipec and Woodbury-Fariña (1991) experienced a similar problem with the translation of DIS for use in Puerto Rico. DIS was created in English and validated in the United States for use in the National Institute of Mental Health Epidemiologic Catchment Area studies. Initially they tried the Spanish translation by Karno, Burnam, Escobar, Hough & Eaton (1983) developed for use among Mexican Americans in California (see also Karno et al., 1987). However, this case showed that a single translation cannot necessarily be extrapolated to other cultural contexts where the same language is spoken. Sixty-four percent of the Karno version had to be modified with synonyms, changes in syntax, division of long or complex items, etc. (p. 10). A significant example was the word *ataque*, used in Karno's translation, which was omitted from the Puerto Rican translation because of its possible association with a culture-bound syndrome known as *ataque de nervios* consisting of trembling, sudden aggressivity and subsequent unconsciousness in the Spanish-speaking area of the Caribbean (Cuba, the Dominican Republic and Puerto Rico) (p. 11).

Other studies and attempts to validate instruments have encountered similar difficulties. For example, while Kinzie et al. (1982) were working on a Vietnamese-language depression rating scale, they observed that shame and dishonor were categories associated with this disorder, but the inclusion of guilt feelings made it impossible to distinguish psychiatric cases from nonpsychiatric cases.

Generally speaking, these examples show that linguistic translation of a questionnaire is insufficient to adapt it to a particular cultural context. Not only does the language have to be translated, but also the cultural code through which symptoms are expressed. This requirement acquires even greater importance if we keep in mind that while the reliability of instruments of measurement, like that of diagnostic criteria, can be established, there is no way of corroborating their validity. Given this limitation, epidemiological research remains incomplete without ethnographic analysis of local cultural knowledge. However, this too is problematic. From an anthropological point of view, the translation of local world view is the final goal of ethnography, but epidemiology considers this kind of information to be preliminary and anecdotal, an exercise in "background."

The endless variety of culturally distinctive patterns of illness and distress points to a problem that in most cases remains latent: the commensurability or incommensurability of codes for expressing suffering, of symptoms and of diagnostic categories. This question poses a considerable challenge, not only for the construction of measurement instruments, but also for the stability of contemporary psychiatric nosology.

NOTES

1. In epidemiology, prevalence refers to the frequency of cases of an illness over a period of time, while incidence refers to the number of new cases.
2. For an evaluation of epidemiological research in the psychosocial era, see Mishler and Scotch (1963), Bastide (1965) and, to a lesser extent, Prior (1993). For a discussion of more contemporary debates, see Kleinman (1988b), Bibeau (1997) and Kirmayer (1997).
3. This idea does not correspond precisely to the orientation of the later Kraepelin (1992a), for whom pathogenicity is the underlying pathophysiological process which shows that symptoms and signs (pathoplasticity) vary according to such variables as age, sex and social class. In fact, pathogenicity and pathoplasticity are all-purpose terms, the meaning of which depends on how they are used by different authors.

CHAPTER 6

The Limits of
Psychiatric Observation

In an article entitled "Depression, Buddhism and the Work of Culture in Sri Lanka," Gananath Obeyesekere, one of the most representative defenders of the hermeneutic approach in anthropology, introduces a simile which constitutes one of the most controversial critiques of contemporary psychiatric nosology:

> Take the case of a South Asian male (or female) who has the following symptoms: drastic weight loss, sexual fantasies, and night emissions and urine decoloration. In South Asia the patient may be diagnosed as suffering from a disease, "semen loss." But on the operational level I can find this constellation of symptoms in every society, from China to Peru. If I were to say, however, that I know plenty of Americans suffering from the disease "semen loss," I would be laughed out of court even though I could "prove" that this disease is universal. The trouble with my formulation is that while the symptoms exist at random everywhere, they have not been "fused into a conception" (such as semen loss) in American society. Yet if I were to employ the methodological norms implicit in the several Diagnostic and Statistical manuals and apply them from a South Asian perspective to the rest of the world (as Western psychiatrists do for depression), then it is incontrovertible that "semen loss" is a disease and is universally found in human populations (1985, p. 136).

This passage represents a simple ethnocentric inversion: finding depression in India is as methodologically possible as finding "semen loss" in the United States, but if categories lose their context, their cultural frame of reference, they also lose their labeling capacity. The argument, in sum, is that nosologies cannot aspire to universal applicability, because what legiti-

113

mates them is not simply their ability to distinguish groups of symptoms in space and time, but their linkage to particular cultural and historical traditions.

The writing is reminiscent of classic anthropological arguments in which the critique of Western nosologies is based on the idea of the cultural relativity of criteria for normality and abnormality. Indeed, Obeyesekere appears to be taking up an old question in the manner of the most skeptical culturalism, locating the fundamental problem not in the difficulty of discerning invariable, universal features among the diversity of symptomatological forms and content, but in the very precariousness of Western nosologies, of syndromes (ensembles of signs, symptoms and courses) defined as depression, anxiety, schizophrenia and so forth. But Obeyesekere's dilemma is original in that, unlike other relativist critiques, it attempts to invalidate the universalist logic from within, using the methodological procedures of psychiatric and epidemiological theory. This strategy deserves some comment.

First of all, his brief definition of the signs and symptoms of the semen loss syndrome, also known as *dhat* (from the Sanskrit *dhatu*), *jiryan* or *sukra prameba*, is a little perplexing. In Ayurvedic medicine it is a nosological type based on on a conception of seminal fluid as one of the four basic humors of the human body, both male and female, whose loss can lead to illness and death. Surprisingly, and not without a certain irony, Obeyesekere departs from ethnographic discourse to introduce us to a landscape of bodily and psychic phenomena which evokes, in its parsimony and exactness, the measured descriptions of Western medicine. The symptoms of the *dhat* syndrome (urine discoloration, nocturnal emissions, drastic weight loss and sexual fantasies) are easily observable on a somatic level.[1] With the exception of "sexual fantasies," all the rest can be regarded as signs rather than symptoms, even though they may also be both simultaneously; for instance, when an observer notices that the patient has lost weight, and the patient also complains of weight loss. But what is significant is that, paradoxically, the *dhat* syndrome is more objectively defined than most nosological entities in contemporary psychiatry. The symptoms listed in the DSM-IV definition of dysthymic disorder, for example, are less precise: low self-esteem, poor concentration or difficulty making decisions, and feelings of hopelessness (APA, 1994, p. 349). In comparison with the most ambiguous of the diagnostic criteria for the *dhat* syndrome—sexual fantasies—low self-esteem or feelings of hopelessness are decidedly vague.

If we are dealing with objective signs, we should be able to find *dhat* syndrome in a Western context such as the United States using even the strictest of epidemiological research methods. Indeed, we might conceivably develop a standardized instrument to distinguish cases of *dhat* from non-cases. Since it need only detect physical signs, such an instrument should be highly reliable, maximizing agreement among researchers and minimizing the need for theoretical inference. Subsequently, we should be able to administer this semistructured interview to a particular sample and determine rates of incidence and prevalence for *dhat* syndrome. In short, everything seems to suggest that this disorder could be considered universal in the same way as Western disease categories. Paradoxically, however, Obeyesekere uses precisely this argument to show that these nosologies cannot be universalized, because the categories must first be "fused into a conception." In other words, the validity of a nosology is relative to the tradition to which it belongs: *dhat* in India and Sri Lanka, *koro* in China, *susto* in Central America, most controversially for my purposes here, depression in the West. Otherwise, diagnostic categories would drift away from their true meaning and become methodological artifacts of little validity because, from Obeyesekere's point of view, what makes it possible to identify psychopathology is not the ahistorical and asocial exercise of grouping signs and symptoms according to a naturalist logic, but the social construction of illness. From this point of view, it seems absurd to extrapolate a syndrome such as *dhat* to the North American cultural context, in which semen is not a humor of primary importance and spermatorrhea and sexual fantasies are not necessarily pathological. This experiment in reverse ethnocentrism reveals the limits of treating symptoms, syndromes and mental disorders as universally observable psychophysiological twitches, rather than as winks that must be interpreted locally. Once again, the problem is ontological: the nature of mental illnesses and their manifestations.

For Obeyesekere, mental disorders cannot be analogized to physical diseases. Or rather, they can, but — as his experiment in reverse ethnocentrism shows—at the price of severing their connection to local context and meaning. In Western societies, depression is assumed to be an unquestionably real and universal disease entity. But is this the case in the context of the South Asian tradition, in which feelings of hopelessness, for example, indicate not illness but rather the attitude of a "good Buddhist" whose awareness of this feeling impels him to search for a way of attaining *nirvana* and, therefore, release from suffering? Is this not a religious experience rather than a pathological process? Which is the mistake: interpreting the mood state as a religious experience, or medicalizing it? What is the defining feature of disorders such as depression or *dhat*: their fusion into a cultural concept, or their hypothetical relation to biological processes?

There are no quick, definitive solutions to Obeyesekere's dilemma. If the organic basis of an illness such as *dhat* is doubtful, its validity as a cultural construction is beyond question. And we are still left with an unresolved contradiction between the cultural particularity of *dhat* and the fact that it can be shown, through the use of Western psychiatric procedures, to be universal, as can a long list of folk diseases of which *koro, amok, susto* and *latah* are but a few examples. What we are observing here are the limitations of contemporary psychiatry. The neo-Kraepelinian project is poorly equipped to deal with the so-called culture-bound syndromes, and its resources are even further diminished when a simple inversion makes the "scientific" exotic, and the "exotic" at least operational.

Generally speaking, contemporary psychiatry has responded to dilemmas such as the *dhat* syndrome in three possible ways:

1. The first of these treats this type of syndrome not as a disease, but as the result of people's "ignorance" of pathophysiological processes. The superiority of Western science over cultural beliefs is used to demonstrate this argument.
2. The second response reduces the syndrome in question to a pathoplastic expression of universal psychopathological processes. That is to say, *dhat* is simply another name for depression or anxiety.
3. The third response is to make room in the diagnostic classification for this type of culture-bound syndrome, but with the consequent problem of vague and imprecise definitions.

Let us analyze these different readings more closely.

READING I (SCIENTISM)

In orthodox psychiatry, "depression" is a scientific category, but *dhat* is not considered a disease because it does not correspond to any organic dysfunction as defined by Western medicine. On the contrary, depression would be regarded as the paradigm case of a disease on the threshold of definitive medical knowledge. Evidence of the biological constitution of depression would include, for example, possible pathophysiological mechanisms such as neurochemical alterations in the serotonin receptors. This approach would attempt to invalidate any supposed likeness between the clinical features of depression and categories lacking any scientific basis, such as *dhat* syndrome. The defining characteristic of a disease is not the world of beliefs and concepts surrounding it, but the point at which it is anchored in biological reality.

Singh has recently defended this stance, alleging that what underlies an entity such as *dhat* is neither a disease nor a culture-bound syndrome, but only "ignorance" about sexual relations and associated pathologies (1992, p. 280). In his view, this opposition between science and belief, between depression and *dhat*, exposes what is wrong with Obeyesekere's experiment in reverse ethnocentrism: the terms involved are of an essentially different and non-comparable nature. As impregnable as Singh's argument may seem, it has two weaknesses: on the one hand, its excessive organicism ignores the psychological, social and cultural factors that give rise to disease; and on the other, it fails to recognize that to this day, despite experimental studies, the psychiatric diagnosis of depression is based on its phenomenology and course, not on known etiological processes. In fact, because there is no biological point of anchorage except on a purely hypothetical level, the distinction between scientific knowledge and cultural belief begins to break down. The procedures used to diagnose depression belong more to the realm of appearances than to supposed neurochemical causes and, as I have pointed out above, the signs characteristic of the *dhat* syndrome are anything but lacking in objective definition.

In the final analysis, this reading shows the dangers of what Habermas called "scientism" (1989, p. 13): the faith that science has in itself, the conviction that science should no longer be regarded as one form of knowledge among others, but as knowledge itself; a type of scientistic fundamentalism which allows psychiatric (and biomedical) categories to be understood as *the* (definitive) representation of reality and not as *a* (possible) representation. But the image of scientific objectivity, rationality and neutrality cannot explain why nosologies from other medical systems such as Ayurveda can be found using the research methods of psychiatric epidemiology. The distinction between science and belief does not even address this problem, much less solve it. Only the appearance of a solution is achieved by treating the resemblance between depression and *dhat* as an aberration; the enigma remains.

READING II (UNIVERSALITY)

Fundamentalism aside, another of the most frequent strategies has been to shift the emphasis from categories to empirically observable realities. From this point of view, *dhat* is merely a different name for the same phenomenon.

Bottéro (1991), who is not a staunch positivist, has produced an interesting critique of Obeyesekere. Symptoms, he argues, are always interpreted according to a particular cultural model, but diseases have a prior and independent existence. On the basis of his own fieldwork in northern India, he suggests that Obeyesekere's list of disorders is too short compared to the richness of the phenomenon. The *kavirajas* (Ayurvedic professionals), he says, treat *dhat* syndrome as a hodgepodge of signs and symptoms including spermatorrhea, but also persistent fatigue, apathy, inattentiveness, anxiety about possible physical decline, and cases of unexplainable madness (*pagala*). Thus *dhat*, according to Bottéro, is in essence an amalgam of disorders condensed into a unitary cultural conception of the importance of seminal fluid and its possible loss. In the final analysis, however, these elements can be shown to correspond in each case to depressive disorders, anxiety disorders, etc. (p. 316).

This analysis is partially supported by some epidemiological studies. One of the most recent was carried out by Mumford (1996), who found a strong association in Lahore, Pakistan between *dhat* and depressed mood, fatigue symptoms and a DSM-III-R diagnosis of depression. He concludes that *dhat* is not a culture-bound syndrome but a "culturally determined symptom associated with depression" (p. 165).

A similar conclusion can be drawn from a study by Chadda and Ahuja, two psychiatrists from the Indian subcontinent who found an association between *dhat* syndrome and, in decreasing order of importance, neurotic depression, anxiety neurosis, psychogenic impotence and gonorrhea. Curiously, however, they state that several cases were simply *dhat*, and they conclude that *dhat* syndrome is a culture-bound sex neurosis of the Indian subcontinent (Chadda & Ahuja, 1990, p. 577).

A few years later, one of these two authors, Chadda, confirmed this last result. In a study comparing 50 *dhat* syndrome patients with 50 controls, Chadda (1995) shows that some of the patients could be diagnosed according to DSM-III-R as having a major depressive episode (20%) or a generalized anxiety disorder (2%), but most (66%) were given an unspecified diagnosis. In conclusion, the author suggests that the *dhat* disorder can be seen as a distinct clinical entity, although it should be researched in more detail, particularly through longitudinal studies (p. 136).

Another study by Bhatia, Bohra and Malik (1989) yielded a similar result in a group of 48 males with *dhat*. Many of them had high scores for neuroticism and depression (64.6%), neurotic depression (39.5%) and anxiety neurosis (20.8%), and responded well to anti-depressant drugs. However, the most interesting result is that 31% of the patients could not be diagnosed using Western nosologies. They simply suffered from *dhat*.

Unlike these studies, which support the utility of the authochtonous nosology (*dhat*) (Bhatia &Malik, 1991; Chadda, 1995), Bottéro and Mumford reiterate the classic interpretation of transcultural psychiatry also shared by some contemporary psychiatric anthropologists such as Hughes;[2] that is to say, the application of the pathogenicity/ pathoplasticity model to resolve the contradiction between a rich phenomenology and an impoverished nosology. In the case of *dhat* syndrome, the pathogenic element would be the depressive or anxious clinical picture, among other things, and the pathoplastic element would be the characteristic symbolic content associating mood changes with a progressive loss of seminal fluid. However, this stratigraphic and reductionist model in which local meaning is merely epiphenomenal does not provide a solution to the enigma of reverse ethnocentrism in its methodological aspect, for two reasons:

1. Some cases of *dhat* resist classification according to Western biomedical psychiatric categories such as depression or anxiety. That is to say, the Western nosology does not cover all situations.

2. In the absence of knowledge about disease etiology, it is impossible to determine whether the translation of different nosologies accurately represents biological reality (*denotatum*).

In other words, there is no reason why Western psychiatric nosology should possess greater validity than Ayurvedic categories, since a skilled *kaviraj* can also test the cross-cultural applicability of his conceptual system of bodily humors (*dosas*) and his etiological principle of the possibly dramatic consequences precipitated by uncontrolled discharge of the most refined vital substance. The empirical bases for arguing that *dhat* is a culturally determined syndrome associated with depression are practically identical to those that would enable us to argue that depression is a culturally determined symptom associated with *dhat*. In fact, we can challenge the presumptive universality of depression in contrast with the supposedly localized nature of *dhat* by showing that the association between semen loss and a general worsening of health exists in a wide variety of cultures along both shores of the Mediterranean, in northern Europe, and elsewhere. However, substituting one totalizing argument with another would create distortions similar to those that exist in contemporary psychiatry. Because neither *dhat* nor depression is totally independent of cultural context, they cannot be reduced to simple biological dysfunctions. This may be illustrated more clearly by another example.

Between 1984 and 1985, there was an epidemic of *koro* which affected about 2,000 individuals in Guangdong, a region of the People's Republic of China. In accordance with the phenomenology known as *koro*, all those affected thought that their penis would gradually get smaller until it would eventually recede into the abdomen and cause death. The epidemic gradually disappeared, although in 1987 there was a similar one in the Leizhou peninsula (Tseng et al., 1988). It is unlikely that 2,000 individuals would be affected simultaneously by a cerebral disorder of short duration. A more probable explanation is a cultural reaction of generalized panic or, as Sheung-Tak (1996) rightly points out in a recent article, "a social malady maintained by cultural beliefs that affect the whole community" (p. 67). In this case the *koro* syndrome, which has been interpreted on many occasions as an exotic expression of anxiety (Tan, 1988), cannot easily be adapted to Western nosology.

Koro could be understood in much the same way that Mumford and Bottéro interpreted *dhat*; that is, as a phenomenon which can conceal many different disorders because, although symptoms vary, diseases remain the same. But how elastic must Western nosologies be in order to make room for so much symptomatic diversity? What is most significant here: *koro* as a reality in itself, or the possibility that it reflects universal pathological processes? To what extent is it possible, in the absence of any etiological knowledge, to translate forms of affliction from other local worlds into our supposedly universal nosologies ? How will knowledge be advanced by substituting *koro* for anxiety if we do not know its causes? In operative (and objective) terms, would *koro* or *dhat* be as exotic for a Westerner as depression would be for a Sri Lankan, or Type A personality for a Nambikwara?[3]

The difficulty with the pathogenicity/pathoplasticity model is, precisely, that in the absence of etiological knowledge, something which is regarded as an unproblematic process of designation or diagnosis becomes a translation. A bad translation, in fact, in which the language of the categories from other local worlds is always epiphenomenal, and the universal language is that of Western psychiatric categories. Local meaning is thus pushed into the background in favor of invariable forms of pathology. Kleinman and Kleinman (1991; see also Kleinman, 1995) have recently raised the question of whether the horror experienced by survivors of genocide should be re-phrased in terms of depressive disorder, post-traumatic stress or sociopathic personality disorder. Something is obviously lost when one speaks of post-traumatic stress instead of genocide, of anxiety instead of *koro* or of depression instead of *dhat*: namely, the frame of reference, violent or peaceful, in which *dhat* or *depression* acquire meaning.

READING III (INDETERMINACY)

Another possible reading has been put forward along theoretical lines similar to the pathogenicity/ pathoplasticity model. The strategy is to postpone the translation of the categories by making room for exotic phenomena within the nosological apparatus but without questioning the psychiatric categories themselves or engaging in a throughgoing methodological critique. One example of this option is the inclusion of *dhat* syndrome in one of the first Spanish versions of the International Classification of Diseases tenth edition (ICD-10). Here, under the heading "other specified neurotic disorders," we read:

> Included in this category are mixed behavioral disorders, beliefs and emotions of unknown etiology and nosology which present in some cultures with particular frequency, such as DHAT syndrome (unfounded anxieties concerning the debilitating effects of semen loss).

The definition continues with reference to two other culture-bound disorders:

> Koro syndrome (fear that the penis will invaginate itself into the abdomen and cause death) and Latah (mimetic and automatic behavioral responses). The behavior itself, and the close relationship of these syndromes with accepted belief in particular cultures in specific regions, suggest that they should not be considered delusional (WHO, 1992b, p. 215) [4]

Not only is the definition ambiguous enough to permit the extrapolation of "*dhat* syndrome" to any other part of the world, but its brevity and simplicity are striking in a document which attempts to define psychopathological conditions and their course, outcome and differential diagnosis with precision. If the quotation from Obeyesekere that opened this chapter is compared with the one above, we are surprised by the contrast between a definition in which physical signs predominate, and one in which the same syndrome is described in terms of symptoms rather than signs. Concern about the pernicious effects of semen loss is, clearly, a reality of a different order than urine discoloration or drastic weight loss. Furthermore, in this new definition of *dhat* syndrome there is an appraisal which breaks with mere phenomenological description and introduces a judgment which is not the patient's but the researcher's or the psychiatrist's: the concern is unfounded. In other words, the concern in question is something like an erroneous conception of pathophysiological processes. This is important, because it is precisely this lack of foundation (in biomedical truth) which renders concern about the effects of semen loss indicative of a state that is not physical but psychopathological.

Because of the introduction of this biomedical value judgment, of this pathological meaning, the references to cultural contexts, "accepted beliefs" or "behaviors" appear here as spurious variables whose only clinical utility is to differentiate between a delusional (and thus idiosyncratic) idea and a normative concept. It is of little real importance that the syndrome in question is linked with a tradition in which semen is a youth-giving substance, irreplaceable because it cannot be regenerated. Neither is it important that about twenty percent of those who consult a *kaviraj* are either diagnosed by him or self-diagnosed as suffering from *dhat*, nor that this category condenses a world of sensations and emotions organized through shared meanings. What is important from the psychiatric point of view is that these sensations are not grounded in changes in the physical body. Seen in terms of a scientific and Western, or Westernized, world view such as the one expounded by Singh in Reading I, such beliefs can only be erroneous and inaccurate. In fact, introducing the "unfounded" judgment transforms an interpretation that could be the patient's ("concern about the weakening effects of semen loss") into that of the observer ("unfounded concern about the weakening effects...").

However, the drawbacks of the WHO definition are not limited to the appropriation of local meaning by means of value judgments. The very definition of *dhat* is problematic, because it does not distinguish between "concern" as a cultural representation and "concern" as an individual experience. This is what Devereux has called the confusion of "traditional belief" with "subjective experience" (1973, p. 47) the same way that there is a difference between believing that a traumatic experience can lead to depression, and experiencing trauma and subsequent depression personally, there is also a considerable difference between sharing a cultural belief in the dangers of semen loss to health, and feeling that one is getting weaker because of the loss of seminal fluid. In the case of *dhat*, both possibilities involve concern, but one is in the experiential domain and the other is on the cultural plane of expectations about the dangers of sexual excess. This difference is not clear in the brief ICD-10 definition, probably because the symptom is excessively formalized.

Furthermore, the ICD-10 definition shows a striking lack of interest in specifying the cultural and historical traditions within which *dhat* occurs and acquires its distinctive character. On the contrary, *dhat*, like *koro* and *latah* are a sort of hodgepodge whose provisional nature is indicated by the notion of "unknown etiology and nosology." Although its existence in "some cultures" is emphasized, the definition does not specify which ones, nor does it describe the relations between the concern in question and other associated factors. This indeterminacy makes *dhat* a clearly problematic syndrome, because not only can it be identified in the context of Southeast Asian societies, but also in less exotic circles, such as those in which Tissot wrote in the eighteenth century and Esquirol in the nineteenth. Both of these European authors—among many others—believed the progressive loss of seminal fluid to be a fundamental etiological condition for the development of dementia, melancholy and physical debilitation (Bottéro,1991).

In short, the WHO definition of *dhat* syndrome is so vague and imprecise that it recognizes no historical or cultural limits. But this is not all. Talk of "unfounded concern" is something like speaking of sudden weight loss without regard for its cultural location and the meaning this concern has for the person who is experiencing it. In other words, the ICD-10 invalidates the implications of the code and annuls its local meaning in favor of a pathological meaning provided by the classification itself. As in the Kraepelinian project, this methodology eliminates the possibility of surprise because its purpose is not to discover the cultural system in which *dhat* is situated, nor systematically to open up its local world of meaning and experience, but to constitute an acultural and supposedly aseptic nosological model. In short, this definition reveals the contradiction between a totalizing, empirically based and asemiotic logic of symptoms and a reality rich with meanings which resists narrow definitions. It is true, nonetheless, that the ICD-10 attempts to recover something of the native's point of view. Unlike the other two readings, the ICD-10 treats the category of *dhat* as a valid nosology, if only as an exotic referent. Nevertheless, this immersion in vernacular categories is accompanied by greater use of psychiatric jargon, with decontextualizing effect: lack of specificity in defining cultural context, the introduction of value judgments, vague and superficial description, reification and formalization of symptoms, etc.

Fortunately, this bias has been partly (and only partly) rectified in the glossary of culture-bound syndromes which DSM-IV includes in one of its appendices. Here the definition is also brief, although it avoids the excessively formalizing tone of the ICD-10. The entry reads:

> Dhat. A folk diagnostic term used in India to refer to severe anxiety and hypochondiacal concerns associated with the discharge of semen, whitish discoloration of the urine, and feelings of weakness and exhaustion. Similar to *jiryan* (India), *sukra prameba* (Sri Lanka) and *shen-k'uei* (China) (APA, 1994, p. 846).

This is certainly an improvement. Despite its brevity, at least DSM-IV refers to the cultural contexts in which *dhat* occurs and is named or diagnosed. However, we should not allow ourselves to be deceived. The category of *dhat* is still anecdotal in nature and marginal within the totalizing structure of DSM-IV. The problem is not exclusively one of recognizing the existence of culture-bound syndromes, but the way in which these are observed and understood. Obeyesekere's dilemma reveals that in psychiatric epidemiology, as in sleight of hand, the secret lies not in what is apparent but in how the observer is distracted.

NOTES

1. Other symptoms associated with the *dhat* syndrome are: weakness, loss of energy, fatigue, vague aches and pains, loss of libido, distortion in the shape of the penis, impotence, premature ejaculation and anxiety or depressive symptoms. See Chadda (1995, p. 136).
2. See especially Hughes (1985) where the author, in a somewhat forced fashion, attempts to interpret the *nangiarpork* or *kayak angst* syndrome (an Inuit syndrome characterized by feelings of anguish and anxiety during journeys by kayak) in terms of pathoplastic modifications of DSM-III categories such as panic disorder or simple phobia (p.18).
3. An application of the notion of culture-bound syndromes to Western societies can also be found in Ritenbaugh (1982) and Cassidy (1982). For a critique of the excesses of culturalism in some approaches to culture-bound syndromes, see Hahn (1995).
4. Fortunately, in a subsequent Spanish version of the ICD-10 (WHO, 1993) this type of definition was eliminated in favor of a glossary of culture bound syndromes.

Part Two

... And Anthropological Understanding
Symptoms as
Symbolic Constructions

A *Symbol* is a Representamen whose Representative character consists precisely in its being a rule that will determine its Interpretant. All words, sentences, books, and other conventional signs are Symbols

—Charles Sanders Peirce
Collected Papers

By symbol I mean all those meaningful structures in which a direct, primary, literal meaning also has another indirect, secondary, figurative meaning which can only be understood through the first. *This delimitation of expressions with a double meaning constitutes the hermeneutic field itself.* [italics in original] [my translation]

—Paul Ricoeur
Le conflit des interpretations

CHAPTER 7

Toward an Anthropology of Symptoms I: Four Pre-Interpretive Approaches

In 1964 Philip Newman described with considerable precision the behavior of an individual suffering from "wild man" —also known as *Wild pig, AhaDe idzi Be* or *longlong*[1]—among the Gururumba of New Guinea (1964).

Gambiri, the name by which Newman calls the person in question, had refused to give food to the children who were playing in the village. As the ethnographer had observed many times previously, this was a game of demands and negotiations characterized by the insistence of the youngsters and the apparently patient and calm response of the adult. However, this daily scene gradually began to acquire a strange tone. Gambiri wanted to be given back a bowl that one of the children had snatched from him and, clearly mistaken, accused the ethnographer of having taken it. Then, Gambiri found a plastic pot used as a toilet by the ethnographer's children and said, "There is my bowl. I can take it and throw it away in the forest. It is not heavy." Gambiri's sentence contained a conventionalized message: the moral career of the wild man had begun.

While Newman watched, the villagers began to gather around Gambiri, saying, "*Gambiri ahaDe idzi Be*" ("Gambiri has turned into a wild man"). To the ethnographer, this situation seemed to be not unlike a theatrical production in which the actor plays his part and the audience hangs on his every word and gesture. Apparently, however, the relation between actor and audience was in this case even closer. Newman writes, "When Gambiri made threatening gestures toward them they ran off laughing or screaming in mock terror" (p. 2). In one of these intermittent and contrived rushes, the wild man managed to grab hold of a young girl and take a net bag that she was carrying. Then, in the ethnographer's words:

> Gambiri sat down on the ground, removed the contents of the bag, found a piece of soap, which he gave to an onlooker, and a small knife, which he gave to me, saying that it had been given to him by an Australian Patrol Officer for being a good worker on the government road. After gathering up the contents of the bag he then made a series of demands on me, asking for a loin cloth, a tin of meat, and some tobacco. Each denial was answered with a shouted "Maski" [Neo-Melanesian for 'no']...This particular episode was ended when he again accused me of stealing his bowl and was then told by an onlooker that a young boy who happened to be passing by at the moment had taken it. The onlooker also suggested that Gambiri ought to shoot the boy, a suggestion he took up with gusto as he put an arrow to his bow and ran after the intended victim (p. 3).

Following the account of this performance, Newman describes Gambiri's subsequent behavior during the following sixteen days: he visited nearby villages where he stole a number of small items which he considered to be gifts from imaginary people; he was always aggressive and defiant; he shot arrows at people who were too far away to be wounded; he collected numerous objects he traveled to more distant villages which did not belong to the area of his own subclan; he disappeared into the jungle, where he scattered the objects he had acquired; and finally he returned to the village and, surprisingly, to everyday normality. His extensive repertoire of "bizarre," strange behaviors were also, nevertheless, conventionalized forms of deviation which enable Newman to speak of a wild man pattern among the Gururumba.

BEHAVIORS

Newman's description is not new. The ethnopsychiatric literature is full of references to deviant behaviors, patterns of misconduct, folk mental illnesses, culture-bound syndromes or similar phenomena otherwise named.[2] However, some elements of Newman's description and analysis of the wild man are particularly striking. At first, the wild man process is initiated with a phrase which is complemented with a *"Gambiri ahaDe idzi Be"* from the onlookers. This sets off a whole chain of behaviors, forms of expression and attitudes which the ethnographer reconstructs, focusing especially on the analysis of behavior and behavioral sequences. Although present in Newman's description and analysis, Gururumba forms of expression are clearly of secondary importance compared to Gambiri's behavior: the collection of objects, petty thefts, return to the village, etc. Newman's article emphasizes these behaviors at the expense of Gururumba discourse. Ethnographic observation seems to be more important than listening to his informants. The transcription of behavior emerges, then, as paramount, and the words of the actor and his audience are relegated to a merely supporting role when the wild man disturbs the calm of village life (which is not, however, without its tensions). Newman rarely analyses the complaints and questions that are the wild man's typical forms of expression, but focuses primarily on the behaviors and behavioral sequences that take place in a perfectly orchestrated fashion for sixteen days. In short, the message of Newman's ethnography is that the principal object of study is behavior. This behavioral focus is so all-consuming that it tends to behavioralize the game of questions and answers; that is to say, local discourse.

In Newman's analysis, behavior is seen as the result of a combination of social, cultural and psychological determinants. Newman traces this idea back to North American culturalism, acknowledging his intellectual debt to Kluckhohn's analysis of Navajo witchcraft (Newman, 1964, p. 8). The author thus places himself in the culturalist tradition, although this does not prevent him from asserting that the case of the wild man, like any other deviant behavior, is not only the mechanical result of "culture using man" but also of "man using culture." What is of interest here is that the reciprocal relation established by the author between the categories of "culture" and "the individual" is determined by the dynamics of the interaction between cultural patterns and behavior.

First of all, the description of the wild man removing objects from a bag, threatening other people, or roaming from village to village and carrying out small unconnected thefts is reminiscent of the way in which the more recent versions of DSM arrange diagnostic criteria. Think for a moment about the similarities between the description of the wild man and the DSM criteria which define antisocial personality disorder: "fails to conform to social norms with respect to lawful behavior;" "is irritable and aggressive;" "repeatedly fails to honor financial obligations;" "fails to plan ahead, or is impulsive," among others. These criteria form patterns of behavior not significantly different from the stereotyped sequences of the wild man's behavior. However—and this is important—these patterns of behavior are anchored, in one case, to social convention and, in the other, to a supposed psychobiological pathology. But there are other elements which prevent Newman's description from being assimilated in any simple way to this mixture of reification and universalization of symptoms so characteristic of contemporary neo-Kraepelinism. Newman proceeds differently; he does not read behavior as a physical sign pointing to a preexisting diagnostic category nor does he treat behaviors as forms of expression whose meaning depends on the observer. Instead, the observer must be attentive, and the important thing, the first step, is to record the native version. This version is seen as a dimension of reality which, because it expresses more than just unintentional and mechanical bodily movements, cannot be apprehended only by using a priori concepts and categories. For neo-Kraepelinism, access to the emic dimension is practically impossible, but in Newman's description the analysis from within is viable, even though he is less interested in meanings than in deviant behaviors.[3]

Newman reconstructs the complexity of the cultural system in which the action unfolds. In other words, he is discovering the (cultural) system, not applying a previously developed model which already contains the keys for understanding the behavior. In great detail he describes the obligations of Gururumba married couples, the social pressure on men in their thirties (who are also those affected by the wild man syndrome) and their desire to acquire power and prestige. Gambiri, he says, is in an awkward situation: he hasn't paid the bride price and the deadline has come and gone. What is more, his wife is expecting a second baby and he will soon have to remunerate his affines for the new child in accordance with the customary obligations of the Gururumba. Gambiri's outburst, therefore, seems to be the result of exogenous, but extremely powerful forces which overwhelm his capacity to absorb them: he only has one pig with which to pay off his increasing debt.

The ethnographic description of the wild man emerges out of the anthropological strategy of locating the central focus of observation (here, Gambiri's bizarre behavior) in a sociocultural context which not only provides meaning but also makes it possible to link together a considerable number of variables through holistic reconstruction. At the time when Newman was writing, there was in place a tradition of ethnographic analysis which endorsed his procedure and a set of key concepts which allowed ethnography to reach beyond the mere description of events to explanation. Benedict had already made it possible to speak of normality and abnormality in the context of culture in her controversial *Patterns of Culture*. Toward the end of his life, Boas [1932] (1966) had also developed a model in which the concepts of individual, culture and behavior were essential to the anthropological task. As Boas wrote, it was:

A vain effort to search for sociological laws disregarding what should be called social psychology, namely, the reaction of the individual to culture. They can be no more than empty formulas that can be imbued with life only by taking account of individual behavior in cultural settings (p. 258).

This was a preview of what were to be the interests of the culture-and-personality school from Benedict to Linton and from Mead to Kardiner: the relation between culture and individual through the dynamic tension between cultural patterns and behavior; the importance of psychological and psychoanalytic theories; and the attempt to explain culture by means of a processual approach based not on history, but on the constant feedback through which individual behaviors reproduce traditional norms by means of the so-called process of socialization. This, in sum, is what Newman understands as the process of culture using man.

However, the type of behavior of which Newman speaks is of a special nature. Gambiri's affliction does not represent ordinary and habitual behavior, but the emergence of a deviant, abnormal or dysfunctional form of behavior, to use the words current in the anthropology of the early 1960s. Strangely enough, though, this is deviant behavior reproduced according to a standardized protocol. What Newman observes is not genuine incoherence, but the performance of what Devereux calls "ethnic disorders" (1973, p. 56) and Linton "patterns of misconduct" (1937). There is a sort of cultural message which tells the affected individual: "Don't do this, but if you must, do it this way." Newman also started from the same assumption and, like Linton and Devereux, observes while it is possible to establish a repertoire of sociocultural determinants, it is difficult to answer the question, "Why do some individuals within a group opt for this sort of behavior and others do not?" It may be that social pressure is more intense in some cases than in others, or that some situations are more likely than others to trigger the wild man syndrome, but the final answer to this question lies in the domain of temperament, constitution, hypothetical intrapsychic conflicts or preexisting personality characteristics of the affected individuals. The culturalist and behavioralist model seems to reach its limits here: it introduces the reproduction of cultural norms and the interaction of variables, but it barely scratches the surface of a complete explanation. Nor can contemporary psychiatry complete the picture; in refusing to accept the social origins of illness, it loses its connection to sociocultural context. Newman's culturalism works the other way round, from the exogenous to the endogenous, but it does not completely unravel the enigma of how such phenomena are produced. Here, the psychological dimension is a sort of camera obscura which allows us to discern only snippets of the processes within.

At this point we may ask ourselves: "Is it possible to make headway by analyzing sociocultural and psychological variables until we achieve detailed and precise knowledge of syndromes such as wild man, or should anthropology have more modest objectives?" Contemporary anthropological theory has, in fact, partly abandoned, or at least postponed, the goal of answering the question "How is it produced?" with all its implications. In contemporary medical and psychiatric anthropology it is easier to find attempts at translation and interpretation than more ambitious projects designed to explain the relation between cultural, social and psychological variables (not to mention the biological variables, which were somewhat marginalized by the culture-and-personality project). This state of affairs is traceable in large measure to a shift of interest from the function, role, nature and motivation of behavior to the meaning of symptoms. In medical anthropology, this is reflected in a shift from concepts such as function, behavior, deviant behavior, normal/abnormal, cultural patterns, patterns of misconduct, to terms such as meaning, text, illness semantic networks, idioms of distress, illness narratives, embodiment, experience, and so forth.

This change in expectations may reflect the impossibility of constructing a totalizing explanation for the phenomenon of sickness, or it may simply be the consequence of a paradigm shift in anthropology; or it may be some combination of the two. In any case, anthropological knowledge has come to consist of the interpretation of meaning—including the interpretation of behavior as a vehicle of meaning—rather than the explanation of behavior as such. In short, anthropology has substituted the decoding of semiosic and discursive constructions for the observation of behavior.

This point can be taken further. Only when anthropology developed an interest in "meanings" and "significations" did the concept of symptom acquire anthropological relevance, for a very simple reason. As Canguilhem notes, a concept cannot become part of the framework of a discipline until it is seen as "true" and consistent with the other concepts, theories and hypotheses of the discipline. Thus, in medicine, the concept of "reflex" is introduced when the physiological assumption of unidirectional movement from the center of the nervous system is abandoned. That is to say, when physiology begins to formulate the idea that the relation between center and periphery may involve a process in both directions, the concept of reflex, which emerges from an an analogy between life and light, can be taken up (Canguilhem, 1955, p.6).

The concept of symptom came into anthropology, then, just as the concept of reflex came into medicine: only when anthropology acquired its interpretive character could the symptom, as a construction of meaning, become ethnographically relevant. In this connection it is especially important to remember that we are dealing specifically with the conceptualization of the symptom as a transmitter of meaning. We have seen that psychopathology had already attracted the attention of culturalists like Newman, but his analytic concepts were consistent with the culturalism of the 1960s: "deviant behavior," "dysfunction" or "abnormal behavior" (p. 1). This is not to say that the word *symptom* was absent from the anthropology of this period. Newman does not use it, but some other studies do (see Parker, 1962; Schooler & Caudill, 1964). In these cases, however, the term does not refer to the construction of meaning, nor is it even an anthropological notion. As Canguilhem tells us, concepts and words are different things. In fact, the same word may contain different concepts. A concept is a discipline-specific analytical notion; defining a concept, therefore, involves delimiting a problem (Canguilhem, 1955, 1989). In this case, the problem is the meaningful nature of symptoms, understood as discursive and symbolic forms of expression.

Let us take as an example Seymour Parker's study of Inuit psychopathology, published two years prior to Newman's work. "Symptoms," he writes, "will be viewed not simply as a reflection of socio-environmental pressures, but as they function in the personality and social systems in which they appear" (1962, p. 76). "Function" and "personality" emerge here as key elements to which another extremely important variable must be added: "social systems." What, exactly, does Parker understand by symptoms? And what do Schooler and Caudill understand by symptoms in their well-known comparative study of the symptomatology of Japanese and North American schizophrenic patients (1964, p. 172)?

When these authors use the term "symptom," they have in mind a conventional psychiatric category in use at the time. Thus Parker says: "the most frequent psychopathological symptoms are morbid depressions, anorexia, and obsessive and paranoid ideation" (1962, p. 77). In Schooler and Caudill's case, the word "symptoms" refers to "withdrawn," "sleep disturbance," "emotionally labile," "euphoria," "apathy," etc. (1964, p. 173). That is to say, symptoms are neither constructions of meaning nor forms of expression used by the patient, but generalizations resembling the diagnostic criteria of the psychiatric manuals. Here symptom is not a category of anthropological theory but a loan from the terminological arsenal of psychiatry. There is no conceptual reformulation or emic analysis of symptoms here, only a dovetailing of disciplinary interests.

As we shall see in the next chapter, this situation has changed in recent years. First, anthropological interest in meaning rather than in function has allowed expressions of illness to become an ethnographic object. This has been facilitated by the development of symbolic and interpretive anthropology. However, in the case of medical and psychiatric anthropology, the development of ethnoscience and ethnosemantics has also been of considerable importance. Before analyzing the ethnoscientific approach to symptoms, however, we must take account of two theories which, like Newman's culturalism, are pre-interpretive ethnographic models. One of these is Goffman's approach, which straddles the ideas of symptoms as representations and symptoms as forms of social deviance. The other is that theoretical island in the ocean of anthropology, classical psychoanalytic anthropology.[4] This paradigm not only attempted to maintain the viability of Freudian orthodoxy in the face of the more heterodox approaches of the of culture-and-personality school; it also continued to strive for a synthesis between cultural variables and intrapsychic processes. In this, as in Freud's works, the term *symptom* had a certain importance.

SYMPTOMS AND THE UNCONCIOUS

Unconsciously, we always believe that victories can be achieved on the basis of past victories and that the world will take the mother's place.

—G. Róheim
Magic and schizophrenia.

Although Géza Róheim was one of the principal defenders of Freudian orthodoxy in anthropology, here I will use as an example of this theoretical position the work of another author who was no less influential: George Devereux, the teacher of such outstanding ethnopsychoanalysts as François Laplantine and Tobie Nathan.[5]

It does not take much ingenuity to deduce that Devereux would consider the case of the "wild man" to be an ethnic disorder of the same kind as the Malay *amok* and *latah*, the Algonquin *windigo*, or "Crazy-dog-wishing-to-die" among the Plains Indians of North America. It is a form culturally patterned by the message: "Don't do this, but if you must, do it this way." Devereux's work, however, is not limited to the analysis of ethnic disorders in these terms. He also developed an ethnopsychiatric theory in which the relationship between psychoanalytic and ethnological models is not merely additive, but complementary (1975). This characterization may seem odd, since certain passages in Devereux's work use psychoanalytic and anthropological models in a way that is primarily additive; for example, the conceptual splitting of the unconscious into an "unconscious segment of the ethnic personality" and an "idiosyncratic unconscious," two objects that are not totally independent, but interact with each other (1973, p. 28). This distinction is more additive than complementary, affecting the very integrity of the object of study (the unconscious). It is also a typology Devereux uses to develop a classification of disorders that does not contradict the diagnostic classifications of psychiatry, although here his intellectual genius seems to undermine his own orthodox intent.

Devereux speaks of four different types of personality disorders: the sacred or the shamanic; the ethnic; those which are dependent on social structure; and finally, the idiosyncratic. Some of these are of interest for my purposes here.

The first of these disorders (the sacred) is based on intrapsychic conflicts located in the ethnic segment of the unconscious rather than in the idiosyncratic unconscious. This does not prevent Devereux from asserting that the shaman himself is sick, unlike Ackerknecht who describes this behavior, in a somewhat awkward and ambiguous way, as both autonormal and heteropathological: normal within the cultural system, and pathological from the viewpoint of medical science (Ackerknecht, 1943; Devereux, 1973).

For Devereux, the shaman is sick, but he is a special kind of sick person, since the psychopathological picture is structured according to a cultural convention. In other words, in the shaman, cultural belief becomes subjective experience. Why, then, does Devereux consider the behavior of the shaman abnormal? First, because it is recognized as such by the group to which he belongs; and second—and this is the most significant part of Devereux's approach—because it reflects tensions and conflicts of a psychopathological nature. For Devereux, the universality of psychodynamic processes takes precedence over any sort of cultural relativism or particularism, whether it emerges from ethnological theory or from what he irreverently refers to as: "That gang of neo-and pseudo-Freudian 'culturist psychoanalysts' who not only boast of greater subtlety and a better ethnological nose, but also claim that their points of view are more useful to ethnologists than those of classical psychoanalysis" (1973, p. 102) [my translation].

Given Devereux's broad-spectrum anti-relativism, it is not surprising that what he calls ethnic disorders combine basic universality with the appearance of cultural specificity. *Amok* or crazy-dog-wishing-to-die are cases which, according to Devereux, use "the defenses and symptoms provided by culture" (1973, p. 70) in the same way as sacred disorders. The precipitating cause, however, is not necessarily cultural but may also be psychic or even biological; for instance, an attack of malaria can trigger *amok*.

Ethnic disorders are, in fact, patterned forms of resolving numerous psychic conflicts and pathologies from "a single complex of symptoms" (1973, p. 73). Nevertheless, Devereux is aware that this may be a stumbling block to the identification of the key symptoms of a psychopathological picture, as well as a point of friction with the defenders of cultural relativism.

In principle, an ethnic disorder such as crazy-dog is a particular manifestation not easily generalizable to other societies, and this requires Devereux to distinguish between cultural behaviors and psychiatric symptoms: the former belong to the "cultural axis" and the "ethnological domain," while the latter belong to the "neurotic axis" and the realm of psychiatry and psychoanalysis. The case of transvestism is used here as a paradigmatic example:

> Among the Plains Indians, the solution for cowards was to become transvestites, while for the Tanala of Madagascar, transvestism is the refuge of the sexually deficient man who, if he were to marry, would find that his unsatisfied wife would announce his impotence publicly. The fact that two different individuals under stress resort to the same type of deviant behavior shows that transvestism is still a symptom despite being culturally structured and framed (1973, p. 76) [my translation].

This passage clearly shows that, despite their cultural variability, symptoms can be identified crossculturally or metaculturally. Nevertheless, Devereux's notion of symptom is free of the waxen rigidity of the concept used by Kraepelin and the neo-Kraepelinians, whom he dismisses as the promoters of an elegant but superficial procedure for producing statistics (1973, p. 128). Moreover, Devereux's use of the concept of symptom varies. Sometimes symptoms are ethnically specific behaviors and cannot be extrapolated to other cultural contexts, such as crazy-dog-wishing-to-die which, like the hysteria observed by Charcot in the Salpêtrière, is likely to vanish in historical time or crosscultural space. But in other cases such as that of transvestism, symptoms seem to possess a degree of crosscultural validity, although the entire symptom complex may not necessarily be universal. This is of particular importance in Devereux's work:

> Why should we be surprised by the fact that the whole set of psychiatric symptoms is rarely found in a single society while we calmly accept that an Eskimo will never suffer from malaria nor a native of the Congo from snow blindness or frostbite? (1973, p. 67) [my translation].

Curiously, this identification between symptoms and signs at the biological level is in conflict with the author's own interests, since for Devereux, as for Freud, symptoms are "an attempt to reconstruct personality according to the logic of the unconscious" (p. 112). Such a reconstruction originates in a psychic and emotional conflict which remains concealed, tacit, and whose only manifestation is symptomatic. Behaviors such as nail-biting illustrate the point. According to Devereux, people may bite their nails simply for the technical reason that they do not know that there are such things as nail clippers, but "in our society, this is often a neurotic symptom complex, and the actual nail biting is only the nucleus of the behavior" (p. 111).

Here, symptoms are but the tip of an iceberg. But Deverux warns readers of the dangers of trying to deduce the structure of the submerged part from the parts that are showing: a symptom of hysteria may conceal schizophrenia, while a symptom of schizophrenia may mask hypomania. Symptoms of different psychopathological types may also coexist when a type disorder such as the schizoid structure of Western society happens to coincide with an individual disorder such as idiosyncratic hysteria (p. 265).[6] In these cases, Devereux believes that the sick individual should produce symptoms of both hysteria and schizophrenia, and attributes the resistance of Western patients to psychotherapy to psychiatric ignorance of the existence of overlapping and complexly intertwined dimensions of personality.

In this relation between psychopathology and symptom, Devereux finds further mysteries to illuminate. Behind an appearance of normality or, in his words, "a beautiful cultural facade," there may lurk the threat of a completely unexpected but serious psychiatric disorder. What appears to be well-balanced and consistent with cultural context may be normal in form but not necessarily in "its function" and "substance." Drawing on his training as a classical scholar, he asserts that Euripides is mistaken, since Hippolytus' difficulty is not that he is excessively chaste, but that he is suffering from a sexual phobia (p. 261).

Devereux's problem here is that of how to distinguish between the manifestations of psychopathological processes. If the symptoms of different illness types can coexist, the manifestations of one type can mask another type, and psychopathology can be concealed behind an appearance of normality, what, then, is the procedure for determining mental illness? Devereux's tactic here is to use holistic terms to view the entire panorama of symptomatological forms. Like an aerial photograph, a complete vision of the phenomenon would enable the observer to distinguish the topography of personality, the structure of psychic processes, relationships and interconnections, behaviors and symptoms. Order would be found among seemingly unrelated elements, laying bare the logic of the implicit underlying conflict, and in this manner, the incomprehensible would be rendered comprehensible (p. 191). But is this the task of ethnography?

At this point I should clarify that what Devereux understands by symptom belongs strictly to the domain of psychiatry or to a form of ethnopsychiatry which aims to distinguish between the normal and the pathological. The meaning of symptoms, then, is the pathological meaning assigned by the psychiatrist or psychoanalyst, while the local meaning that can be revealed by ethnographic analysis is pushed into the background. Thus, the difference between cultural behavior and symptom is simply the distinction between ethnography and psychiatry. Devereux attempts, on the one hand, to extract as much observational and interpretive value as he can from each of the theories he uses, but the weight of his psychoanalytic training leads him to use ethnography as a means to understanding, and psychiatry as a means of identifying preexisting pathological truth. As a follower of the Freudian tradition, he introduces into his analysis objects of study which are in principle alien to psychiatry—folklore, mythology, and dreams—but always with the aim of discerning unconscious psychic processes and endowing their representations with a meaning that goes beyond the local context in which they were created and expressed (1941, 1961). His contribution, however, is the introduction of ethnographic diversity and flexibility into the psychoanalytical model, and the construction of an approach that in many aspects is more additive than complementary, since it is formed by segmenting objects of analysis: the unconscious, the basic axes, types of disorders, personality, etc. His is a Herculean effort to understand the complexity of the relation between culture and the individual, without at the same time losing sight of classical psychoanalytic theory. If on occasion the tension between these two perspectives causes Devereux's psychoanalytic orthodoxy to founder, it is not because he lacks the capacity to be surprised by psychopathological phenomena, but because he has it in excess.

DEVIATIONS AND TRANSGRESSIONS

Although Goffman is famous for his microsociological forays into such disparate arenas as mental hospitals, prisons and daily life, his innovative way of interpreting symptoms has aroused little comment. The reason for this is that his best-known works deal at best tangentially with this problem. However, there is one interesting exception. In his 1969 article "The Insanity of

Place," he explicitly takes up the interpretation of symptoms, and provides us with one of the best examples of the application of the game analogy to what he calls "mental symptoms."

Devereux sees in symptoms the manifestations of a psychopathological order intimately related to cultural context. Goffman, however, finds in "mental symptoms" a whole complex of rules, actions and deviations which do not have the same referent as "medical symptoms" and imply social values, infractions and offenses. For Goffman there is a world of difference between medical symptoms and mental symptoms. Of the former, he says:

> Signs and symptoms of a medical disorder presumably refer to underlying pathologies in the individual organism, and these constitute deviations from biological norms maintained by the homeostatic functioning of the human machine. The system of reference here is plainly the individual organism, and the term "norm," ideally at least, has no moral or social connotation (1969, p. 362).

This definition is reminiscent of Sydenham's, several centuries earlier, in which symptoms were defined as the mechanical consequence of a dysfunction in the human machine.

However, the probable organic causes of some psychoses aside, Goffman's "mental symptoms" are forms of deviation from established norms which lead back to the very substance of social obligations. For this reason, deviation in these cases is not the deviation of the tuberculosis patient or the disabled person, but rather a transgression of social norms, a game in which there are offenders and offended, inappropriate and bizarre actions, behaviors destructive of social obligations and, of course, a great deal of unawareness on the part of the patient. Here, mental symptoms do not emerge as things in themselves, but as acts both constructed and interpreted from social material. This is why Goffman is not interested (as Devereux is) in the psychopathological meaning of symptoms. In fact, his main interest is not even the meaning of symptoms for the patients themselves. Instead, what occupies him is ferreting out the meaning of symptoms for the "other" players in the social game. Mental symptoms are violations of the organization of public places, streets, neighborhoods and shops. They also disrupt the organization of work, particulary highly formalized and rationalized work. In the domestic context they can lead to conflicts that upset daily life and force the family into an uncomfortable position between the patient and the community. In all these considerations, what so attracts Goffman is not the symptom from the point of view of the sender of the message, but the relation between the sender and the receiving group, the forms of social control that the group and/or the institution develops, the coalitions established between family members against the disruptive agent, and also the way in which the game of behavior and the behavioral responses of others models the symptomatological expressions of the patient. Hence, Goffman's aim is "to sketch some of the meanings of mental symptoms for the organization in which they occur, with special reference to the family. The argument is that current doctrine and practice in psychiatry have neglected these meanings" (p. 385).

What characterizes Goffman is precisely this ability to discuss symptoms in a way that locates their primordial meaning not in the organic or even in the psychic order, but in a broader social and organizational order. What justifies this analytic strategy is that the formation of the symptom is fueled by the same complex of social obligations and social positions that allows it to be recognized as a transgression and not as an appropriate or excusable action. In this way he establishes an alternative reading of symptoms, one that differs from the psychiatric reading. Goffman's model is not, however, without its weaknesses.

Let us go back for a moment to his definition of "medical signs and symptoms." Somewhat hastily, Goffman distinguishes mental symptoms from medical signs and symptoms, associating the former with the transgression of social norms and the latter with underlying pathologies in the individual organism and the absence of "moral or social connotation." One of the main problems here is that not all mental symptoms—or, for that matter, all mental disorders—imply a form of deviation, an "infraction of social rules," of a different type than that produced, for example, by migraine or indigestion. For example, where should we place feelings of hopelessness, which are psychological in nature but without strong moral connotations? Where should we put psychosomatic symptoms? It is clear that the infractions generated by these mental symptoms are practically identical to those precipitated by the so-called medical symptoms. When Goffman speaks of mental symptoms, he means those symptoms of a psychotic and disorganized nature, bizarre and transgressive, those sudden accesses of madness that are quite distinct from the signs and symptoms of, say, tuberculosis or some other physical disease. But what, then, of these other psychological manifestations? Goffman does not address them because they are beyond his range. His model for distinguishing mental symptoms is that of madness, with all its transgressive impact.

However, the problems do not end here. Goffmann's typology is also controversial because the manifestations of physical diseases are not exempt from moral considerations, and the manifestations of mental disorders cannot be hastily dismissed as non-biological forms. In other words, not all the manifestations of physical diseases are twitches, and not all mental disorders are winks. Any health professional knows that clinical pictures are a tangle of objectifiable and non-objectifiable manifestations. The former reflect the logic of physical signs, while the latter reflect the logic of symptoms. These symptoms arouse feelings of unease which are difficult to identify as either physical or psychological, because they are often both. Some psychopathologies involve such physical signs as trembling and palpitations. How, then, can we differentiate medical signs and symptoms from mental symptoms? Goffman seems unaware that the difference between mental disorders and physical diseases is not exclusively a question of different symptoms, but of the fact that the former mainly consist of symptoms and the latter of signs, to which we can add the above mentioned difficulty of locating an organic point of anchorage not only for the symptoms but also for many of the signs of mental disorders. We are not dealing here with differences in the nature of phenomena, but with the different interpretive and explanatory possibilities offered by biomedicine on the one hand, and psychiatry on the other. As Young (1976, p. 14) lucidly pointed out several years ago, "In 'physical' illnesses as well as 'mental' ones, symptoms are shaped in ways that cannot be explained by biophysical causes."

What I want to stress here are the limitations of transgressive behavior as the principal criterion for separating physical disease from. It only reveals a segment of the symptomatological spectrum, and it is valid only for distinguishing between situations that contrast sharply; for example, a skin rash as opposed to the storing of tons of rubbish at home; or a chest X-ray showing pulmonary emphysema versus publicly declaring oneself to be a KGB spy when one is neither Russian nor a secret agent.

In other words, the distinction is possible when physical signs are compared with symptoms which involve a transgression of social norms. When the contrast is not so obvious, however, Goffman's concepts begin to break down. Consider, for example, two symptoms: "my head aches," and "I feel down." In both cases, the transgression of social obligations is neither completely present nor completely absent, and is therefore useless as a distinguishing feature. Neither is it valid to say that one is exclusively a social product since, independently of their diagnostic contexts and possible biological referents, they are both semiosic and cultural constructions, and as such, they conceal moral and social worlds of affliction. In short, both are symptoms.

THE NAMES OF DISEASES

A review of the anthropological literature over the past one hundred years shows that studies of local medical systems have always been part of the discipline, even though this was not initially a major area of research. From the early article by Washington Matthews (1888) on the prayers of a Navajo shaman to Charles Frake's well-known study on the diagnostic categories of the Subanun[7] of Mindanao (1961; see also 1980), the problem of folk definitions of illness has been a field of activity both for anthropological theory and applied research. However, there seems to be a turning point after studies such as Frake's. His article on the Subanun is, in fact, one of the first attempts to apply ethnoscientific theory to the analysis of local diagnostic categories.

Frake's study of Subanun medical categories was a bit fortuitous since his fieldwork was initially focused on social structure. This medical system turned out to consist of no less than 186 "disease names" with their corresponding etiologies, diagnostic criteria, complexes of signs and symptoms, and therapeutic formulae. Frake pays particular attention to one set of categories: the terminology of skin diseases. Each category is analyzed from an essentially emic viewpoint, since his aim is not to construct generalizations beyond the cultural boundaries of the Subanun, but to discover their cognitive domain. His ethnoscientific methodology was already well-represented in Goodenough's work on componential analysis, as well as in Conklin's study of color classification among the Hannou (see Frake, 1961).

Frake is mainly interested in Subanun names for diseases, rather than and not so much in their etiologies or possible therapeutic alternatives. From his point of view, diseases are a valid object of study for ethnoscience not only because they are experienced and treated, but also because they are labeled and conceptualized. Subanun establish their taxonomies of skin diseases in the same way that English speakers use a discrimination axis to distinguish between a dog and a cat, and a generalization axis to establish taxonomic hierarchies such as poodle-dog-animal. "Sores" (*beldut*) contrast with both "ringworm" (*buni*) and "inflammation" (*neyebag*). Within the category "sores" (*beldut*), there is a contrast between "distal ulcer" (*telemaw*) and "proximal ulcer" (*baga*). In turn, within the subdomain "distal ulcer" there are other types such as "shallow distal ulcer" (*telemaw glai*) and "deep distal ulcer" (*telemaw bligun*). It is no coincidence that this taxonomy is reminiscent of botanical classifications.

One of the major premises of this ethnoscientific exercise is that diseases belong to a preexisting order of reality. It is difficult to imagine how this could be otherwise, since Frake's object of study was skin diseases, a paradigmatic example of what is observable, the evident domain of physical signs. Given this, few readers would find it surprising that he chose to focus his analysis on the domain of objective symptoms.

Frake regards native taxonomies as the simple exercise of giving names to things, real objects that already exist independently of any exegesis on the part of the Subanun or, for that manner, the Hannou, the Lacandón, or any other group. Following this logic, the meaning of a diagnostic category is the disease itself as a biological and pathophysiological reality. But how applicable is this model to the more controversial domain of mental disorders? Here physical signs are less important than symptoms, and this requires a change in ethnoscientific methodology. A sore may be categorized either as a monosymptomatic disease, or as a physical sign, but it is after all a sore, and culture intervenes only in the social conditions of its production, in the way a certain social group constructs categories to account for it, and in therapeutic efforts to get rid of it. A symptom such as "I have a headache," however, is from the very first a semiosic construction. What is the meaning of the symptom in this case? Is it the head as an anatomical territory, or the head as a linguistic construction referring to a range of cultural meanings, a specific native encyclopedia? If Frake does not address this issue, it is because pathological signs on the skin, like physical diseases, are not problematic in this way. They are simply there, not as an exegesis but as a natural occurrence.

A different problem emerges, however, from other ethnoscientific and related forms of interpretation using both signs and symptoms. This is the case of Fabrega's work in Chiapas on Zinacantecan medical terminology (1970; see also 1974, chapter 8). Fabrega's later criticism (1987) of the analogy between botanical classifications and psychopathological taxonomies notwithstanding, in this early article he seems to work from precisely this logic. His aim is to establish a taxonomy of Zinacantecan diagnostic categories and their symptomatological components, and to compare the degree of similarity or difference between lay and professional knowledge using a set of terms such as *pumel, cuvah, takicamel, mévinik, sarampio*. Each category consists of a list of signs and symptoms. What commands our attention about these lists is that emic diagnostic categories are treated as cultural constructions, but the outward manifestations of distress as natural elements. In many cases they are, but in others they are not. Clearly physical signs such as "feverishness," "blood in urine," "pruritus," "coughing," and "blood in stool" appear alongside such symptoms as "crying and sadness."

Because Fabrega's point of departure is the assumption that Zinacantecan diagnostic constructions reflect objective reality, he is faced with inexplicable folk configurations in which different diagnostic categories are characterized by almost identical clusters of symptoms. Not surprisingly, his analysis founders precisely on such symptoms as "crying and sadness" or "weakness," because they appear consistently in the eighteen folk categories he analyzes (1970, p. 308). Should these symptoms be interpreted as natural manifestations, or as cultural forms for the expression of suffering?

Apart from the criteria used in a particular culture to group different signs and symptoms, there is in fact a clear difference between the process culminating in fever and the expression of "crying and sadness." In fever, cultural context is contingent in the same way that history (in its most social sense) is for ants. The same, however, cannot be said of "crying and sadness," since people express their emotions in culturally different ways and in equally diverse situations. In this case, neither cultural tradition nor history is contingent. As a small test of this, think for a moment of the *Iränengruss* or "tearful greeting" of the aboriginal Australians, the equivalent of which would be our "social smile" (Devereux, 1973, p. 271). Fever is fever, but something as apparently universal as "crying" may refer to a whole cultural universe of meanings.

Arguing along similar lines, Byron Good has suggested that one of the weaknesses of the ethnoscientific approach is its evident intellectual debt to the empiricist theory of language, in particular the premise that the meaning of words lies in their direct relationship with the objects named. Developing this argument further, Good (1977) has deconstructed some of the implicit assumptions of medical ethnosemantics; for example:

1. Diseases are discrete pathological conditions, which can be adequately described in biochemical and physiological terms.
2. These diseases are categorized differently in different societies, using various discriminating principles (p. 51).

I have noted briefly that these conceptualizations affect the understanding of illness. In fact, there is little difference between the assumptions underlying ethnosemantic studies of medicine, and the linguistic empiricism of contemporary biomedicine and psychiatry. The ethnoscientific task seems to project the taxonomic rationality of Western medical knowledge onto the local cognitive domains, which are then structured according to the principles of naming and classification. The aim here is to know the names of diseases, their taxonomic order and the internal hierarchies established by this classificatory scheme.

This rationality becomes precarious when symptoms, complaints and other forms for the expression of distress are introduced. The empiricist approach may be useful for developing native taxonomies which show how signs like "fever" or "coughing" are classified, or how, in a particular cognitive domain, a superficial sore may be contrasted with another kind of sore that penetrates deeper into the skin. What seems less evident, however, is the applicability of this approach to symptoms. This is why ethnoscientists reduce symptoms to objective forms which reflect a sort of native DSM in which symptoms are signifiers whose meaning is the pathology itself. But at this point our suspicions are aroused because, as in Fabrega's case, symptoms like "crying and sadness" seem to defy the ethnographer's classificatory logic.

Medical ethnosemantics is based on the reproduction of ideal cognitive domains. From an emic standpoint, it has addressed forms of cataloguing, hierarchies of concepts, and contrasts between categories. If biomedical empiricism is constructed on this implicit ideal of classifying and naming, ethnoscience has made these processes its object of study without questioning the assumption that meaning resides in the link between word and object. Symptoms, complaints and expressions of distress are not analyzed as they arise in the flow of social life, but are instead isolated and subjected to a form of laboratory analysis detached from their context of use. However, ethnoscience is not the only theory concerned with the linguistic dimension of illness and its forms of expression. For some time now other ethnographic models have been available for the analysis of symptoms, models that take account of symptoms in social and cultural context.

NOTES

1. Wild man has also been associated with amok. See Langness (1965), among others.
2. Here I have used Newman's work. However, any article of the period would take a similar approach. See especially Harris (1957), Mischel & Mischel (1958), Langness (1965) and Parker (1960).
3. Pike was also thinking more in terms of behaviors than in terms of meanings when he formulated his famous emic/etic dichothomy.
4. By classical psychoanalytic anthropology, I understand the more orthodox positions of Róheim and Devereux, among others. Although Marvin Harris (1968) identifies these two authors as members of the culture-and-personality school,

they are separated from it by their critique of cultural relativism. The term "classical" enables us to differentiate between their approach and Obeyesekere's (1990) and Crapanzano's (1992) contemporary works, which are more hermeneutic in nature, although other contemporary works, such as those of Tobie Nathan and Laplantine, may also be described as "classical."

5. See Laplantine's *L'Ethnopsychiatrie* (1973) and Nathan's *L'influence qui guérit* (1994), both dedicated to George Devereux.

6. Devereux considers that Western culture is basically schizoid and relates this condition to the typical properties of the *Gesellschaft*, although he turns not to Tönnies to define it but to Parsons instead. According to Devereux, this schizoid structure is a "type" disorder produced by social structure. Nevertheless, it may be compatible with psychopathological processes on other levels: "ethnic disorder" and "idiosyncratic disorder" (1973, p. 97).

7. A history of the ethnographic study of indigenous ethnomedical systems is beyond the scope of this book. However, interested readers may wish to consult some important early works; for example, Frank Russell's (1898) magnificent description of an Apache healing ritual and the role of the *sotli* or healer. See also Grinnell's work (1905) on Cheyenne ethnobotany, undoubtedly one of the first interdisciplinary studies in this field; Arthur Parker's study (1909) of the secret medical societies of the Senecas, a functionalist analysis *avant la lettre* which advances some serious criticisms of Morgan's early work on the Iroquois; Wilson Wallis' article (1922) on the medical system of the Micmacs; and Albert Reagan's collection (1922) of Chippewa healing songs. Other works of interest include the much-quoted comparative studies of Rivers (1924) and Clements (1932), and, especially since the 1950s, a growing genre of ethnomedical literature (Ackerknecht, 1946, 1947; Erasmus, 1952; Nurge, 1958; Rubel, 1960).

CHAPTER 8

Toward an Anthropology of Symptoms II: Hermeneutics and Politics

Almost thirty years after Newman described the behavior of the Gururumba wild man, Matsuoka Etsuko (1991) approached a case of *Kitsune-Tsuki* (fox possession) in Japan in a markedly different manner.

Michiko, Matsuoka's informant, began to hear strange voices after the death of her parents. These became more frequent after she visited the "spiritual mountain" where she had attempted to communicate with them through a shaman. The voices became so insistent and loud that she sought help at a psychiatric hospital. However, her seven-month stay in the hospital did not solve her problem because, according to Michiko, "the medicine was no help, but it's natural that spirits can't be cured by medicine and doctors would never understand spirit possession" (p. 456).

Subsequently, Michiko turned to several different shamans—seven in all— who suggested a variety of possible diagnoses and treatments. Depending on the version, she was possessed by either a snake, a mountain spirit, or a fox. The last interpretation seemed to Michiko to be the right one, to the extent that she identified the source of the voices as being the spirit of a fox killed by one of her ancestors. The special feature of this spirit was that it provided her with true information about the world and about her past. "I'm not cheating you, so listen carefully," the fox told her before proceeding to recite her life story. The fox informed Michiko that she was of aristocratic origin and that some of her ancestors were even connected to the imperial family. He also told her about matters that were not part of her personal

147

history; for example, that the Chernobyl nuclear power disaster had been caused by a curse placed on the Soviet Union for shooting down a South Korean plane, and that Ronald Reagan had put a bomb on another plane, a Japanese plane, which caused a terrible accident. But the voices mainly spoke of unexplained incidents from Michiko's past: the fire that burned down her parents' house, the suspicion that their neighbor might have been involved, and the family's subsequent economic difficulties. According to Michiko:

> The fox says that it will not go away until I prove the arson, because it has possessed me to let me know the truth. It is not an ordinary fox but a box fox. And the fox is a follower of the fox deity, so it should know everything (p. 457).

Over the years, the voices did not disappear, but Michiko experienced a change of great significance. After several failed attempts, she became a shaman in a Buddhist sect (*shugendo*) in a desperate attempt to cure herself. In her own words:

> I finally had the first client. A brother or a sister of a friend of my colleague suddenly disappeared. The spirit behind me told me to search for him/her. So I guessed the place. I didn't receive any money because he or she is not yet found...I still work on religious practice every day. I'll keep on doing it because it has made me what I am (p. 459).

Matsuoka's account of this case is important not only for its portrait of Michiko's experiential universe, but also for the way it is presented in ethnographic context. Articles of this kind—like Newman's, which opened the previous chapter—are not unusual in anthropological literature. However, when Matsuoka's analysis is contrasted with Newman's, some interesting divergences in their ethnographic styles emerge. For instance, Michiko speaks extensively in the first person, whereas Gambiri tells us hardly anything in his own words. In fact, these two articles construct affliction in markedly different ways. Whereas Newman behavioralizes Gambiri's discourse, Matsuoka discursivizes Michiko's behavior. In Matsuoka's article, in fact, the patient's narrative is at the core of the ethnographic analysis. The central issue is not behavior and sequences of behavioral response, but the significance of indigenous discourse, to such an extent that behavior is accessible only through the informant's narrative. This not only affects the transcription of Michiko's narrative, but also the analytic concepts that the Japanese ethnographer uses to unravel the case and develop a coherent interpretation of it. Matsuoka does not speak in terms of patterns of misconduct, ethnic disorders, the ethnic unconscious, social deviance, or folk taxonomies, instead treating Michiko's illness as a metaphor with a number of possible interpretations: shamanic, psychiatric, and anthropological (which includes the sufferer's narrative).

This range of possible interpretations does not reproduce Newman's analytic strategy using different variables. Matsuoka's aim is not to construct a definitive explanation, but simply to juxtapose different readings of the same case. Of course, this juxtaposition is not gratuitous; she means to show us that one of these readings is likelier than the others to shed the most light on the curious case of *Kitsune-Tsuki*. A causalist or etiological model, she observes, is much less productive than an interpretive approach, which gives the informant's symptoms their "metaphoric" and polysemic nature. In other words, she does not attempt to explain away possession as a pathoplastic form of a disease—which in this case could easily be schizophrenia—but ventures into the domain of meaning, placing the informant's illness narrative in relation to a larger frame of reference. And what she finds, first of all, is a plural universe of meanings which Michiko uses alternately, and even simultaneously, reflecting a context in which different medical systems coexist. Second—and more importantly for my purposes—she also finds that fox possession is a reflexive symbol which provides Michiko with an opportunity to think about her geneaology and ancestors. This symbol—which is also a symptom—turns the fox into a liminal agent which voices the truth of a life; a local, cultural instrument for reflection.

We are led to the conclusion that Michiko's symptoms are like winks which cannot be understood outside the cultural context in which foxes and the memory of ancestors acquire meaning. What is less clear, although also true, is that Matsuoka's analysis cannot be understood outside the universe of knowledge in which it was produced; that is to say, outside the framework of an interpretive medical and psychiatric anthropology concerned with tracing the meanings of illness and symptoms through such concepts as symbol, metaphor, narrative, idioms of distress and so on. Unlike pre-interpretive theories, this approach is not a coolly distanced appraisal of behaviors and functions, patterns of misconduct or taxonomies, but retains all the immediacy of culturally specific forms of expression.

Interpretive approaches, however, are not the only alternative theories within anthropology which have problematized symptoms. Alongside hermeneutic and semiotic theories, other paradigms have emerged: phenomenology and materialist trends. This is not a new intellectual development. The polarization of contemporary North American anthropology represents a revisitation of the almost perennial confrontation between hermeneutics and

Marxist-oriented critical theory. Thus we find, on the one hand, what has come to be known as the meaning-centered approach, which is simply the application of hermeneutics and semiotics to the domain of illness and its forms of expression. On the other hand, a critical approach has been formulated which employs, in a somewhat heterodox fashion, the European Marxist approach and, almost always unknowingly, some of the basic arguments that have characterized Italian and Latin American anthropology since the 1950s:[1] for instance, the idea that cultural categories and meanings conceal hidden structures of power and domination. Let us take a look at these two approaches in greater detail.

HERMENEUTICS

Two Harvard scholars, Arthur Kleinman and Byron Good, have played a leading role in the development of the meaning-centered approach, the main principles of which are applied in Matsuoka's article: the hermeneutics of the emic dimension of affliction through close readings of illness narratives and symptoms; textual analysis; the use of linguistic and semiotic models; and the critique of neo-Kraepelinism and the biomedical model in general. Although many other anthropologists are also associated with this paradigm, I will limit myself here to these two. Not only are they the most representative of this approach, they have also made the greatest theoretical contribution to the study of symptoms in medical anthropology. First I will comment on the writings of Byron Good and then move on to discuss the work of Arthur Kleinman.

I believe that Good's work cannot be completely understood without taking into account the influence of his professor, Victor Turner, from whom he took the idea of "dominant ritual symbols." Turner developed this concept in *The Forest of Symbols* (1967) to refer to those meaningful elements in Ndembu ritual with a central role in ritual processes. These symbols are characterized by such fundamental properties as polysemy, condensation of meaning, the unification of diverse meanings in a single symbolic formation, and the polarization of meaning in two extremes, one of which is orectic or sensory, while the other is normative or ideological. An example of this type of symbol is the *mudyi* or "milk tree", which has a central role in rituals like *n'kanga* (puberty ritual for young Ndembu girls). Turner traces its range of meaning from mother's milk (sensory pole) to the Ndembu principle of matrilineality (ideological pole) (Turner, 1967, p. 21).

In her prologue to the posthumous *On the Edge of the Bush,* Edith Turner (1985, p. 6) has related Victor Turner's principle of condensation to the work of the well-known linguist and anthropologist Edward Sapir, and the idea of polarization to the work of Freud. In *The Forest of Symbols,* Victor Turner himself seems to speak exclusively of Sapir as the source of his inspiration (1967, p. 29), although in subsequent writings he recognizes the influence of Freud's intellectual style on the development of his own thought. More recently, Oring (1993) has traced these associations back to their origins, concluding that in Sapir's work, the concept of condensation is irrelevant, and the principle of unification altogether absent. He interprets Turner's curious amnesia as a sort of intellectual repression of Freud's work which is similar to the Ndembus' denial of their ancestors (p. 278).

Without going into further detail on this matter, what is certain is that both Turner's idea of condensation and the notion of polarization are not new. Although Freud does not speak explicitly of sensory and ideological poles, the idea that ambivalent meanings can be concealed and unified in a single representation (symptoms, dream symbols, etc.), and condensation as a centrally important concept, are among the fundamental contributions of *The Interpretation of Dreams.*

However, Turner is critical of psychoanalytic interpretations of ritual symbols:

> Furthermore, they [the psychoanalysts] tend to look upon ritual symbols as identical with neurotic and psychotic symptoms or as though they had the same properties as the dream symbols of Western European individuals. In effect, their procedure is the exact reverse of that of the social anthropologists who share the views of Nadel and Wilson. This school of anthropologists, it will be remembered, considers that only conscious, verbalized, indigenous interpretations of symbols are sociologically relevant (1967, p. 34).

And he is right to be critical; consciously or unconsciously finding inspiration in psychoanalysis for his own theories is not incompatible with rejecting the hypotheses, not to say dogmas, of some psychoanalysts. But let us for a moment concentrate on what he is saying: he is articulating the abovementioned conflict between those interpretations that search ritual symbols for pathological meaning, and those that focus on local cultural meaning. What Turner is criticizing is the appropriation of meaning, the hasty generalization, and the monosemic style characteristic of Freudian exegesis. He is not denying the identification between symptoms and ritual symbols, but rejecting the extrapolation of totalizing psychological interpretations to the terrain of ethnography:

> Such psychoanalysts claim to recognize, in the structure and action context of
> ritual symbols, material derived from what they consider to be the universal
> experiences of human infancy in the family situation (1967, p. 34).

Here Turner adopts the correcting tone of the ethnographer criticizing
psychoanalytic claims. But the correction is directed less at the familiarity
of symbolic objects (ritual symbols and symptoms) than at a very specific
type of approach: the search for pathological meaning, the totalizing treatment of all types of winks as twitches. It is also clear that when he speaks of
neurotic and psychotic symptoms he is not conceptualizing them as a potential field of ethnographic study—not because such objects are of a fundamentally different nature than symbolic forms, but as a consequence of
established anthropological criteria for defining ethnographic objects. Good,
among others, was to dissolve these criteria.

In a 1977 article entitled "The Heart of What's the Matter: The Semantics
of Illness in Iran," Good attempts to formulate a new approach to illness and
also to develop a new theory of medical language which neither reifies illnesses nor restricts semantics to mere naming. To this end, he develops the
concept of "semantic illness network" based on Turner's idea of "dominant
ritual symbols" as well as on other approaches, such as Fox's notion of "core
terms" and Izutsu's "focus words" (Good, 1977). The idea is that an illness
is not only a set of predefined signs, but:

> rather a 'syndrome' of typical experiences, a set of words, experiences, and
> feelings which typically 'run together' for the members of a society. Such a
> syndrome is not merely a reflection of symptoms linked with each other in
> natural reality, but a set of experiences associated through networks of mean-
> ing and social interaction in a society (p. 27).

Insofar as an illness is also a set of meanings and social interactions, it
contains dominant symbols which condense multiple meanings for the members of a given society. The study of semantic networks, then, provides an
alternative to the assumptions of what Good calls the "empiricist theory of
language" and, more specifically, to what he later called the "empiricist theory
of medical language" (Good, 1994, p. 185, see note 3). Good is interested
neither in pathological meanings—whether in biomedical form or in sociological translation as social deviance—nor in folk taxonomies based on the
idea of a direct relationship between category and objective reality, but simply in what these forms of expression mean for the social actors themselves.

The ethnographic example which Good uses to illustrate the potential of
this approach is *"narahatiye qalb"* or heart distress. This is a folk category
resulting from the unequal influence of different medical systems: Arabic-

Galenic medicine, biomedicine, and local medical concepts in Maragheh, a Turkic-speaking town in the province of East Azerbaijan in northwest Iran. Following a brief cultural and historical analysis, Good explains how he gradually became aware of the importance of this category in the life of the town. Women, much more than men, complained of *"qalbim vurur"* (My heart is pounding), *"qalbim tittirir"* (My heart is trembling), or *"qalbim narahatdī"* (My heart is uncomfortable, upset, in distress, uneasy or in disease). To find out the meaning of this form of expression—which I would call a symptom—Good carried out a survey in Maragheh and its surrounding area, and found that the frequency of "heart distress" was forty percent, and that most sufferers were women between the ages of 15 and 44 years old. For my purposes here, what is most interesting about Good's work is not so much the statistical results of his survey, but the more qualitative information that he provides. Underlying the complaints associated with heart distress there are four fundamental emotions and feelings: *qus* or sorrow, *quam* or sadness, *fikr* or worry and *xiyalet* or anxiousness. Each is specific to particular personal and social circumstances; for example, grief and sadness at the death of a relative; worry about one's financial affairs; or anxiety induced by conflict with one's mother-in-law or insufficient living space at home. But the matter does not end here. Good discovers that "heart distress" condenses even more meanings: a belief in the pernicious effects of oral contraceptives, palpitations, cold, lack of blood, and nerves, among others. A wide range of symbols, situations, afflictions, diseases, events and emotions are condensed in a single public image, in the collective representation that is *narahatiye qalb*. Not all of these associations of meaning are culturally explicit; there is also a deep-lying implicit or unconscious dimension which must also be an object of ethnographic interpretation.

Although Good's analysis is interesting, he does not take advantage of all the potential inherent in Turner's model of dominant ritual symbols, on which his own model appears to be based. Here I have in mind Turner's idea that these symbolic formations do not only condense but also polarize meaning. The sensory and ideological poles of meaning about which Turner writes bear more than a passing resemblance to the type of polarization evident in Iranian "heart distress." Good himself, in fact, shows us that the symptom of "heart distress" can condense meanings ranging from palpitations (sensory pole) to the mother-in-law conflicts that arise from rules governing postnuptial residence (ideological pole). Further exploration of this analytic pathway suggests the possibility of a stratification of polarized meanings which would situate the literal meaning of "heart distress" at the sensory pole, while the second- or third-order meanings are located at the ideological pole. It detracts nothing from the value of his contribution, however, that Good himself does not pursue this line of analysis. He is, after all, one of the first social scientists to approach symptoms as meaningful constructions. A number of earlier efforts paved the way for Good's work on Iranian "heart distress;" for example, Zola (1975) studied Italian and Irish patients' complaints in relation to eye, ear, nose and throat diseases, and Ann Parsons (1961), with considerable analytic skill, addressed the relationship between symptoms and cultural values in her ethnographic portrait of Giuseppina, a southern Italian woman diagnosed as having schizophrenia. "The Heart of What's the Matter," however, has had a greater impact on subsequent research, for a number of reasons.

Good's work gives force to the notion that illness has a local dimension which can be studied in hermeneutic terms, using the concept of the semantic network to gain access to a system of meanings based on a dominant symbol: the symptom as an expression of distress. This approach challenges the close association that medical empiricism establishes between symptom (complaint) and pathophysiology, and displays some of anthropology's potential: the interpretation of illness and its expressions.

In his first article, Good is reluctant to use the term "symptom" to refer to the complaints of his informants. However, if we consider, as Canguilhem once said (1955, 1989), that a concept is not a word but an idea or a problem, we can recognize Good's interest in expressions of illness as semiotic constructions even though he does not use the word "symptom". Moreover, the use of this term is quite clear in his subsequent work; for example, his article co-authored with Mary-Jo DelVecchio Good entitled "The Meaning of Symptoms."

In this article, the authors take a more pragmatic approach, proposing a hermeneutic and interpretive model as an alternative to the clinical procedures of biomedicine. Here there is no doubt about the role of symptoms in their theory:

> Symptoms do not reflect somatic abnormalities in any simple way, and the relationship among symptoms does not mirror a set of mechanistic or functional physiological relationships. Symptoms are irreducibly meaningful (Good & Good, 1981, p. 191).

Unfortunately, the Goods make no distinction here between signs and symptoms; they simply assume in a general way that the expressions of illness are meaningful. In this respect, their approach is more radical than mine, perhaps because they do not explicitly state what they understand by symptoms, or because they use the term in a wide sense embracing both signs and symptoms. What is most relevant here, however, is not only their argument that symptoms "do not reflect biological abnormalities in any simple way," but their approach to this new object of analysis, the symptom as a condensation of meanings. Both authors are clear on this point. Where the biomedical model seeks somatic or psychophysiological lesions, the hermeneutic model investigates the construction of meanings: "the illness reality of the sufferer" (1981, p. 179). Clinical practice requires physical evidence of disease; hermeneutics decodes semantic networks. The biomedical model "dialectically explores relationships between symptoms and somatic disorder;" the hermeneutic model interprets symptoms as texts in relation to the wider context of semantic networks. In short, while biomedical knowledge takes the form of explanation (*Erklärung*), hermeneutics opts instead for knowledge as understanding (*Verstehen*) (p. 179).

In his more recent *Lewis Henry Morgan Lectures* published under the title *Medicine, Rationality and Experience: An Anthropological Perspective* (1994), Good introduces in passing the distinction described here between signs and symptoms. The former are "physiological abnormalities that can be measured"—and, I would add, observed—using clinical and laboratory procedures. In contrast, the latter are "the expressions of the experience of distress, communicated as an ordered set of complaints" (p. 8). While some of these are physical, others are culturally and linguistically coded. Although this distinction is not subsequently applied in the rest of the book, a careful reading suggests that Good suspects that the problems associated with symptoms are quite complex, and this is evident not only in the more theoretical parts of the book, but in the analysis of cases as well. For instance, a physical sign such as "rectal bleeding" is identified as a symptom, concretely as a "primary symptom" which forms part of a complex, semiotic order of possible patient associations (p. 93). This does not necessarily contradict the above distinction between signs and symptoms, because any physical sign may also be converted into a symptom: a message expressed linguistically and culturally, referring to an observable reality which causes suffering to the sender of the message. The important thing here is that the conversion of a physical sign into a symptom introduces a symbolic and narrative dimension which goes well beyond the simple organic referent. For instance, Good discovers in the symptom of rectal bleeding a local universe of affliction and even a conflict between biomedical treatments and religious loyalties: the informant is a Jehovah's Witness and is reluctant to accept a possible blood transfusion. Further, in an attempt to relate his semantic approach to the

structuralism of Lévi-Strauss, Good analyzes the different elements underlying the patient's primary symptom, and discovers that these are expressed
in a play of oppositions between health and sickness, purity and contamina-
tion, "blood as life" and "blood as something foreign and unclean," "the
baptismal life" and "the old life of Satan," "Jehovah's family" and the rest of
the world (p. 94-98). In a surprisingly formalist tone, he concludes: "Symptoms are given meaning within cultural systems relationally, by the position
they occupy within complex symbolic codes" (p. 99).

Of course, complaints and illness narratives may be subjected to structural analysis of the kind Lévi-Strauss applied to myths.[2] Where Lévi-Strauss
saw mythemes or contrasting units similar to phonemes, we can identify
symptomemes. We can even attempt to apply to symptoms the structuralist
idea that there is a syntagmatic plane (a level of contiguity and concatena-
tion of language) and a paradigmatic plane (a domain in which appropriate
categories are selected by their similarity or difference in relation to other
categories within a system). In fact, we can reproduce some of the binary
oppositions derived from the syntagmatic/paradigmatic dichotomy, and speak
of the metonymic level versus the metaphoric level (Jakobson, 1980), the
order of events versus the order of structure (Lévi-Strauss, 1962a, p. 46),
parole versus *langue* (Lévi-Strauss, 1962b, p. 300),[3] sign versus symbol
(Leach, 1976, Chapter II) or displacement (*Verschiebung*) versus condensation (*Verdichtung*) (Lacan, 1981, p. 317). However, Good does not take his
flirtation with structuralism to these lengths, probably because he is aware
that excessive formalism reduces the meaning of illness and its expressions
to mathematical permutations, and converts the local worlds of meaning
condensed in a symptom into mere transformations of a panhuman binary
logic.[4] Nevertheless, throughout *Medicine, Rationality and Experience*, he
does try to reflect on the limits of his semantic and hermeneutic approach.

In the last chapter of his *Lectures*, entitled "Aesthetics, Rationality and
Medical Anthropology," Good revises his concept of "semantic network"
and finds that "while core symbols in a medical lexicon may indeed condense or hold in tension a powerful network of meanings, the process of
synthesis is not only semiotic, but social, dialogical, imaginative and political. And so too should be our analyses" (1994, p. 173). True enough: the
process of constructing, condensing and synthesizing meaning has many
facets, one of which is political. As Marxist medical anthropologists have
been suggesting for several years now, meanings also conceal forms of domination, and biomedical categories conceal forms of mystification (Singer,
1990; Taussig, 1980; Frankenberg, 1988). But does this invalidate hermeneutic analysis in the study of illness and its expressions?

Of course, any form of human experience can be reduced to language only with great difficulty. In the same way that Freud suspected that it was impossible totally to subsume the force of desire in language, illness and suffering cannot entirely be reduced to a set of meanings, among other reasons because they transcend them and may even be prior to them. Thus, to a hermeneutics of illness we can add a phenomenology of suffering and a politics of affliction. We can even include an "energetics" of the production and synthesis of meanings, and of the different forces (social, instinctive, political) that combine to make a symptom what it is: a semiosic expression that condenses a world. However, despite the fact that the intellectual fashions of medical anthropology are at present striking off in different directions (embodiment paradigm, postmodernism, neo-Marxism) we should not forget that an ethnography of symptoms and affliction should above all be hermeneutic or, using different terminology, it should interpret complaints in terms of a code which is not the receiver's but the sender's, even if this code is implicit, deep-lying, or unconscious. This task is clearly an interpretive one, although later it may provide access to a world of oppression, social inequalities, torture and social misery. In fact, without a true hermeneutics we run the risk of silencing the voice of the sufferer, so often ignored, and therefore of introducing a new and subtle form of domination.

The dynamics of Arthur Kleinman's work are very similar to those of Good's. Kleinman is one of the few to acquire the status of a classic author in medical anthropology, probably because he is one of the scholars who has contributed most to the intellectual conditions for the development of this field. Despite the diversity of his writings, I believe that we can do him justice if we start by looking at what he likes to define, not without a certain irony, as one of his main "errors": the concept of "explanatory models" (EMs), which is one of the contributions of *Patients and Healers in the Context of Culture* (1980). This "error" has been extremely useful not only for research in medical anthropology, but also in its application to the analysis of clinical communication. But let us begin at the beginning: what exactly are EMs? Kleinman says:

> Explanatory models are the notions about an episode of sickness and its treatment that are employed by all those engaged in the clinical process. The interaction between the EMs of patients and practitioners is the central component of health care. The study of practitioner EMs tells us something about how practitioners understand and treat sickness. The study of patient and family EMs tells us how they make sense of given episodes of illness, and how they

choose and evaluate particular treatments. The study of the interaction between practitioner EMs and patient EMs offers a more precise analysis of
problems in clinical communication (1980, p. 105).

It is evident that not only the notions of patients and their families, but
also those of specialists, are included in this definition. The cultural domain
of lay people and folk knowledge is given equal standing with that of a
group of practitioners which includes biomedical and psychiatric professionals. However, the EMs of professionals, patients and their relatives are
not isolated notions; they form part of what Kleinman calls a health care
system (HCS), which can contain not only a body of medical concepts but
also multiple systems of knowledge. The example he uses is that of the Chinese health care system, in which Western-style practitioners, Chinese-style
doctors, bone setters, fortune-tellers, physiognomists, geomancers and others coexist on the professional level (p. 1.). The exchange and borrowing of
knowledge among different universes of medical practice becomes a reality
at the moment of clinical communication (p. 50), the moment in which the
different EMs interact.

In an attempt to provide clinicians with a useful tool for analyzing the
interaction of the illness concepts of professionals, patients and their families, Kleinman defines five areas which may be involved in EMs: etiology,
time and mode of onset of symptoms, pathophysiology, course of sickness
and treatment (p. 105). These axes of analysis are obviously drawn from the
biomedical model: a reminder that Kleinman is also a psychiatrist. However, on a different level, EMs are also instruments which provide knowledge about the emic dimension of patient's illness concepts. This interest is
clearly distinct from the purposes of biomedicine, implying as it does the
possibility of an ethnography of symptoms.

But the contribution of *Patients and Healers* is not restricted merely to
introducing the new concept of explanatory models. Its significance is much
greater: it is a foundation work in medical anthropology. In my view, the two
most important contributions of *Patients and Healers* are the turning of the
ethnographic gaze to biomedical terrain and the consolidation of an interpretive analysis of suffering and affliction. Although the latter contribution
is more relevant to my purposes here, the former also deserves comment.

Most scholars would probably agree that anthropology has traditionally
not considered biomedicine or Western science to be ethnographic territory.
It is certainly true that authors such as Caudill or Goffman devoted themselves to the ethnographic study of Western psychiatric institutions, and that
Erasmus (1952), among others, analyzed the similarities and differences

between Western scientific logic and indigenous ethnomedical logics. The traditional approach, however, was based on tacit acceptance of the distinction between folk beliefs and scientific knowledge. On the one hand, there was the universe of appropriate ethnographic objects: traditional and folk medical systems, folk illnesses, etc. On the other, there was the world of scientific rationality and the ethnographically forbidden territory of biomedicine. Kleinman's primary contribution was helping to dismantle this distinction, taking inspiration from another hermeneutically-oriented anthropologist whose work is of an order of importance comparable to Turner's: Clifford Geertz. In particular, Geertz' notion of "cultural systems" opened up possibilities for the study of medical systems very similar to those created by the notion of "dominant symbols" in the analysis of illness.

Building on Geertz's studies of religion and art as cultural systems, Kleinman regards biomedicine as a cultural system that is both a model *of* and a model *for* reality. In other words, it is a system of double aspect, simultaneously endowing illness with meaning, and shaping the illness to itself through its diagnostic and therapeutic practices. However, neither the categories and meanings (the "model of" aspect) nor the various forms of medical intervention based on the codification of this already-named reality (the "model for" aspect) make biomedicine superior either to other medical systems or to the conceptions of patients. The "cultural system" model of biomedicine is grounded in a sort of conceptual symmetry or epistemological relativism which shapes a new territory of what can be approached ethnographically by demystifying biomedical knowledge. The way in which Kleinman uses the concepts of disease and illness reaffirms this symmetrical structure. He departs from the contrast between "illness" as a reference to the patient's point of view and to folk medical knowledge as opposed to "disease" understood as a biological event or process, developing a notion of "disease" as simply one more explanatory model among many others. In his words, "disease and illness are explanatory concepts, not entities" (1980, p. 73). This idea implies placing Western disease categories (tuberculosis, cancer, depression) alongside *susto, amok, koro* and *wiitiko*, and therefore making them ethnographically accessible.

The second great contribution of *Patients and Healers* is, from my point of view, the consolidation of what has come to be known as the meaning-centered approach. This approach involves the recognition and analysis of the native's point of view within the symmetrical structure of notions about and conceptions of health and sickness discussed above. Accordingly, Kleinman asks his patient-informants questions such as: What do you call your problem? What do you think has caused your problem? How does it work? etc. That is to say, he *listens* to the illness narratives and then, like Good, interprets them in accordance with a meaningful context, one dimension of which is cultural in the broad sense, and the other of which is the medical system, which is cultural in a specific sense. But the matter does not end here.

Kleinman identifies a process of cultural construction and modeling which enables the recognition of some states as illness and others as normality. In fact, it is even possible for there to be disease without illness:

> For instance, an individual, for entirely personal or sociocultural reasons, may evaluate early symptoms as not worth worrying about, minimal, natural or not part of sickness but representing some other state, or he may deny their potential significance (1980, p. 75).

Conversely, there may also be situations of illness without disease. As a result, symptoms may "represent the insidious onset of a number of discrete diseases or might be associated with no disease at all" (1980, p. 76).

Independently, however, of whether or not symptoms refer to a biological disorder, or whether they can be recognized as such by a biomedical practitioner, expressions of affliction contain a whole domain that escapes purely biological definition to form part of a local world of meaning. Kleinman's approach, like Good's, allows us to understand symptoms and complaints as messages, and gives us access to the meanings they have for their senders and not only for the health professionals who receive them. However—again, like Good—Kleinman does not always make it clear exactly what a symptom is.

For example, if we analyze the first of the above quotations, we read that an individual "may evaluate early symptoms." Here, "symptoms" probably refers to signs and sensations which are perceived by the sufferer and may or may not be a cause for concern. I say probably because it is always possible that sufferers will evaluate not physical signs, but their own complaints and expressions of distress in a self-reflexive fashion. The simplest way of interpreting this quotation is that Kleinman is referring to signs and sensations which are not constructions of the patient, but parts of an illness or the illness itself, although in many cases these are accessible only to the patient. At this point, however, we should recall that according to medical definitions a symptom is "a specific manifestation of a patient;" or, in the words of Julian Leff "what patients tell you about their abnormal experiences" (1988, p. 3); or, to return to Byron Good, "the expressions of the experience of distress communicated as an ordered set of complaints" (1994, p. 8). In other words, symptoms are more the expression than the experience of distress. Kleinman's apparently simple statement that individuals "may evaluate early symptoms" has, then, two possible interpretations: either he is saying that they evaluate their own expressions of distress; or he is relegating symptoms to the status of objects which have an existence independent of and prior to the patient's perception of them. This ambiguity points to a central problem in the analysis of symptoms: that of the relation between experience and its expression. Experience evokes intrasubjective worlds not limited to the meaningful possibilities of symptoms and other forms of expression. When Kleinman says that individuals "may evaluate early symptoms," he is, in effect, introducing this experiential dimension, without saying so explicitly. But why does he call these sensations "symptoms" instead of "illness"? Why does he not recognize that a symptom is a semiotic expression and not the experience of illness or a natural part of it? Or is Kleinman perhaps making an excessively psychiatric use of the concept of symptom?

Clearly, in *Patients and Healers* Kleinman uses the term "symptom" in its psychiatric sense, not in its ethnographic sense. As in the pre-interpretive anthropological literature examined in Chapter 7, a symptom is not an expression of distress, but a state or a malaise such as depression, anxiety, sleep disturbances, etc.; or part of a sickness whose objective reality precedes any interpretation by the sufferer. My purpose in criticizing this approach is not to call attention to its limitations—indeed, *Patients and Healers* opened so many new doors that we could hardly ask it to open any more—but simply to situate it as representative of the earliest period of the meaning-centered approach. Good's reluctance to characterize Iranian "heart distress" as a symptom in "The Heart of What's the Matter" is of the same nature as Kleinman's conceptualization of symptoms in *Patients and Healers*: in both cases, symptoms are limited to physical signs and sensations. In subsequent works, however, Kleinman modified his approach in a way that distanced him from psychiatry and brought him more fully within the anthropological orbit. Curiously, it was *The Illness Narratives*, written primarily for an audience of health professionals, that signaled this change.

In this book Kleinman is clearly repositioning himself within the framework of interpretive anthropology. He tells us, for example, that "Symptoms, too, can carry cultural significance" (1988a, p. 23), from which it is understood that symptoms, insofar as they are or can be bearers of meaning, acquire the cultural and linguistic form of the complaint. At this point there is a leap forward. A symptom is no longer a sensation interpreted after the fact by the sufferer, but a message which, like a wink, is meaningful for the sender prior to any interpretation by its recipient.

In this work, he devotes a whole section to the analysis of symptom as meaning in which we can detect an implicit identification between the concepts *symptom* and *illness complaint* or *illness idioms*. Here, symptoms recover their great expressive variability:

> Think of the many ways to complain of headache in North American society: 'My head hurts,' 'My head really hurts,' 'My head is pounding,' 'I'm having a migraine,' 'It's only a tension headache,' "I feel a fullness and heavy feeling in my temples,' 'It feels like a ring of pain is constricting my forehead,' 'My sinuses ache,' 'My scalp is tingling,' 'When I move my head I feel dizzy, as if a veil were passing before my eyes' (1988a, p. 11).

Kleinman observes a performative intention in symptoms which is manifest in rhetorical diversity, not only among different cultures but in a single culture among different social groups and between individuals. A symptom is a communicative artifact which tests the sufferer's skill in mobilizing his social network or in negotiating certain privileges with his interlocutor. In this approach, symptoms are dynamic rather than static. In a continuous feedback process, the receiver(s) interpret(s) the sender, who interprets both himself and the receiver. In this process, the symptom itself is transformed:

> I hear you say your headache is a migraine, or a tension headache owing to too much 'stress' or that it is 'beastly', 'awful', 'pounding', 'throbbing', 'boring,' 'aching,' 'exploding,' 'blinding,' 'depressing,' 'killing,' and I interpret something of that experience and how you feel and want me to feel about it. (You also interpret your own language of complaining and my response to you, which will affect your symptoms) (1988a, p. 15).

Although Kleinman is sometimes ambivalent about whether symptoms are physical sensations or semiosic realities, in *The Illness Narratives* he is clearly treating symptoms as meaningful constructions, not as physical signs. Although the concept of symptom is not central in his writings, his approach to illness is clearly interpretive, aimed at the exegesis of the personal and local meanings of affliction. Though he stops short of developing a theory of symptoms, Kleinman's work in general has contributed to the problematization of symptoms.

The contributions of Kleinman and Good are often cited in medical anthropology, and have been applied in a wide variety of research contexts. For example, Fried (1982) analyzed the EMs of black lung disease among Appalachian coal miners. Parsons and Wakeley (1991) used this construct to study somatic responses to the pressures of everyday life among the Australian middle classes. Ying (1990) investigated the relation between EMs and health-seeking behaviors among Chinese-American women suffering from major depression. Pugh (1991) found heuristic value in the concept of semantic networks for the interpretation of meanings associated with pain in Indian culture. Blumhagen's work (1982) on hypertension combines the contributions of Kleinman and Good, using one concept (explanatory models) to extract information and the other (semantic networks) to systematize it graphically.

But explanatory models and semantic networks are not the only concepts which the meaning-centered approach has contributed to medical anthropology. Analytic notions such as *idioms of distress* (Nichter, 1982), *idioms of misfortune* or *illness narratives* have enriched not only interpretive approaches, but applied work as well. However, possible applications aside, the interpretive approaches have also had a decisive impact on the theoretical development of medical anthropology and the critique of the biomedical and neo-Kraepelinian model, shaping the epistemological shift that brought into clear focus the meaningful dimension of symptoms, making the voice of the sufferer, so sensitively depicted by Matsuoka, ethnographically accessible.

With the passage of time, the meaning-centered approach has undergone several transformations. For example, Kleinman's later writings (1992, 1995, 1997) evidence an enviable reflexivity concerning the shortcomings of a hermeneutic vision of illness and its expressions. Kleinman's most recent work, like Good's, introduces two concepts—"power" and "experience"— which combine with "meaning" to yield a broad vision of sickness and suffering. Since the next section of this chapter is devoted to the concept of power, I will end this section with a discussion of "experience."

In some of his recent articles, Arthur Kleinman, sometimes writing with Joan Kleinman, has developed a phenomenological analysis in which the notion of experience or, alternatively, "interpersonal experience," is used as a more all-encompassing notion than "meaning" (1991, 1995). The ideas of suffering, resistance and delegitimation have also emerged in several of his publications (1992, 1995, 1997). As one of its most active creators, Kleinman has come to represent a theoretical trend in medical anthropology grounded in an interpretive approach to illness but moving toward a phenomenology of suffering and a critical theory of forms of affliction. In the corresponding conceptual transformation, analytic notions such as meaning, illness narratives, idioms of distress, semantic networks, etc., give way to others: embodiment, experience, suffering, body politics, social body, mindful body, resistance and many others. In fact, in recent years medical anthropologists have hurriedly been abandoning the ship of hermeneutics in favor of the more promising phenomenological paradigm. Only a few short years ago, Csordas (1994) was able to say that "in anthropology, phenomenology is a poor and underdeveloped cousin of semiotics" (p. 11), but now this poor cousin is growing steadily in importance. We need only glance at international literature to become aware, for example, of the tremendous impact of the embodiment paradigm (Csordas, 1990, 1993, 1994; Pandolfi, 1990, 1991; Scheper-Hughes & Lock, 1987; Ots, 1994; Desjarlais, 1992). I have no doubt that this approach has a great deal to say about experiences of suffering, but even so, I believe that it may be both incomplete and methodologically clumsy if totally dissociated from hermeneutics.[5] As Ricoeur points out, while hermeneutics almost always implies phenomenology, understood in a non-psychological sense, phenomenology always presupposes hermeneutics (1974, p. 223). I raise this matter not simply to reproduce some of the arguments which, as Csordas notes, have been recurrent themes in the debates between semiotics and phenomenology; for example, the question of what we can know of the experience (i.e. illness, suffering) of others without access to their expressions of distress (i.e. symptoms, complaints, laments) (1994, p. 11). Rather, what I wish to emphasize here is that the phenomenological approach in anthropology must be conscious of its intellectual debt to hermeneutics. This is important not only because these forms of expression are the means of access to the forms of suffering that are the stuff of ethnographic analysis, but also because of another principle of equal importance: the potential of hermeneutics for avoiding ethnocentrism and misreadings. The hermeneutic method seeks the code for interpreting illness not in technical and philosophical jargon, but in the speech of the sufferers themselves, and thus acts as a corrective to the universalizing tendencies of certain varieties of phenomenology (i.e., the existentialism of Sartre and Merleau-Ponty, or Husserl's phenomenology). This role is possible because, as Gadamer (1975, p. 217) points out, hermeneutics is located "between" (*Zwischen*) the feeling of strangeness (*Fremdheit*) or alienation (*Verfremdung*) from one's own tradition and the feeling of belonging (*Vertrautheit*) or closeness (*Zugehörenheit*) to it. This position does not totally free anthropologists from their own prejudices, but it is, nevertheless, the best path of access to other worlds of experience.

POLITICS

In the early 1980s, the growth of interpretive approaches stimulated a series of responses and controversies in medical anthropology, with the result that the field became theoretically richer. For instance, during this period Young (1981, 1982) was an outspoken critic of the individualism, medicalism and instrumentalism which, in his opinion, were the ultimate products of the explanatory models construct. Although Kleinman had originally developed this construct as part of a broader analysis of the organization of medical systems, it quickly became a convenient tool for managing the microsocial dimension of interaction between medical professionals and patients.

For Young, the larger social context of illness was just as important as illness narratives, symptoms, illness concepts or the problems of clinical communication. Medical anthropology, he argued, should not only be an analysis of how a disease enters into the consciousness of the individual (which he defines as an anthropology of illness), but also of what he calls "sickness," or "the process for socializing disease and illness" (1982, p. 270). This process involves social, economic, political, ideological and other forces which anthropological analysis disregards at its peril. Thus, medical anthropology becomes an anthropology of sickness, a study of the social relations and conditions that produce both disease and illness, and includes the analysis of what Young calls "the social conditions of knowledge production" (1982, p. 277). His own work on the social determinants of scientific knowledge among "stress researchers" (1980) and his analysis of how ideology shapes clinical knowledge in the case of post-traumatic stress disorder (1993, 1995) furnishes some lucid and penetrating examples of this type of research.

Here, however, I wish to focus on his critique of the explanatory model approach, which contains some surprising elements. For example, Young tells us that the EM approach greatly resembles biomedicine in its individualism; concretely, he says that "both views take the individual as their object and the arena of significant events." In this respect, Young believes that the EM approach "is not so different from the biomedical model as its advocates seem to believe." This raises some questions. Don't Kleinman's concerns go beyond the individual to the nature of health care systems? Isn't Good's use of the category "*narahatiye qalb*" a way of approaching not an individual expression of distress, but an entire cultural tradition? What I find in Kleinman's and Good's early writings is not so much a pronounced form of individualism as a sort of culturalism reborn in an interpretive paradigm more interested in meanings than in the psychology of the informants. In his haste to discredit the EM approach, I believe that Young has forgotten the fundamental epistemological difference between:

1. a biomedical approach based on the position of the practitioner as a "knowing subject" for whom the knowledge and expressive code of the patient is irrelevant; and

2. an interpretive ethnographic approach in which the investigator is the one who lacks knowledge because the code for understanding an illness narrative is located in the sufferer and not in a particular technical jargon.

In fact, as Young points out, the first of these approaches denies the social relations which produce sickness and, therefore, desocializes and dehistoricizes it. However, the second approach, correctly applied, involves entering into the universe of meanings and social relations present in the sufferer's narrative. This sort of approach does not individualize the social, but reveals what is social in the individual.

Young's other criticisms of the EM approach, medicalism and pragmatism, also deserve some comment. As far as medicalism is concerned, in Kleinman's and Good's early studies there seems to be a good deal of conceptual borrowing across the frontier between anthropology and biomedicine. This is counterbalanced, however, by a highly explicit critique of the empiricism, universalism and biologicism of biomedicine. I see this less as medicalism than as a double objective on the part of the defenders of the meaning-centered approach: (1) finding clinical applications for ethnographic knowledge and (2) expanding the terrain available for ethnographic research and extending anthropology's range of influence by critiquing the shortcomings of the biomedical model.

Young is closer to the truth in his critique of instrumentalism, since it is undeniable that in the United States the analysis of explanatory models has developed into a minor industry which has come to be known as "clinically applied anthropology." Though clearly influenced by Kleinman's and Good's ideas, this branch of applied anthropology seems to me to be more eclectic than hermeneutic, since it makes use not only of the concept of EMs, but also of social network analysis, cultural domain analysis, the technique of focus groups, and the concept of "sick role," depending on the specifics of any particular applied project (see Chrisman & Johnson, 1990; Chrisman & Maretzki, 1982; Trotter, 1991). This eclecticism marks a difference between clinically applied anthropology and the meaning-centered approach, although the so-called critical medical anthropologists have tended to identify the one with the other.

Critical medical anthropology, which draws inspiration from various Marxist and neo-Marxist trends, is characterized by the inclusion of political-economic variables in the terrain of sickness and healing (Baer, Singer & Johnsen, 1986; Singer, 1990). This has been a salutary development in

North American medical anthropology, calling our attention, for example, to the effect of social and economic inequalities on morbidity and mortality rates, and the way in which biomedicine re-presents poverty and misery as tuberculosis, cholera, dysentery, and other diseases. Nevertheless, at times the political agenda of critical medical anthropologists has led them to paint distorted portraits of other approaches, identifying hermeneutics with the subordinate role of anthropology in relation to biomedicine, or reading uncritical pragmatism into cultural interpretation.

Of course, not all critical medical anthropologists are guilty of such excesses. Critical medical anthropology is not a monolith, but a variety of different approaches which can be grouped into at least two larger and well-differentiated trends. The first of these, which I will call "hard materialism," is devoted to investigating the role of economic and political forces in the functioning of medical institutions and the unequal distribution of sickness (Waitzkin, 1981; Morsy, 1981; Singer, 1986; Morgan, 1990). Using dependency theory, this approach develops a critique of the badly-concealed association between the global distribution of wealth and the global distribution of sickness, and is characterized by the use of macro-sociological data and economic variables. Ideology is thus subordinated to the social relations of production, and therefore the meaning-centered approach is deprived of explanatory power, relegated to an epiphenomenal area of study. Consequently, neither symptoms nor illness narratives can be important objects of investigation, since the priorities clearly lie elsewhere.

The second of these large-scale trends, "soft materialism," seems at first glance to be similar to the "hard" variety, but in fact is theoretically and methodologically distinct. It also makes use of political-economic variables and neo-Marxist theories, but priority is given to a type of critical analysis which opens the door to an exegesis of illness representations. Because the sources of inspiration are different—the more "idealist" Marxisms of Lukács or Gramsci, and Foucault's critical archeologies of knowledge—ideology or superstructure is not viewed as merely epiphenomenal (Taussig, 1980; Scheper-Hughes & Lock, 1987; Frankenberg, 1988; Lock & Scheper-Hughes, 1990). An interesting example of this approach is Lock's research in Canada on the complaints associated with the category *nevra* among immigrant Greek women employed in the garment industry. Lock's analysis is not exclusively materialist, but one in which symptoms, laments and narratives, on the one hand, combine with social, political and gender inequalities on the other (Lock, 1990).

I have led the reader through this account in order to point out that strangely, despite much heated discussion, the emergence of all these approaches in medical anthropology has not given rise to a debate on the the the role of symptoms in anthropological theory. One of the reasons for this theoretical vacuum is that the discussion has centered not so much on symptoms as on how sickness should be approached, and the role of medical anthropology in relation to biomedicine. There are, however, some important exceptions to this. Here I will focus on two of these: the debate between Michael Taussig on the one hand, and Eisenberg and Kleinman on the other; and the polemical contributions of Nancy Scheper-Hughes. I will begin with Taussig.

In an article published in 1980, Michael Taussig applies Marxist theory to the problem of sickness and symptoms in a most opportune and heterodox fashion. Following Lukács' work (1969) on the problem of reification and the consciousness of the proletariat, he discusses reification and the consciousness of a 49-year-old working-class patient/informant with a diagnosis of polymyositis (a muscular disease). His intentions clearly go far beyond the ethnographic specifics of the case when he argues that the signs and symptoms of a disease such as his informant's signify something more than biological dysfunctions:

> I am going to argue that things such as the signs and symptoms of disease, as much as the technology of healing, are not 'things in themselves,' are not only biological and physical, but are also signs of social relations disguised as natural things, concealing their roots in human reciprocity (1980, p. 3).

Taussig perceives symptoms and signs as meaningful realities which condense critically sensitive and contradictory components of culture and social relations. "The manifestations of disease are like symbols," he writes, pointing out that health practitioners make diagnoses with "an eye trained by the social determinants of perception" (p. 5). However, biomedicine and its practitioners reject this view in favor of an orientation which allows the illness experience to be dehistoricized and desocialized; that is to say, it is reified with the aim of reproducing a particular social order: the capitalist system.

To support his argument, Taussig uses Luckács' clever argument that the Western notion of "objectivity" was in fact an illusion created by capitalist relations of production; instead of piercing this illusion, Marxist authors such as Lenin and Engels accepted it uncritically, and perpetuated it in their writings (p. 3). In its refusal to recognize the social component in the signs and symptoms of illness, Taussig argues, biomedicine reifies human relations, which in turn gives rise to what Luckács defined as a "phantom-objectivity," a mystification through which capitalist political ideology is reproduced in the name of a supposed objectivity, of a "science of real things" (p. 3).

Seductive though it is, however, Taussig's analysis passes lightly over such centrally important concepts as reification and symptoms. Young raises the question of whether Taussig is referring to a type of reification distinct from the objectification that is an inescapable feature of any form of symbolization, or whether he was thinking in narrower, more specific terms (Young 1982, p. 276). Taussig does not, in fact, clarify the sense in which he understands reification, probably because Lukács himself was not very explicit on this point either. Since Lukács later recognized this ambiguity as a problem in his own work (see Arato, 1972), it is not difficult to understand Taussig's conceptual imprecision.

The conceptual problems in Taussig's work do not, however, end here. Taussig passes up the opportunity to address two issues of great theoretical import. First, in failing to distinguish between signs and symptoms, he misses the chance to demonstrate precisely how biomedicine converts symptoms into natural signs with the aim of obscuring the social relations of sickness. The second issue is one raised by Marx in Volume I of *Capital* : capitalist relations of production not only lead to the reification of people but also, no less importantly, the personification of things (Marx, 1976, p. 1054). This idea is also present in Lukács' theory: the mutual reification of both subject and object leads to the objectivization of the subject and the subjectivization (that is to say, personification) of the object (Lukács, 1969, p. 111). However, this dialectic is absent from Taussig's work. Although he is deeply aware of the reification of patients and human relations, the personification of things—rooms, spaces, services, machines, reports, instruments and, of course, diseases—seems to escape his notice. For instance, when one physician remarks to another, "Today I have treated three cirrhoses and two malignancies," disease and its manifestations are the primary object of this dual dialectic. First, the disease is reified—dehistoricized, desocialized and disengaged from the sufferer by the mind/body dualism that reifies and objectifies the patient as well. Second, the disease (though not the patient) is personified as a new character endowed with subjective identity in the symbolic and imaginary universe of biomedical rationality. Taussig, however, applies only the first part of the analysis, not the entire dialectic.

According to Taussig, all sick people ask themselves, "Why me?" "Why now?"— existential questions which can be addressed by philosophers but not by physicians (1980, p. 4; see also Young, 1982, p. 275). Biomedicine can explain the "how," but not the "why." In Taussig's words:

> It can point to chains of physical cause and effect, but as to why I am struck
> down now rather than at some other time, or as to why it is me rather than
> someone else, medical science can only respond with some variety of prob-
> ability theory which is unsatisfactory to the mind searching for certainty and
> for significance (1980, p. 4).

Unlike other medical systems such as that of the Azande, which fuses the
how and the why, biomedicine separates the facts (how) from the values
(why), and therefore disengages diseases and their manifestations from the
social nexus which gives them life. Thus, the manifestations of disease are
regarded as things in themselves, separate from history and society. Whereas
sickness and suffering inevitably challenge the complacent and daily acceptance of conventional structures of meaning (the why), biomedicine obscures
this critical awareness through a science and epistemology of "real things"
(the how) that holds out the promise of a stable world. In this way, clinical
practice becomes a mechanism of political and social control, offering security in exchange for obedience, "certainty" in exchange for acceptance by
both patients and practitioners of "common sense," or what Taussig calls the
conventional structures of meaning (p. 13).

Given this highly critical perspective, it is hardly surprising that Taussig
regards as almost heretical the early project of Kleinman, Good and Eisenberg
(1978) for humanizing medical care by using knowledge of the "native's
point of view." In Taussig's view, any such application of anthropological
knowledge can only enhance biomedicine's ability to manipulate the patient. In Taussig's words:

> In this regard, it is a scandal and also self-defeating to appeal to Anthropology
> for evidence as to the power of concepts like the 'patient's model' and the
> difference between the 'how' and the 'why' of 'disease' and 'illness.' For the
> medical anthropology of so-called 'primitive' societies also teaches us that
> medicine is preminently an instrument of social control (1980, p. 13).

Given the harsh and caustic tone of Taussig's critique, the response was
not long in coming. Only a year later, in an article entitled "Clinical Social
Science," Eisenberg and Kleinman (1981) argue that the excessively abstract nature of Taussig's analysis has caused him to lose contact with reality, and that:

> In its obsession with power relationships, it entirely ignores the central fact
> that the patient comes to the doctor in search of relief from distress, a relief
> which can only be obtained if effective medical measures are available and if
> the patient agrees to apply them (p. 18).

An extended analysis of the critical/clinical debate in medical anthropology is beyond the scope of this chapter. I bring up this particular episode, however, in order to point out that Taussig's argument, taken to its logical extreme, ends in paradoxical situations of the kind described by Johnson (1995), who, in a flash of irony and humor, imagined a physician telling his patients, "I cannot treat you because I will be reproducing social inequities!" or a patient arguing, "Forget the pain, Doc...let's talk about the sociopolitical impact of my illness" (p. 109). Humor aside, Johnson's point is not that Taussig's analysis is worthless, but that it should be more nuanced. Our ability to discern in biomedicine the dehistoricization of disease or a sophisticated form of social and political control should not necessarily lead us to renounce all forms of medical practice. Some of the representatives of nineteenth-century German social medicine were already well aware of this. For instance, in his famous "politico-ethnographic" report of 1847, Virchow proposed treating a typhus epidemic in Upper Silesia with "radical social reform," "full and unlimited democracy," "education," "liberty," and "welfare" (Rosen, 1947). As a social analyst, Virchow was conscious of the social relations that produced typhus, but as a doctor he did not hesitate to prescribe a treatment, however unconventional.

An approach similar to Virchow's can be found in some anthropological traditions which have approached professional practice and critical awareness as two inseparable, not opposite, realities. This is the case of the Latin-American tradition of "investigation-intervention-participation," or the Gramscian approach of the *Centro Sperimentale di Educazione Sanitaria* in Perugia (Italy), directed by Tullio Seppilli in collaboration with other anthropologists such as Bartoli and Romizzi. The strategy of these two approaches is not to assume an advisory role, proposing minor adjustments to the biomedical model with the aim of consolidating its hegemony, but to help biomedicine recognize its own dominant position with respect to forms of popular knowledge and make it possible for social actors themselves to have a role in the transformation and development of medical doctrines. This is a possibility that Taussig's trained eye prevents him from seeing.

Taussig's work is not, however, the only contribution that critical theory has made to the study of that occult ethnographic object in medical anthropology, the symptom. Among the works that shed some light on this problem, although in a more tangential fashion than Taussig, is Nancy Scheper-Hughes' magnum opus, *Death Without Weeping* (1992). She dedicates the whole of Chapter 5, entitled "Nervoso: Medicine, Sickness and Human Needs," to an analysis of the processes through which hunger in the *favelas* of northeastern Brazil is masked and medicalized. Here the task of ethnography is clearly one of developing a critical consciousness of biomedical mystification.

Bringing all of her considerable literary skill to bear on this issue, Scheper-Hughes suggests that there is a clear juxtaposition in the emic universe of her informants between *fome* (hunger) and *nervos* (nervousness) (1992, p. 167). At one point she writes:

> If food and sex are idioms through which the people of the Alto reflect on their social condition as *os pobres*, nerves and nervousness provide an idiom through which they reflect on their hunger and hunger anxiety (p. 169).

However, this association is denied daily by the agents of the state, the biomedical practitioners and intellectuals who reproduce hegemonic culture and common sense by converting hunger into a biomedical disease. On this point, Scheper-Hughes says:

> *Nervos*, a rich folk conceptual scheme for describing relations among mind, body and social body is appropriated by medicine and transformed into something other: a biomedical disease that alienates mind from body and that conceals the social relations of sickness (p. 169).

This argument seems clearly inspired by Taussig's, as well as by the work of Gramsci and other Marxist theorists, to which there are explicit references throughout the book. In fact, it is this position between the critical and interpretive approaches so characteristic of Gramsci which enables her to interpret *nervos* which are both symptom and folk category simultaneously.

Scheper-Hughes asks her informants: "What are your symptoms?"; "Is there a cure for overworked nerves?"; "Are *nervos* and *fome* the same thing?"; "Why are you treating your nerves and not your hunger?"; and "Which is worse—hunger or *nervos*?" And she finds that *nervos* is a polysemic expression which condenses tiredness, weakness, irritability, headaches, anger and resentments, grief, parasitic infections and, not the least, hunger. Scheper-Hughes does not, in fact, equate *nervos* exclusively with hunger, but she does believe that hunger is one of its essential meanings. Oddly, however, her own informants do not agree, arguing that *"Nervos* is one thing and *fome* is another" (p.177). But she does not let this stop her.

At one point in her account, Scheper-Hughes describes her interview with Seu Tomás, an informant suffering from *nervos* who says that he has "weakness in his lungs," "tiredness," "coldness in his head," "pain in his stomach," and "paralysis in his legs." As a result of his illness, he has been unable to work in the canefields for two years, and takes several different medications: antibiotics, painkillers, worm medications, sleeping pills, vitamins and antidepressants (p. 183). In response to the ethnographer's awkward questions (Why doesn't he treat his hunger instead of his nerves?) the informant seems to deny any association between *fome* and *nervos*. However, Scheper-Hughes' certainty that the idiom of *nervos* is also an idiom of hunger is such that she even goes so far as to feel her informant's thin legs in order to conclude that the "paralysis" is partly physical (the weakness of hunger) and partly metaphoric or symbolic. In this metaphor Scheper-Hughes finds two contradictory meanings. On the one hand, the informant's paralysis expresses "lying down, sinking, yielding, succumbing, giving up," which also applies to his position in a semi-feudal economy where the nervous-weak body of the cane cutter is the metaphor and metonym of the "weak position of the rural worker in the current economic order" (p. 186). In the case of Seu Tomás, she argues, "the language of the body is the language of defeat" (p. 183). On the other hand, however, she finds that paralysis and *nervos* seem to be something more than just surrender and defeat, and represent a "drama of mockery and refusal" (p. 186). That is to say, the refusal to stand up is also an act of political resistance, which she likens to the behavior of another of her informants, Black Elena, who, following the murder of her husband and eldest son by the death squads, "sits outside her hut near the top of the Cruzeiro, dressed in white, and she shakes and trembles and raises her clenched fists in a paroxysm of anger nerves" (p. 187). These two cases, among many others, enable her "to recuperate and politicize the uses of the body and the secret language of the organs that play such a large part in the lives of many anthropological subjects" (p. 185).

Scheper-Hughes' interpretation has great appeal, since by describing Seu Tomás' paralysis is partly physical and partly metaphoric or symbolic, she is pointing to the existence of two poles of meaning in the symptom: one which is physical, sensory and literal, and another which is ideological and symbolic. However, the intelligence of this approach is overshadowed by an unfortunate tendency to overinterpretation. The meaning that Seu Tomás attributes to his own symptoms is discarded in favor of the ethnographer's theory-driven interpretation. Is there really defeat and surrender in the paralyzed legs of Seu Tomás, or is the ethnographer simply reading into them the moral coordinates of her own world, where there are winners and losers, mice and men? We know what is most important: *fome* exists, an intolerable *fome* that pricks our conscience, but as a reader I am uncomfortable when anthropologists allow their own concerns to overwhelm those of their informants. This critique detracts nothing, however, from the powerful human appeal of this sad ethnography, and I introduce it here not gratuitously, but as a starting point for developing a re-synthesis of political and hermeneutic approaches.

TOWARD A CRITICAL HERMENEUTICS

In this chapter I have argued that there are two ways in which anthropologists have viewed symptoms. The first approach analyzes symptoms as linguistic facts dependent on a local world of meaning and experience. The second stresses the social and political-economic conditions that may underlie a complaint, as well as the strategic power concealed in the biomedical reification of illness. However, the key concepts that identify these approaches —"meaning" and "power," respectively—complement rather than oppose each other. Both Taussig and Scheper-Hughes see symptoms as linguistic in nature, but they suggest that "something else" conditions this language: the system of social relations within which the symptom is produced. Good himself recognizes that the process of synthesis or condensation of semantic networks in symbolic forms is not exclusively linguistic, but also social and political. A symptom, then, is enormously complex, more than just a symbolic construct whose primary biological referent is joined to secondary and tertiary cultural meanings; the very process that brings it into being is also political and economic in nature. Symptoms condense realities of various types which are activated at the moment of their expression, bridging nature and culture via highly emotive language. As an expression of distress, "Oh, my God!" fuses together language, emotion, existential uncertainty and religious belief in a mere three words.

But if symptoms go beyond the level of language in the strict sense to evoke a whole world, the key to this world is inescapably linguistic. It is precisely for this reason that the hermeneutic method is necessary for an anthropology of symptoms, and for this reason also that Nancy Scheper-Hughes' excessively theory-driven interpretation is objectionable, because it risks ethnocentrism and flies in the face of the anthropological commitment to understanding the native's point of view, a cornerstone of ethnographic practice at least since Boas and Malinowski. Curiously, this interpretive style is significantly out of keeping with Scheper-Hughes' own proposal, together with Margaret Lock, for a critical-interpretive paradigm in medical anthropology (1990), a much more balanced approach that avoids both extremes: a strict culturalism that leaves out any consideration of forms of power and domination; and a heavily politicized approach in which supposedly fundamental realities crowd out the meanings sufferers attach to their own distress.

In other words, a true interpretive critique, a critical hermeneutics of symptoms and affliction, cannot afford to disregard either local worlds of meaning or the social inequalities and forms of political oppression that are foremost among the factors conditioning the synthesis and condensation of meanings. An accounting of the power relations underlying all forms of language should not annul the meaning of expressions of distress and illness narratives. In an anthropology of symptoms, the role of politics should be to develop reflexively critical theory, which should in turn use hermeneutics to ensure that the voice of the patient, all too often ignored, is not silenced again in a new and subtle form of domination. It is here that politics and hermeneutics endow each other with significance. The former contributes its radicalizing potential and the humanity of its critical conscience. The latter, in contrast, takes a more distant and relativizing tone that mitigates the tendency toward ethnographic hubris. However, hermeneutics has one modest advantage which anthropology should never lose sight of: understanding other worlds of experience without misreading them.

NOTES

1. See De Martino (1983 [1959]), who developed an extraordinary synthesis of Gramsci's theories and the anthropological approach in the late 1950s. See also the more recent writings of Tullio Seppilli in Italy (1983, 1989) and Eduardo Menéndez in Mexico (1981), both of whom are clearly influenced by Gramscian thought.
2. See Lévi-Strauss (1964) for an application of the structuralist method to the terrain of myths.
3. Although in *Le Totémisme aujourd'hui* (1962a) and *La pensée sauvage* (1962b) Lévi-Strauss skillfully associates the categories of syntagmatic level, parole and event on the one hand, and the paradigmatic level, langue and structure on the other, I believe that this conceptual relationship is more than debatable because it means that the order of contiguity and combination (syntagmatic level) of language is not prior to speech, but is formed during "parlage"—the act of speaking—itself. However, the possibility of expressing language in significant and significative sequences (the syntagmatic order) is prior to the event in the same

way that the paradigmatic level is. We could even say that it is the potential time of the structure just as the paradigmatic order is the "incorporeal" space of language.

4. Someday the seamless universalism of Lévi-Strauss, his genius notwithstanding, should be studied in the light of French centralism and jacobinism. His attempt to reduce cultural diversity to an invariable and universal logic is reminiscent of the ideal that all French schoolchildren should be taught the same subjects at the same time in all the villages, towns and cities throughout France.

5. In fact, the contributions to a recent collection of essays representative of the embodiment paradigm—*Embodiment and experience*, edited by Csordas (1994)—are mostly combinations of hermeneutics and phenomenology. In several cases, hermeneutics is the fundamental analytic approach; where it is not, it remains the means of access to lived experience.

CHAPTER 9

Semiotic Incursions

If we are to believe Gilles Thérien (1985), Peirce was not only one of the founders of modern semiotics, but also a shrewd clinician who, by analyzing his own signs and symptoms, was able to make a diagnosis with little chance of error.[1] Although Thérien warns us against drawing from this example the inference that medicine may be replaced by semiology, the anecdote retains a certain evocative power: at the moment in which Peirce made his self-diagnosis, a medical semiology which can be traced back to the Hippocratic tradition was present simultaneously, albeit momentarily, with the new principles of a semiotic theory of signs.

Even though these two disciplines are at present far removed from each other, linguistic and medical semiology seem to have a common origin. Eco (1984, 1996) has shown that the Greek word *semeion* (*signum*, sign) emerged as a technical and philosophical term with Parmenides and Hippocrates, and more than two thousand years later came to constitute the etymological basis of modern semiotics. This discipline has preferred to adopt the name of semiotics and not semiology, as Saussure proposed in his *Cours de linguistique générale* (1974), in order to avoid confusion between the science of linguistic signs and medical semiology.

It may seem at first glance that this terminological distinction has a certain logic. Both for Hippocratic medicine and contemporary Western medicine, signs are indications, natural signals, evidence and symptoms—understood as physical signs—which only seem to find their meaningful nature in logical inference, and they are distinct from what Saussure considers to be signs in social life (language, symbolic rituals, military commands, etiquette), messages which require a human sender (1974,

p. 33). However, on closer inspection, we observe that signs have not always been compartmentalized into intentional signs for semiotics and natural signs for medical semiology. And there are reasons for this. Not all authors seem to agree with limiting the field of semiotics to intentional signs originating in a human source. We need look no further than another great precursor, Peirce, whose work contrasts with that of Saussure and whose broad definition of the object of semiotics not only includes signs produced by a human sender, but all those that mean something for a receiver (Collected Papers of Charles Sanders Peirce [CP], 2.228). From this point of view, natural indications, physical signs or natural signals become semiotic realities, even though this may only take place in the cognitive processes of the receiver. In fact, in semiotics Saussure's and Peirce's points of view have existed side by side: the former requires the intentionality of a human sender, while the latter only requires a receiver. Despite significant differences on this point, these two semiotic traditions have always shared similar notions about what a symptom is.

As we shall see below in greater detail, the two traditions have regarded symptoms as physical signs, natural indications, indices or traces whose meaning depends on a human receiver. However, this assumption appears to have undergone a gradual change. In the analysis of symptoms, what we might call the new medical semiotics (distinct from medical semiology) seems to have found one of its most important challenges: the distinction between physical signs and symptoms; between the amorphous sounds made by the internal organs, and the dynamics of complaints and laments (Staiano, 1982; Honkasalo, 1991; Johnson, 1994). Let us take this step by step.

SAUSSURE, BARTHES AND FOUCAULT

Despite the considerable influence of positivism on his work, Ferdinand de Saussure introduces a definition of signs which is considerably at odds with the most classical assumptions of linguistic empiricism. A sign is not the result of joining a name to a thing, he asserted, but of linking a concept (*concept*) to an acoustic image (*image acustique*). After hesitating between terms such as soma and sema, image and concept, form and idea, he settled on two familiar words to name these two aspects of a sign: the signified (*signifié*) and the signifier (*signifiant*). The signified of the word "tree" is not, therefore, the tree as a thing in itself, but the idea to which this sign refers in the context of a particular social code. The signifier, for its part, is not the purely material sound, but "the psychic print of this sound, the representation of it that our senses provide, is sensory"(1974, p. 98) [my translation].

For Saussure the sign emerges from the bonding of signifier and signified, but he also says that the relationship between concept and acoustic image is artificial and arbitrary. In other words, there is nothing in the signifier "tree" which leads us to its signified. Saussure considers this to be one of the keys to the definition of signs as opposed to other meaningful constructions, such as symbols:

> By nature symbols are not always completely arbitrary; they are not empty, there is a rudimentary natural link between the signifier and the signified. The scales, the symbol of justice, could not be replaced by anything, a cart for example (1974, p.101) [my translation].

Obviously, a cart has little to do with justice in our intellectual universe. However, it is not very clear why for Saussure the signifier "scales" does not have an artificial and socially conventional quality similar to the signifier "tree." Is there really such a big difference between the signifier "tree" and the image of a set of scales in terms of the arbitrariness of their relation with the signified? A cross-cultural analysis of the signifier of the concept of justice would almost certainly show us that the signifier "scales" is more arbitrary than Saussure thinks it is, and therefore more of a social convention. My aim here is not to sort out a rather confusing example which Saussure merely sketches. What is of interest in it for my purposes is the principle which enables him to define the relation between signified and signifier in the sign: arbitrariness. This principle is important because it contains the keys for differentiating between what can be considered to be a sign and what cannot. The latter group contains such phenomena as indications, traces or physical signs which emerge as natural signifiers and not as conventional forms in social life.

The narrow definition of the sign (*signe*) also has implications for Saussure's discussion of the scope of semiotics (what he calls "semiology"). Paradoxically, he uses the Greek terminology of *semeion*, a concept which is closer to natural signs than to artificial ones: "So it is possible to conceive of a science which studies the life of signs in social life; it would be part of general psychology; we shall call it semiology (from the Greek séméion, 'sign')" (1974, p. 33) [my translation].

In the simple sentence "the life of signs in social life," writers such as Eco have perceived, again, the Saussurean restriction of semiotics to those signs produced by a human sender. Since the sign is the object of semiology, only artificial signs will be included and natural and unintentional manifestations excluded (Eco, 1968, 1977). From an orthodox Saussurean perspective, then, there is no place in semiotics for the analysis of such physical signs as fever, skin rashes, or abdominal swelling, just as there is no place for natural signs such as the column of smoke that indicates fire or the gathering clouds that precede a storm. There is, however, a place for what we understand as symptoms: the range of laments, expressions, verbalizations, gestures and even somatic complaints that reflect a universe of meanings. Those who expect to find an analysis of this type in Saussure will, nonetheless, be disappointed. His work makes no reference to symptoms (as Peirce's did), partly because his effort is directed toward the more urgent task of defining the new field of semiology, but also for another reason: in all likelihood, Saussure categorizes symptoms as physical signs, and therefore excludes them from the field of semiotics (his "semiology").

Despite the clear boundary which relegates natural signs to an extrasemiotic order, Roland Barthes (1985), a well-known author in the structuralist tradition whose work was strongly influenced by Saussure's, explored the domain of symptoms and physical signs in an attempt to locate parallelisms between medical semiology and general semiology, between "medical signs" and "linguistic signs." I want to examine his work in some detail, because Barthes' distinction between sign and symptom is diametrically opposed to my own.

Barthes confesses that he searched the medical semiology literature in vain for a theory of medical signs, and that given this vacuum, he has no choice other than to put forward "an ingenuous picture" of the similarities between general and medical semiology. It is, perhaps, for this reason that he uses one of the sections of Foucault's *Birth of the Clinic* to reinforce his own arguments.

According to Foucault, the medical tradition of the eighteenth century makes a clear distinction between symptom and sign. The symptom is the form in which disease presents, the closest thing to its essence, that which makes the disease visible. Coughing, fever and pain in the side are not pleurisy itself, but forms that allow us to detect its presence; that is to say, natural and definitive signs of pleurisy. Signs, on the other hand, involve something more than this, as Hippocrates long ago noted with respect to the three temporal dimensions of symptoms. Foucault tells us that signs announce what is going to happen (prognosis), analyze what has happened (anamnesis) and bear witness to what is happening at the present moment (diagnosis) (Foucault, 1972, p. 89-90). Signs, therefore, indicate what lies beneath the surface of things—life, death and time—but they also imply an observer's gaze, unlike symptoms, which are the motionless, timeless, natural expression of the pathological.

In a somewhat cryptic fashion, Foucault demonstrates that the emergence of the clinical method is related to the pre-eminence of a "grammar of signs" over a "botany of symptoms." Here he is probably referring to the emergence of a medical consciousness which permits a reordering of pathological manifestations in which symptoms, as natural signifiers, seem to acquire a new transparency which makes them intelligible and thus transforms them into signs. In other words, Foucault is advancing a conceptualization of symptoms as objective and natural phenomena indicative of illness as a physical state discontinuous with health, while signs are the transformation undergone by this phenomenological reality in the consciousness of the practitioner. Using Landré-Beauvais' 1813 treatise on medical semiology, Foucault writes:

> Signs and symptoms are and say the same; except that the sign *says* exactly what the symptom *is*. In its material reality, the sign identifies itself with the symptom which is the indispensable morphological support of the sign. Thus there is no sign without symptom. However, what makes the sign a sign does not come from the symptom but from elsewhere (1972, p. 92) [emphasis added].

This activity which "comes from elsewhere" is the clinician's perception of pathology, the act of placing a symptom in a meaningful diagnostic set which allows him to examine the temporal dimension of the sickness, while converting the symptoms (which, according to Foucault, are asemiotic) into signs. A page later, Foucault expresses this same idea with greater clarity: *"Le symptôme devient signe sous un regard sensible"* [beneath a gaze that is sensitive...the symptom therefore becomes a sign] (p. 93). Further on, where he outlines the epistemological foundations from which positivist medicine emerged, he writes: "The sign does not speak the natural language of disease; it takes shape and acquires value only within the questions posed by medical investigation" (1972, p.165).

In short, Foucault considers symptoms to be natural realities (coughing, fever, a pain in the side), while signs are the clinical construction of these realities (the association of coughing with pleurisy, for instance). A cough or a fever, in and of itself, has no semiotic (or even semiosic) qualities. As signs of pleurisy, however, they become meaningful in the process of clinical inference; that is to say, in the conceptual and logical structures of anamnesis, diagnosis and prognosis.

Here, the distinction between symptom and sign becomes operative, a tool for analyzing medical knowledge, for as the subtitle of *The Birth of the Clinic* suggests, Foucault's primary purpose here is formulating an archeology of the medical gaze. However, important questions remain. Where in this scheme can we situate symptoms as complaints, "subjective" symptoms, or patients' expressions of distress? What is the place of local meaning and illness narratives?

Without realizing it, Barthes found himself in the same conceptual morass as Foucault. Here he introduces one of the few definitions of sign and symptom that he had found in his travels through the medical literature:

> A differentiation was made between objective symptoms, discovered by the physician, and subjective symptoms, identified by the patient. If we retain this definition—and I believe that it is important to do so—the symptom would be what is apparently real or really apparent; that is to say, what is phenomenal [*le phénoménal*] but not in the slightest semiological or semantic. The symptom would be the disease itself in its objectivity and discontinuity. (1985, p. 275) [my translation].

Later, however, Barthes turnes his attention from symptoms to signs:

> In contrast to the symptom, the sign which is part of the definition of medical semiology is really nothing more than a symptom subjected to the organizing consciousness of the doctor. Foucault insisted on this point: the sign is a symptom due to the fact that it is located within a description, it is the explicit product of language due to the fact that it is part of the preparation of the clinical picture of the practitioner's discourse. Thus the practitioner transforms the symptom into a sign and the fact that he does so through language is, I believe, an essential point. If we accept this definition, then we pass from the phenomenal to the semantic. (1985, p. 275) [my translation].

Barthes starts with the same distinction that appears in the first chapter of this book: the difference between the subjective symptoms revealed by the patient and the objective symptoms observed by the practitioner. From this point on, however, his argument is exactly opposite to mine: symptoms are phenomenological. Here "phenomenological" is defined narrowly, as "not semiological," rather than broadly interpreted to include the patient's voice and gestures. But since the symptoms are what "the patient says," Barthes' argument is self-contradictory. Symptoms cannot be both patients' complaints, and asemiotically phenomenological at the same time.

Barthes proceeds in the same way as Foucault, the only difference being that his aim is not to formulate an archeology of medical knowledge, but to establish whether or not symptoms are of a semiosic nature. The voices of patients in all their diversity, the universe of meanings condensed by a (subjective) symptom such as "*qalbim vurur*" (My heart is pounding) or "I have ants crawling around in my brain," are missing from Barthes' approach. Barthes' position is even a little more extreme than that of a biomedical professional: what comes from the patient is a brute fact, the meaningless voice of the pathological, unmediated by cultural, historical, or biographical context. Symptoms are, then, the raw phenomenological material of the signifier which only acquires its signified in the physician's consciousness, in the sign.

Barthes' definition of signs is equally problematic, since it is framed as the opposite of his definition of symptoms. The clinician, he argues, transforms symptoms into signs, the phenomenological into the semantic. In the first part of this book, I addressed the problems inherent in the tendency of clinical psychiatry to treat symptoms as signs, and for this reason the reader may assume that my position shares more conceptual territory with Barthes' than is in fact the case. The illusion of similarity evaporates as soon as it becomes obvious that we are using the same terms to talk about different concepts. For Barthes, symptoms are purely phenomenological, while signs are semiotic because they are constructed as such by the receiver. My own position, however, is that symptoms are semiotic because they are messages constructed by a sender (e.g., "my head aches") and signs are physical because they are natural (e.g., eczema) and only acquire meaning in the consciousness of a receiver. The problem I am describing here is that of misreading winks (intentional and cultural) as twitches (involuntary and natural). But Barthes does not raise this issue. Like biomedical empiricism, his approach reifies symptoms as natural signs, and semioticizes signs as the logical inference drawn from them by a specific type of receiver: the medical practitioner. Do not misunderstand me: I am not denying that clinical inference involves a semiosic process, but observing that a patient's complaint also has a logic and a conceptual structure of its own, and is therefore equally semiosic in nature. Why this exclusive focus on the inferences of the receiver? The answer to this question lies in Barthes' stated purpose of using the concept of the sign to bring general semiology closer to medical semiology. This strategy colors his entire argument with respect to symptoms and medical signs.

Medical signs, Barthes asserts, can be compared to those elements of a sentence that are purely structural: that is to say, the syntax that expresses and organizes the signifiers. Another possible analogy is that of a linguistic system using concepts such as the opposition between paradigm (or paradigmatic plane) and syntagma (or syntagmatic plane). Just as in French there is an opposition on the paradigmatic plane between *p* and *b*, because in French "*boisson*" (drink) is not the same as "*poisson*" (fish), Barthes finds a similar opposition between medical signs. However, he is finally forced to acknowledge the limitations of the analogy: unlike language, medical signs require a "bodily support" in order to carry out their function (1985:277).

Barthes also finds similarities between language and medical semiology on the syntagmatic plane. There is a syntax of medical signs. Just as single-word phrases or interjections which have meaning in themselves are found in language, so we can find typical signs in medical semiology which in themselves signify a particular illness. But the comparison does not end here. Barthes constructs a curious analogy between syndromes and stereotyped syntagmas, or groups of two, three or four words which, though they take the form of a phrase, function as a single word. In French, "*pomme de terre*" (potato), he writes, is really only one word, albeit a special one, because it represents an intermediate stage between the purely paradigmatic plane (since it functions as a single word) and the syntagmatic plane (since formally it is a succession of words). The syndrome or regular groupings of signs is, from his point of view, similar to the stereotyped syntagma ("*pomme de terre*") because, even though the signifiers may be ordered syntagmatically, this order is always stable and refers to a signified that is always the same (1985:279). What is this signified? Disease, but obviously not disease in itself, since Saussure has already established that the signified is not the thing but the concept. For Barthes the signified of medical signs or of their syndromic groupings is the place of disease in a nosological category, the name of the disease. This idea enables him to draw a new analogy between medical semiology and language: both are based on the role of "dizzying reversibility": the signified always refers to another signifier, thus generating the infinite circuit of the game of meaning. At this point, we not only encounter Saussure and Barthes, but also Peirce's idea of unlimited semiosis and Lacan's theory that, without recourse to new signifiers and chains of signifiers, the meaning of a word remains forever out of reach (Lacan, 1966, 1973). Lacan, however, is a psychoanalyst, and consequently takes a different view of symptoms, arguing consistently that the unconscious is structured like a language (1973, p. 28) and symptoms undoubtedly depend on this structuring.[2] For Barthes, by contrast, symptoms are not located in the terrain of meaning; it is the sign that he locates in the dynamic through which the signified is trapped in an unlimited succession of signifiers.

In an attempt to force an analogy between the medical sign and the Saussurean sign, Barthes abandons his initial understanding of the symptom as that which the patient points out and the sign as the objective evidence discovered by the practitioner, reducing symptoms to the formal appearance of signs. But there is a world of difference between, for example, the gestures of courtesy and American Sign Language on the one hand, and the bodily signs of pregnancy or allergy: in the former there is intentionality while in the latter there is not, just as there is intentionality in symptoms but not in signs. Foucault and Barthes seem, strangely, not to distinguish between the two; to recognize that while the physician observes fever, cough or eczema, the patient constructs complaints, laments and gestures. As in the biomedical perception, the patient has been reified and, ironically, Foucault's maxim— all forms of knowledge are also forms of power—demonstrated.

PEIRCE AND ECO (OR, SYMPTOMS AS NATURAL PHENOMENA)

As mentioned above, both Peirce's definition of signs and his conception of the scope of semiotics are much broader than Saussure's. According to Peirce:[3]

> A sign, or *representamen*, is something which stands to somebody for something in some respect or capacity. It addresses somebody, that is, creates in the mind of that person an equivalent sign, or perhaps a more developed sign. That sign which it creates I call the *interpretant* of the first sign. The sign stands for something, its *object*" (Peirce, CP 2.228) [emphasis added].

It will come as no surprise that this definition has caused many a headache, especially given the complexity of Peirce's work in general and his signic typologies in particular.[4] A careful reading of this definition leads us to the terms of the triad that generates the process of signification, which cannot, Peirce consistently argues, be generated by paired terms. The elements of this triad are *sign* (or *representamen*), the *interpretant* and the *object*.

A sign refers to something that is not the sign itself, but its object. But the Peircean relation between sign and object is by no means direct: the interpretant lies between the two. What is this interpretant? Peirce defines it as the effect of the signified: that is, the cognitive consequence of the sign's presence. Thus the interpretant is the signified, in relation to the sign that produces it[5], but this is only possible insofar as the interpretant is also a sign, albeit created by the first sign. The sign which acts as interpretant in turn refers to another sign which acts as the interpretant of the second sign and so on, until a continuous semiosic process is created (CP, 5.484 and 8.322).

An in-depth analysis of Peirce's work is beyond the scope of this chapter. For my purposes, however, his definition of signs is important because it releases the sign and semiosis from the Saussurean requisite of a human sender. The statement "is something which stands to somebody" does not necessarily assume the presence of an active source of meaning, but relies only on a receiver. This makes it possible to include in the universe of semiotics both natural signals and physical signs, which he calls symptoms.

According to Peirce, a symptom is a kind of *index* (CP, 8.335). Here we should briefly review the best-known Peircean classification of signs, the one that the author himself considers to be the most fundamental (CP, 2.275): the "second trichotomy" which is based on the relation of the sign with its object (CP, 2.247).

Depending on its object, in Peirce's scheme a sign may be an *icon*, an *index* or a *symbol*:

1. If it is an icon, there is a similarity between the physical properties of the object and the properties of the sign (as signifier). The icon would be, curiously, what Saussure called a symbol and defined as exempt from arbitrariness.

2. The index would be a type of sign that "denotes" its object by virtue of an automatic link or connection; it is physically related to its object. Here the term *denote* is important because Peirce considers the relation between sign and interpretant to be one of meaning, while the link between sign and object is one of denotation. One example of an index would be smoke as a sign of fire.

3. Finally, the symbol would be, paradoxically, the Saussurean sign in which there is no natural relation between sign and object, only an arbitrary and conventional relation or, in Peirce's words, the sign is related to its object "by virtue of a law" (CP, 2.247).

Peirce tells us that symptoms are indices because they have a nonarbitrary relation with their objects and, therefore, have a "real relation" to them (CP, 8.335). Symptoms are, then, the indices or natural signs of an object: disease.

It is evident that Peirce considers symptoms to be natural signs: abdominal swelling indicates a cirrhosis; fever indicates an infection. He does not make a distinction between physical sign and symptom, or between subjective and objective symptoms; all symptoms fall into the same category of what I would consider to be physical signs. Nervertheless, Peirce's semiotic model offers considerable possibilities for the analysis of signs and symptoms. Let me focus for a moment of the categories of icon, index and symbol.

The first category is the most controversial but, as Szasz (1970) has noted, some symptoms of hysteria can be regarded as iconic insofar as they are similar to their object: a fit of hysteria can be regarded as an iconic sign of a real (organic) epileptic fit.

Let us take a look at the other two types. A classic example of an index would be a cough: what I would consider to be a physical sign. Peirce himself endorses this interpretation, classifying symptoms as indices.

The last category, the one that Peirce located beyond the scope of symptoms, is, paradoxically, the category that offers the greatest possibilities since it can be applied to "subjective" symptoms: complaints and laments. "I have the evil eye," "I have a sore throat," or "my head aches," for instance, are arbitrary linguistic expressions whose signifiers (what Peirce would call signs) have no natural relation with their object. Using Peirce's typology, therefore, symptoms could be regarded as symbols.

But Peirce does not apply his signic trichotomy in these terms, although the new medical semiotics would do so later, albeit timidly, as we will see in the next section of this chapter. Peirce's references to symptoms are exclusively to those signs which are indices of a disease, although more can be said about this identification, since Peirce attempts to place symptoms in the context of another of his signic typologies as sinsigns when they occur in a particular case, and as legisigns when they are interpreted as a specific example of a law or a general rule. Concretely, he writes: "The Symptom itself is a legisign, a general type of a definite character. The occurrence in a particular case is a sinsign" (CP, 8.335)

This assertion is based on his first trichotomy of the sign: the domain of the production of the sign or, in other words, the relation of the sign with itself (CP, 2.243-246). According to Peirce there are *qualisigns*, *sinsigns* and *legisigns*. The qualisigns are included in the sinsigns which, in turn, are included in the legisigns. For this reason we are dealing with a hierarchy rather than a typology of signs:

1. A qualisign is "a quality which is a Sign. It cannot actually act as a sign until it is embodied" (CP, 2.244), and therefore it is the very material or substance of the sign, the sign in its firstness.[6]

2. Sinsigns, for their part, refer to a single occurrence of the sign, in one particular case.

3. Legisigns involve a convention, law or general rule.

Applying this hierarchy to the example of the definite article ("the"), Peirce explains that "the" may appear on a page fifteen to twenty times on a single page, and in each case it would be a sinsign. On another level, however, the word "the" as such is an instance of a general type, and this type is the legisign (CP, 2.246).

A symptom—what I would consider a physical sign—such as a red spots on the skin would be a sinsign when it occurs on one particular occasion, and a legisign in the context of the conventions of medical knowledge, which infers from it not an isolated case but a general type according to which a "red spots on the skin" is a normative element of measles.[7]

For my purposes here, Peirce's highly complex scheme of signic classification can be reduced to the following three ideas:

1. Semiotics is not concerned exclusively with conventionally-created signs and, therefore, symptoms (physical signs) are regarded as a particular type of semiotic sign.

2. For Peirce, a symptom is an index, a sign physically related to its object. Just as smoke is the result of fire, so symptoms are the result of disease.

3. The fact that a symptom is an index does not prevent it from also functioning, at least potentially, as a legisign. In this case, it would be an indexical legisign which only becomes normative in the consciousness of a medical receiver.

Clearly, Peirce's point of view with respect to symptoms is not far removed from Barthes'. For both, symptoms are natural indicators, originally asemiotic physical signs, a definition accepted by other generalist semiologists as well. This is the case of Umberto Eco who, despite his structuralist affinities, is in many respects closer to Peirce than to Saussure:

> Those who reduce semiotics to a theory of communicative acts can neither regard symptoms as signs, nor accept as signs other behaviors, albeit human, from which the receiver infers something about the situation of a sender who is unaware of sending any messages to anyone (Eco, 1977, p. 33) [my translation].

Eco argues here that semiotics need not limit itself to the study of Saussurean signs, but may take up any objects—indices, marks, traces, prints or natural signals—that form part of semiosis or the semiosic process (1977). In this list Eco would include symptoms, which he almost invariably associates with physical signs: fever, cough, eczema, etc. I say "almost invariably" because in *La struttura assente* he makes a distinction that appears to be very similar to the one I am making here. Concretely, in the context of mapping fields of semiotic research, he asserts that medical semiotics is divided into two different areas: the system which gives meaning to natural signs, and the system of linguistic expressions by means of which patients from "different cultural environments and civilizations verbally or kinesically report a symptom" (1968, p. 16). Thus, natural signs are included in the field of semiotics as long as there is a system of conventions (such as those of medical knowledge) which gives them meaning. Eco also alludes to patient utterances, although it seems that the verbal expression of distress is not itself the symptom, but a report of the symptom; that is to say, symptoms are natural constants expressed by patients in the same way, we might say, that a hand clutching one's side expresses pain.

In his well-known *Trattato di semiotica generale,* Eco's assessment is identical to the one he advances in *La struttura assente,* with the exception of a comment on psychoanalysis:

> In the final analysis, even psychoanalysis itself is a branch of medical semiotics and therefore of general semiotics, in the sense that it tends to be the continuous systematic codification or textual interpretation of certain *signs* or *symbols* supplied by the patient, either through his own explanation of the signs themselves or through the syntactic structure and the semantic peculiarities (lapsus linguae, etc.) of the verbal explanation (1977, p. 27) [emphasis added] [my translation].

I have highlighted the words "signs" and "symbols" to emphasize Eco's avoidance of the word "symptom," which is absent here because Eco refers to physical signs as symptoms, and to the patient's speech as signs and even symbols (although he seems to have reservations about this term).

Since Eco has no interest in the problems of clinical communication, he devotes no space to those "expressions that report symptoms." He does, however, discuss symptoms as natural inferences, since he can use them to defend his arguments with respect to the scope of semiotics. In his definition of the polysemic nature of the term "sign," he writes:

> We find a block of linguistic usages according to which the sign is "an evident indication from which deductions can be drawn about something latent." In this sense we speak of signs in the case of medical symptoms, criminal tendencies, or atmospheric indicators (1996, p. 5) [my translation].

For Eco, symptoms are signs since they have a semiosic function which takes one of three forms:

1. A part-for-whole relation in which symptoms are a part of a concealed whole which, like an iceberg, cannot be seen in its entirety because only its tip is visible;

2. A cause-and-effect relation which requires proven and codified causality, such as the relation between smoke and fire, or as in "if he's breathing, he's alive;" and

3. A prediction of the possible effects of a particular cause, as in "this is a fatal wound" (1996, p. 5).

In all these cases, the meaning of a symptom does not reside in the phenomenon itself, but in the inference that a receiver draws in accordance with social convention. This is important because Eco believes that a red spot on the skin is a phenomenon resembling the conditioned salivation of Pavlov's dog: a stimulus independent of any socially determined code. Nonetheless, there is always an observer, a physician who interprets signs of disease or a scientist holding the little bell whose ringing stimulates the dog. Depending on how this receiver conceptualizes and draws inferences from this process, these natural realities (or, in Barthes' words, the raw material of the signifier) acquire one or several meanings according to a preestablished code, and function, as Peirce phrased it, as "signs for someone" (Eco, 1977). In his *Semiotica e Filosofia del Linguaggio,* Eco clarifies this point:

> Symptoms refer to a cause to which they have been linked by a more or less codified experience. Since this link is regarded as being naturally motivated, its relation of inferential necessity is quite strong (1984, p. 65).

Here, symptoms are signs for someone who establishes an inferential relation between the phenomenon and a possible cause. For Eco, who is dealing with natural signs, it could hardly be otherwise. He is aware that there is also a universe of "signs," "symbols" and forms of expression originating with the patient, messages produced by a sender. He also recognises that psychoanalysis, among other theories, locates symptoms in the terrain of meaning. But in the final analysis, he restricts the term symptom to physical signs, among other reasons because, in a semiotics based on a theory of the sign as *genus generalissimum,* or at least as the central object, this option is the most convenient because it minimizes terminological confusion.

THE NEW MEDICAL SEMIOTICS

Though their approaches differ, Barthes, Peirce and Eco all consider symptoms to be physical signs, whether as phenomenological presentations, indices, indexical sinsigns, indexical legisigns or signs resembling prints or traces. Evidently, all three are operating within the area of general semiotics (or semiology) and not within the particular knowledge field of medical semiotics. For this reason they touch only briefly on symptoms, and then only as physical signs, excluding the patient's expressions of distress. Neither Peirce nor Barthes (and to a lesser extent Eco) considers how symptoms might differ from physical signs: artificiality and arbitrariness in contrast to a natural link between sign and object; an original semiosic construction in contrast to the requirement of a receiver's consciousness to transform a natural phenomenon into a sign.

Unlike these great theoreticians, those who do empirical research in the terrain of medical semiotics have focused mainly on the problematic nature of the symptom, a slippery phenomenon that resists definitive classification as either a natural or a cultural object. For analytical purposes, though at the risk of overgeneralization in some cases, these contributions to the literature can be divided into two groups:[8]

1. those that have analyzed the problem of symptom by focusing mainly on the interpretive intention of the receiver; and

2, those that have given priority to the semiosic and productive intention of symptoms, complaints and expressions of distress.

The terminology of literary criticism serves my purposes here: to identify the former with the search for an *intentio lectoris* (reader's intention) and the latter with the *intentio auctoris* and *intentio operis* (that is to say, the intention of the author of the symptoms, and the intention of these symptoms as works). In the first case, symptoms need not be defined as original semiosic expressions since the intention of the reader ensures their semiosic nature; in the second case, however, it is absolutely necessary to understand that symptoms have a communicative and meaningful dimension.

Intentio lectoris

This approach has focused on the problem in terms of how symptoms may acquire or lose meaning according to how they are perceived through medical knowledge or consciousness. Although there is room in this approach for the existence of a sender and the sender's meaning, the *intentio lectoris* or inerpreter's intention clearly takes precedence over other interests. Uexküll —who has made important contributions both to medical semiotics and to medical anthropology (1982, 1991)—was the first to outline the twofold argument that symptoms are (a) affected by psychological variables and (b) may be classified in one of three ways, according to the domain to which they are assigned. In biomedicine (what Uexküll calls "natural-science medicine"), a symptom would be interpreted as an error in the human machine; in psychological medicine, as an error in socialization; and in psychosomatic medicine, as an expressive error through which a psychological conflict takes somatic form (1982).

Uexküll argues that the patient has been systematically excluded from the analysis of the meaning of symptoms in favor of a meaning preestablished by medical knowledge. However, his interests seem to lie less in the direction of recovering the original meaning of the symptom than in rendering it intelligible by juxtaposing these three possible readings of it. In Uexküll's work there is a complementarity principle, the formalization of which recalls Devereux's attempts to proceed along more than than one front simultaneously. Here, however, this complementarity is more clearly an integration of knowledge domains, as Uexküll himself noted in his "Semiotics and Medicine" (1982).

In this combination of gazes, perceptions and interpretations, the symptom as a phenomenon is subdivided into parts which correspond to the respective medical fields: biomedical, psychological and psychosomatic symptoms. However, if the symptom as a phenomenon is accepted as a constant—as Uexküll does, and as do the three fields of medical knowledge that constitute his frame of reference—why not enlarge the list to include the entire repertoire of medical systems: Ayurvedic medicine, traditional Chinese medicine, Azande medicine, and so on? Uexküll's model, clearly, integrates semiotics with Western medicine and not Ayurvedic medicine, but it is also clear that his typology makes considerable concessions to the biomedical model.[9] In fact, to the extent that the integration of Western medical traditions is emphasized, there is little for semiotics to do: a symptom is what three specific domains of Western knowledge say it is. But at some level, Uexküll guesses that a symptom can also be something else: what it is for the patient, and what it is for a particular cultural tradition.

In the same vein as Uexküll, Kahn attempted to formulate a semiotics of diagnosis on the basis of a key concept, diagnostic signs, which is defined through a curious and idiosyncratic adaptation of the Peircean description of signs. In fact, Kahn's definition is a sort of exemplification of Peirce's:

> A diagnostic sign will be explained as "something" (and here the "something" in question could include any of the following: nausea, pain, a feeling of depression, a thought, a skin lesion, an odor, a gesture or facial expression, a verbal utterance or stretch of silence, a fragment of human interaction, a bloodstain on a shirt, a photograph in a medical text book, or an image on an X-ray film) "which stands to somebody" (in this case to any competent witness of such a sign, whether doctor, patient or other) "for something" (the "something" in this case being *some conceivable state of "health" or "disease"*) and "in some respect or capacity" (here, with respect to the witness's evaluative judgement, be it sophisticated or naive, concerning such states). (1978, p. 75) [italics in original].

Paraphrasing Peirce is enlightening because it reveals the possible implications of the Peircean definition of signs in the field of medical semiotics, and concretely, its possible application to what Kahn calls "diagnostic signs," which include patients' speech and behavior as well as the results of, for example, computerized tomography (CT). Of course, a CT scan is a technological product of biomedical knowledge and is therefore different from an observable physical sign or patient utterances, which are givens. This self-evident difference leads Kahn to note the existence of three possible codes which mediate the medical interpretation of symptoms:

1. a technological code of signs created by artifacts such as X-rays;

2. a medical code of signs taught in universities and schools of medicine;

3. a general code of signs sustained by the universe of cultural knowledge and social practice within which professionals and patients interact, which forms the substance of everyday face-to-face human communication (p. 79-81).

There is no need to force the analogy in order to see that the first two codes correspond to physical signs as I have defined them, while the third corresponds to symptoms. Kahn's concern, however, is not the code employed by patients as senders of messages, but how the medical receiver of the message discriminates between codes. This is why, in Kahn's definition of diagnostic signs, the meaning of the symptom continues to depend on the receiver ("to somebody"), since symptoms are semiosic signs to the extent that they are subject to interpretation in terms of a repertoire of codes.

Symptoms become diagnostic signs depending on the specifics of cultural and historical context, but not all diagnostic signs are identical. Kahn differentiates between "normo-signs," which refer to a state of health; "patho-signs," which are linked to a state of illness; and "neutro-signs," whose relation to normal and pathological states remains indeterminate (p. 77). In this scheme, interpreting symptoms is the process of converting them into semiosic forms which constitute diagnostic signs, into texts structured according to a preestablished code which determines whether or not they are pathological. Again, the meaning of symptoms as original semiosic facts is subordinated to medical consciousness as the definitive arbiter of meaning. Kahn does not, however, close all doors to the patient's interpretation of illness, noting explicitly that these signs are "for someone," but this someone is not necessarily the physician. Though she continues to emphasize the *intentio lectoris* of a medical interpreter, Kahn believes that symptoms also have meaning for other receivers or for the patients themselves, since her unusual definition of diagnostic signs makes room for the sufferer. Nonetheless, in Kahn— as in Eco, and in Kleinman's early works—the patient seems to be less a sender than a receiver of messages, since she emphasizes the idea that diagnostic signs are *for* someone rather than created *by* someone, and therefore, patients become special receivers who interpret in their own personal way the illness that threatens them. The patient's meaning enters the analysis because of its diagnostic potential, not because of its potential for creating symptoms. Again, there is a failure to distinguish between physical signs and symptoms, not to speak of the vexed distinction between symptom and experience analyzed in Chapter 8. This failure is problematic, because the distancing that occurs between the unintentional physical sign—a twitch — and the patient as a possible receiver does not exist in the case of symptoms. Physical signs occur in the absence of human consciousness (or unconsciousness), but symptoms, like winks, are produced not only *for* but *by* someone: that is to say, by the patient-sender who is not merely the receiver of his own physical signs.

Like Uexküll, Kahn recognizes the inescapable reality that behind a symptom lies not only a medical consciousness, but also the consciousness of the patient. In the absence of a distinction between signs and symptoms, however, treatment proceeds on the assumption that symptoms originate in physical phenomena rather than as expressions of meaning. There is here a dissociation between the symptom as message and its sender, although the patient is recognized as a privileged receiver who, emulating Peirce, can read his own physical signs. This approach is quite distinct from that of Foucault and Barthes, for whom the patient is a kind of a "passive text" to be read by the active gaze of the physician, not a participant in the interpretation of his own suffering (see Johnson, 1994). Kahn's work recognizes the interpretive capacity of the patient but, paradoxically, only as the receiver of a message, not as a sender, because there is no precise distinction between the production of physical signs in contrast to symptoms; instead the stress is laid on the interpretive intention of the reader.

Intentio auctoris, intentio operis

In contrast to those interpretations focusing mainly on the *intentio lectoris*, some scholars have taken up the matter of the author's intention and the intention of the work. I make this distinction because in literary criticism works are considered to be products independent of their creators, with a life and a meaning of their own beyond that of the author's intention. In the production of symptoms, however, the distance between these two intentions is narrower, if only in the immediacy of the moment when "the said" (*noema*) and "the intention" (*noesis*) are fused in the expression of distress (Ricoeur, 1979, p. 84). Although the intention of the symptom as a text is to some degree independent, its linkage to the author's intention is usually much clearer to an ethnographer or semiotician than, for example, Joyce's intention in *Finnegan's Wake* is to a literary critic or Buñuel's in *Un chien andalou* to a film critic.[10]

An interesting, if timid, contribution from this perspective is Staiano's review of Locker's book *Symptoms and Illness*, in which she uses her ethnosemiotic research in Belize to recover the personal meaning of the patient and the local meaning of ethnomedical traditions. The title of her article, "Medical semiotics: Redefining an ancient craft," is a clear indication of her interest in symptoms (1982; see also Staiano, 1986).

Staiano maintains the distinction I have suggested between symptoms and physical signs, although the terms she uses are "intersubjective symptoms" and "introspective symptoms." The former are clinical, organic, physical and objective signs which are accessible to an interpreter other than the patient. The latter are those signs "presented by the patient," the "subjective" universe of complaints and expressions of distress (1982, p. 335).

Apart from this terminological difference, her concepts share a great deal with mine. However, the definition of "introspective" is not entirely accurate because symptoms are also extrospective and consequently accessible to an interpreter other than the patient. The continual confusion between intersubjectivity and introspection in the distinction between physical signs and symptoms succeeds only in enormously complicating matters. For this reason, I find that differentiating between phenomena that are semiosic in origin—winks—and realities that are not originally semiosic—twitches— is more accurate. In this way we avoid the confusion entailed in denying the intersubjective role which symptoms share with all other semiosic constructions. Let me return now to a consideration of Staiano's work.

Several aspects of Staiano's work are relevant to my purposes here. She begins by attempting to demystify any single authoritative interpretation of physical signs, such as fever, or of medical categories, such as malaria. Using Peirce's triadic model of icon, index, and symbol as representamen, object and interpretant, she shows that in the Garifuna ethnomedical tradition in Belize both the interpretant and the object which the malaria fever refers to are completely different from those of the biomedical model. Whereas for biomedicine the object of a sign or representamen of "malaria" is a microscopic antigen and the etiological interpretant is the "bite of an infected mosquito," in the Garifuna interpretive model the object of "malaria" is the intrusion of a strange element into the body and the etiological interpretant is "exposure to cold or wet while in a hot state" (1982, p. 341). In the interpretive process, a sign such as fever can be constituted (in the patient's discourse) not as (natural and nonarbitrary) indices but as (artificial and arbitrary) symbols according to Peirce's terminology. The reason (which is not made explicit by Staiano) is not that physical signs cease to be indices, but that they have become symptoms and discourse.

This is, of course, an exploration of the possible varieties of an *intentio lectoris*. A physical sign is open to multiple readings, to a universe which becomes polysemic because of its wealth of interpretive systems: biomedicine, Garifuna medicine, patient conceptions, etc. Staiano's approach is fundamentally anthropological, as she herself defines it. The analysis of different interpretive systems is essentially a strategy similar to Kleinman's explanatory models. Although Staiano's approach is based on Peircean semiotics and Kleinman's on the Geertzian concept of cultural system, they share the same basic aim: to foreground nonbiomedical models.

Staiano's analysis, however, is not limited to the ways in which a single physical sign can become many interpretants, but includes concepts which cross the boundary separating *intentio lectoris* from *intentio auctoris* and *operis*, belonging both to the realm of Garifuna physical signs and to the creative and performative nature of symptoms.

Insofar as she distinguishes between intersubjective symptoms and introspective symptoms, Staiano includes in her definition of medical semiotics the interpretation not only of physical signs, but also of complaints as vehicles for the transmission of meaning. These expressions of distress correspond to the cultural dimension of illness, the domain of symbolic expression in the Peircean sense. These episodes of discomfort become narratives and cultural texts in which Staiano implicitly includes symptoms.

Staiano's analysis stops at the threshold of a search for the *intentio auctoris* and *operis*. More recently, Hokansalo (1991) crosses it in her reconstitution of the symbolic meaning of the symptoms and complaints of Finnish production-line workers. Following a brief analysis of the evolution of Western medicine from Hippocrates to the beginnings of the biomedical paradigm, Hokansalo introduces the distinction between symptom and physical sign that I have used here. A symptom, she argues, is subjective evidence or an assessment of a disease: the patient's complaint or expression of pain and distress. A sign, on the other hand, is "an objective evidence of the disease, specially as observed and interpreted by a physician rather than by the patient" (p. 251). However, she does not seem to make clear and explicit use of this distinction. Her knowledge of semiotics seems to generate a kind of inertia that manifests itself in continual beating about a theoretical bush. In reviewing the different approaches to symptoms, Hokansalo discovers that they have been regarded almost exclusively as physical signs, a theoretical vacuum only partially filled by the work of a few others, notably Uexküll and Staiano. Hokansalo does not, however, use this discovery to develop her own critique of the classic semiotic and semiological approaches of Barthes, Eco and Peirce, but instead attempts to combine this tradition of knowledge with a type of empirical work in which there are no medical receivers of messages, only Finnish women workers' expressions of distress.

From this curious mix of high-flying theory and close-to-the-ground semiosic phenomena, she draws some conclusions which contradict the great semiotic theoreticians:

> In conclusion, it can be stated that symptoms are essentially multireferential and polysemous. They can be indexical, pointing to a specific disease or disorder, but they can also be, often simultaneously, symbolic (1991, p. 259).

And also:

> The symptoms in my data were partly indexical, but mostly symbolic. As symbols, the symptoms had objects arbitrarily linked to the representamens. It was in the communication process itself that the symptoms gained their various meanings (p. 261).

Here symptoms acquire a new and different place within the Peircean trichotomy of icon, index and symbol. Although Hokansalo is not very clear on this point, the simultaneity of index and symbol seems to be related to situations in which a physical sign and a symptom converge, as when a patient reports or complains of difficulty in breathing or a sore throat. It also seems to be related to the very nature of complaints, which bear traces of emotionality that make Hokansalo hesitate to characterize symptoms as fully symbolic in nature. At one point she defines symptoms as a sort of "second language," although not fully formed, a type of semiotics—following Kristeva—which precedes the symbolic. Here Hokansalo seems to be arguing that symptoms are constituted in this intermediate territory between language and emotion, culture and experience, the symbolic order and feeling. This interpretation is suggested by her subsequent identification of symptoms and bereavement, that experience of affliction in which stereotyped cultural forms become inseparable from feelings.

To argue that symptoms are wholly symbolic does not, however, necessarily mean denying either their emotional charge or the existence of an underlying pathology. Like the highly stylized women's laments characteristic of Finnish mourning, the symptoms of the women on the production line are symbolic and cultural constructions which organize the experience of affliction and provide one with the opportunity to reflect on the misfortunes of life. In extreme situations in which people cry out in pain, as in the case of onomatopoeia, it is difficult to distinguish precisely between what is indexical and what is symbolic, what is natural and what is arbitrary; or, in other words, between twitches and winks, physical signs and symptoms. However, even in such cases, spontaneous outcries are often culturally distinctive and are generally accompanied by more elaborated forms of expression which condense moral judgements, etiological beliefs and pathophysiological conceptions. For this reason semiotic analysis is more fruitful when the symptom is understood not as an index but as a symbol; this facilitates a much more extensive interpretation of illness narratives. Hokansalo's analysis moves in this direction, although she attempts throughout to maintain a mixed definition of symptoms. In her conclusions, however, the symbolic definition is predominant:

> In becoming a symptom, the subjective sensation must be interpreted in a 'symptomatization' process, through a code profoundly mediated by culture. Factory-women obviously share this kind of code, as my data shows. Symptoms also have communicative functions. They can express disorder or health, problems or pleasures of everyday life, or sorrows and bereavements that would

otherwise find no expression. They can function as a channel for conflicts in the workplace that would otherwise be suppressed. Symptoms can also establish a social group and promote social cohesion among women (1991, p. 265).

In arguing that symptoms have communicative functions, Hokansalo is distinguishing between the semiosic character of symptoms as distinct from physical signs. The patient, in this approach, is the sender of a message and this, in turn, implies the existence of an *intentio auctoris* and *operis* which exists prior to biomedical reception of the message. What we learn from this approach is not unlike what Byron Good was attempting to represent through the analytic notion of semantic networks, or Kleinman through illness narratives. Indeed, in both cases, symptoms condense multiple meanings whose referents are not exclusively pathological but include the pressures of daily life, moral convictions and emotions constituted on the basis of cultural categories that evoke local worlds of affliction. Hokansalo's work (1991) is linked to Good's (1977) by an invisible thread of continuity and similarity which is all the more remarkable because it joins independent creations. The starting point in both cases is an ethnographic concern for local meaning which centers on the intention of the author and the work, and the processes lead to a similar result: the symptom as a semiosic, symbolic construction condensing a whole universe of meanings considered by both biomedicine and by theoretical semiotics to be secondary, anecdotal, contingent or simply nonexistent.

·What separates an Iranian woman's "*qalvim vurur*" from the Monday-morning complaints of a Finnish assembly-line worker is simultaneously what unites them: they are both cultural constructions. Once we recognize this, symptoms cease to be the raw material of the signifier, the merely phenomenological which has yet to become semantic, the expression of physical pathology whose meaning depends on a medical consciousness. Its very substance is the cultural and linguistic materials from which complaints, laments and expressions of distress are constructed. The symptom conceptualized as a message is open to new readings which restore its often-denied original meaning—the intention of the author and of the work. The medical gaze is not enough; in this endeavor, hearing is more important, because what is at stake is not explanation—the artificial production of signs by medical technology, the search for pathological meanings, or therapeutic intervention—but the apprehension of complaints as meaningful constructions. We are no longer in the domain of clinical inference, but of semiotic analysis or ethnographic interpretation.

NOTES

1. See also Thomas Sebeok's and Jean Umiker-Sebeok's (1979) excellent work on the relation between crime, illness and semiotics.

2. Jacques Lacan's conception of symptoms—expressed in somewhat cryptic but occasionally enlightening language—can be found in his *Écrits*. As he sees them, symptoms are part of a sort of "first language," a form of communication without conscious intention, symbols that stand in sharp contrast to physical signs (1966, p. 280). On the subject of psychoanalytic initiation, Lacan states: "What the linguistic conception that the trainee (in psychoanalysis) must have as the base of his apprenticeship will teach him is to expect that the symptom will demonstrate its function as signifier; that is to say, that function which distinguishes symptoms from the 'natural' signs to which the term normally refers in medicine" (p. 280) [my translation]. Symptoms are not, then, natural signs but signifiers. Here, the word signifier should be understood in the context of Lacanian theory, in which the signifier has priority over the signified, to such an extent that there are no *signifiés*, only *signifiants* (1966, p. 516).

3. The numerical references correspond to the volume number and paragraph, in that order, not to the page number.

4. Peirce divides signs up in a rather complex way, into three trichotomies. The first of these is derived from the relation of the sign with itself (qualisign, sinsign and legisign). The second is the result of the sign-object relation and includes the already well-known *icon, index* and *symbol*. The third trichotomy is formed by the link between the sign and the interpretant (*rheme, dicent sign* or *dicisign* and *argument*). Here I will deal only with the first two, since these are the ones he uses explicitly in connection with symptoms. See especially Volume 1, Chapter 2 of his *Collected Papers*.

5. The interpretant does not merely translate the sign, but creates a more developed sign. See Peirce's definition of signs quoted above.

6. Eco writes of qualisigns as expressions which have a "material unicity." Michelangelo's *Pietà*... would be a qualisign, but since its existence is predicated on its having been created at least once, it is also a sinsign (Eco, 1977, p. 269).

7. The trichotomy qualisign, sinsign and legisign is related to Peirce's phenomenological categories of *firstness, secondness* and *thirdness. Firstness* is the possibility of original and independent existence without reference to anything else, and it is related to the qualisign by its "material unicity" (Eco, 1977, p. 269). *Secondness* is this original something in relation to a second thing or person but not to a third. Staiano (1982) considers this to be the interpreter's recognition of something specific, and therefore a sinsign (i.e., a symptom). *Thirdness* would be the presentation of this something in its relation to a specific rule or convention.

8. An analysis of the entire field of medical semiotics is beyond the scope of this chapter. Here my purpose is simply to review some of the most significant contributions to the field of the semiotic analysis of symptoms.
9. In a later article situated more clearly in the domain of medical anthropology than in that of medical semiotics, Uexküll reiterates his integrative model, which is really the so-called biopsychosocial model, but in a tone that gives anthropology greater autonomy with respect to the medical sciences (see Uexküll, 1991).
10. Ricoeur (1979) has shown that in the process through which (spoken) discourse becomes (written) text, the distance increases between the intention of the author and the intention of the work.

CHAPTER 10

Ethnographic Interpretations: Symptoms, Symbols and Small Worlds

A comparison of hermeneutic medical anthropology and the new medical semiotics reveals some surprising similarities. Without forcing the comparison, we can easily see that Hokansalo's description of the complaints of a group of Finnish factory workers is a sort of ethnography reminiscent of Good's work in Iran. Nor can we fail to recognize that Uexküll's emphasis on the semiosic nature of symptoms as constructions, as messages from a sender, points to the emic meaning of symptoms. In fact, both specialties have contributed to the emergence of a relatively new field in which the native meaning of symptoms is recovered through the work of understanding.

As a consequence of this method, an unbreakable link is forged between symptoms and their cultural and biographical context. This relationship is not accessible through clinical inference or exclusively biological approaches. Symptoms are now symbols in the Peircean sense, (linguistic) signs according to Saussure's definition, dominant symbols in semantic illness networks in Good's work, expressions of distress which form part of the sufferer's narrative according to Kleinman and Staiano, "texts" according to Good and Good, metaphors and metonyms of the sociopolitical system in the words of Scheper-Hughes, and even symbolizations which can be understood in the same manner as an art specialist gains insight into a work's creative and performative universe (Devisch, 1991).

These related anthropological and semiotic incursions into a realm traditionally restricted to diagnostic tests, biochemical research, and advanced medical technology furnish yet another example of the sometimes-bewildering discursive indeterminacy that characterizes the refiguration of social thought so neatly captured in Geertz' concept of "blurred genres" (1983, p.19). Suddenly, literary critics are writing about anthropology (Clifford, 1983), and anthropologists are behaving as literary critics (Geertz, 1988), not to repeat the entire litany of examples of blurred genres cited by Geertz (1983, p.19-20).

In a very similar fashion, semiotic and anthropological discourses become blurred in the attempt to deal with so strange an object as the symptom. Is Staiano an anthropologist who uses semiotics, or a semiologist working in the field of ethnomedicine? Is Good a practitioner of hermeneutics, or of cultural anthropology? Is Kleinman a psychiatrist, or a medical anthropologist? Is Uexküll a physician, a medical theoretician, a semiologist or an anthropologist? Is Taussig an anthropologist, a physician or a scholar fascinated by the works of Benjamin and Lukács? We could go even farther and suggest that the anthropological interpretation of symptoms might itself be understood as a kind of "symptom," not of individuals but of an entire discipline. In effect there has been, if not a refiguration, at least a revision of the spaces and boundaries of anthropology. My intention here, however, is not to draw attention to the symptoms of anthropology, but to develop an anthropology of symptoms, although I cannot help suspecting that both are intimately linked.

To return to the subject at hand, we have left behind the notion of the symptom as an index. Having established a clear distinction between physical signs and symptoms, we can no longer naturalize the latter in the manner of neo-Kraepelinian medicine. Between the natural fact of disease and the symptom lies a cultural universe which organizes the experience of suffering: the "symptomatization process" which restored to the complaints of the Finnish workers Hokansalo studied their semiosic nature and communicative power. But how should anthropology respond to this new cultural object? Should we approach symptoms as symbols (in which case, what do we mean by "symbol"?) or as metaphors, as texts or as messages, as winks or as narratives?

The answer to the first question is the easier of the two. I have maintained from the outset that a hermeneutics of affliction must remain independent of the search for pathological meaning and take as its object of study the *intentio auctoris* and *operis* of symptoms, exploring the relation between context and meaning. This is what allows us to see symptoms as winks, meaningful in their own right. They are not parts of a natural whole, related as red spots are to measles, but symbolic constructions which communicate something beyond the disease manifestation: distress. More than merely its physical referents, distress is laden with information about the sufferer's moral, historical, cultural and political-economic condition.

The answer to the second question is more difficult, and leads us to complex conceptual and definitional issues. Terms such as symbol, metaphor, metonymy, sign, text, and narrative each have a number of possible analytic uses and require at least some sort of explanation. Taking linguistically-expressed symptoms as a model, let us examine some of the possibilities.

First, to treat symptoms as metaphors is to take up a position within an analytic tradition that runs from Sontag (1991) to Matsuoka (1991) and can be expressed as the proposition that "illness is a metaphor" or "illness can be apprehended as a metaphor." Sontag uses Aristotle's *Poetics* to point out that metaphor "consists in giving the thing a name that belongs to something else" (Sontag, 1991, p. 5). Metaphor seems to suggest the existence of a figurative meaning, as in the use of "the king of the jungle" to stand for "lion." This kind of rhetorical figure, however, is absent from expressions such as "My heart is pounding," "I hear voices" or, as we shall see below, in a symptom such as "I'm nervous." Eco has shown us that falsehood is at the heart of metaphor (1984). This falsehood makes a literal interpretation of "king of the jungle" impossible, because a king is not a lion, just as a woman is not a swan or a man an ass. However, when an Iranian woman complains of heart distress, she is also talking about palpitations, and therefore a literal, though thin, interpretation of her symptom is possible. If we understand metaphor in this sense (and it is not, of course, the only one), the symptom is not, at least initially, a metaphor, because it can be read literally without running the risk of misrepresentation: no "kings of the jungle" or "asses reading the newspaper." But of course, because symptoms depend on language, they may take the form of metaphor, metonymy or synecdoche among other tropes, sometimes surprising or opaque, such as the Igbo complaint "ants are crawling around in my brain" (see Kleinman, 1988b). If not all symptoms are metaphors, this example suggests that some certainly are.

Second, what, then, is a symptom? Having defined it as a symbol, we must then explain what a symbol is. For Peirce, a symbol is that which signifies something "by virtue of a law;" that is, Saussure's signs of social life (military signals, spoken and written language, ASL and other sign languages, etc.). But to say at this point that symptoms are Peircean symbols contributes nothing new. Verbally expressed complaints are clearly part of the domain of language, although it is also true that, according to Staiano's interpretation of Peirce, we can take this further. For instance, we might suggest that the objects and the interpretants of (Peircean) signs can be very different for patients and practitioners. We could identify the symptom as the original *representamen* which sets in motion a whole constellation of patient interpretants that constitute the narrative itself, a sort of unlimited text that for reasons of interpretive economy will have to be confined to the nearest chain of interpretants. But despite its interesting possibilities, Peirce's scheme is excessively restricted by its formalism and abstraction to the production of signs rather than to the meanings that can be condensed in a particular time-space-group relation. Additionally, Peirce's triadic approach is susceptible to interpretations which place excessive emphasis on the idea of a single first interpretant, when the meaningful dimension of symptom is plural and allows for different and even simultaneous interpretants. As Kleinman warned in his classic *Patients and Healers in the Context of Culture*: "Vagueness, multiplicity of meanings, frequent changes, and lack of sharp boundaries between ideas and experiences are characteristic of lay EMs" (1980, p. 107).

Staiano also admits that on her return from Belize, she found that some of her data resisted her attempts to order and homogenize it. Thus: "I was led to the conclusion that much of the variability I had encountered was valid and not an artifact of the manner in which I had collected the data" (1982, p. 327).

Obviously, this is not a new experience for anthropologists. I bring it up here in order to suggest that this multiplicity of content can also be seen in a symptom, and for this reason a different definition of symbol may prove more useful.

Third, once the broad, Peircean version of "symbol" has been set aside, we must still sort through numerous definitions of this term ranging from Saussure to Lévi-Strauss, from Edmund Leach or Mary Douglas to Freud or Lacan, from Dan Sperber to Todorov. However, in the interest of economy, we can agree with Eco that the symbolic mode, unlike metaphor, permits a second meaning without losing the semantic coherence of its literal dimension (1984, p. 282). Although for some the only meaning of "my nerves are bothering me" is restlessness and agitation, it is fair to say that this statement may also have a literal meaning distinct from expressions such as "to have a glass" or "the king of the jungle." The symbolic mode does not, therefore, deny the literal coherence of meaning, even though—and here Eco would agree with Ricoeur—it may refer to a second meaning which can be the object of interpretation (Ricoeur, 1969, p. 16) or a *depth-interpretation*

(Ricoeur, 1979, p. 97). Following Paul Ricoeur's concepts of symbol and interpretation in *Le conflit des interpretations*:

> By symbol I mean all those meaningful structures in which a direct, primary, literal meaning also has another indirect, secondary, figurative meaning which can only be understood through the first. *This delimitation of expressions with a double meaning constitutes the hermeneutic field itself.* (1969, p.16) [italics in original] [my translation].

And also:

> *...interpretation, let us say, is the thought required to decode the hidden meaning within the apparent meaning to extract the levels of meaning involved in the literal meaning* (1969, p. 16) [italics in original] [my translation].

Fourth, if, following Ricoeur, symptoms are symbols, can the symptom also be a text? This is the approach Staiano and Good have taken, through without elaborating a great deal on Ricoeur's "model of the text," and I find that it not only preserves our understanding of the symptom as symbol, but also allows us to expand on considerations only briefly introduced in the previous chapter. Ricoeur points out, for example, that there is a difference between speech and text, even when both represent discourse (*parole*) as opposed to language (*langue*). In speech, there is considerable overlap between "the said" (*noema*) and the speaker's intention (*noesis*). However, when discourse is fixed through inscription, "the said" is objectified, and a gap opens up between the intention of the author (which is sometimes impossible to know) and the intention of the work. In this way a text acquires a life and intention of its own. It becomes a "human document" intelligible without the physical and/or psychological presence of its author, and even without knowledge of his or her intentions (Ricoeur, 1979, p. 78). Ricoeur thus enables us to endow symptom with "objectivity," not by way of reification or by analogy with physical signs, but through restoring to the object much of its meaningful complexity. This idea also has ethnographic possibilities, since ethnographers are interested in the hierarchies of meaning present within a code, shared meaning rather than individual subjectivity. Ethnography remains the inscription or objectivization of such hierarchies of meaning. We must not lose sight of the fact that it is not the sender of the message who enables the symptom to stand on its own as a work independent of the presence of its author, but the interpreter of the message, who inscribes it. The ethnographer encounters the symptom as gestural or spoken discourse lacking a clear separation between the intention of the author and the intention of the work. The textual analogy acquires its veracity from the action of the interpreter, who artificially separates these two intentions. For this reason it is difficult to maintain that symptoms are texts; it is simpler to say that a symptom can be interpreted as a text, or that it is almost always necessary to textualize a symptom in order to account for it. This leaves us with two propositions: a) symptoms can be regarded as symbolic constructions; and b) because ethnographic procedure requires the textualization of symptoms, the textual analogy can be used although with some caution. Two further points of equal importance should be added here: c) the multiple meanings (both literal and symbolic) of a symptom cluster around two poles resembling the ones defined by Turner for dominant ritual symbols: a sensory or orectic pole, which in this case represents physical and psychological sensations; and an ideological pole, which represents moral, political and cultural categories; and d) just as in textual interpretation, where interpretive conjectures can be tested by whether or not they are supported by the text as a whole (Eco, 1996, p. 41), the considerable polysemic potential of a symptom must be limited by investigating its meaningful relation with its context.

The difficulty here lies in the extent to which a symptom can be approached as a symbolic construction. How sure of this can we be? What polysemy can a symptom contain? What meanings? What is the relation between the symptom and cultural values, norms and categories? Do symptoms really have two poles of meaning?

Below, in an attempt to answer these questions, I present an ethnographic interpretation[1] of a type of symptom and complaint which, at a formal level, can be found in many different cultural contexts but which, nonetheless, acquires specific meanings in a distinctive microcontext. These symptoms are variously expressed as: "I'm a bundle of nerves!"; "I'm getting nervous."; "My nerves won't stand it!"; "I suffer from nerves."; "My nerves are giving me trouble." or, when the past is evoked, "I had a nervous breakdown." or "I did such crazy things, I must have had a minor nervous breakdown." The informants are all people diagnosed with "schizophrenia" or other "psychotic" pathologies according to DSM-III and DSM-III-R in various psychiatric institutions in Barcelona, the capital of Catalonia in northeastern Spain, an industrialized Mediterranean city with a population of about two million inhabitants and a system of psychiatric care structured into three levels: primary mental health care; hospitalization, which differentiates between short- and long-term admissions (acute and chronic disorders, respectively); and centers for psychosocial rehabilitation, which along with recreational clubs and apartments for assisted independent living make up what is called the tertiary level of care. Most of the information presented here comes from this last type of source.

The users of the psychosocial rehabilitation centers and clubs all live in the city of Barcelona, but do not necessarily belong to the majority Catalan ethnic and linguistic group. Many of them represent the characteristic cultural and linguistic diversity of the Spanish state, coming from Castile, Andalusia, Estremadura, the Basque Country, Galicia, the Canary Islands, Valencia, Asturias, etc. while a much smaller minority are immigrants from other European societies, North Africans or Latin Americans. Most of them are male (70%), of low socio-economic status (80%), and of an average age between 27 and 35. They live with their families and usually stay in the rehabilitation centers between 9 a.m. and 7 p.m. from Monday to Friday. Their tasks in these centers consist of what the psychologists call "the development of social skills" and various activities such as bookbinding or photocopying. The treatment they receive is about the same as in any neo-Kraepelinian psychiatric institution: ECT, neuroleptics and psychotherapy (behavioral or cognitive). However, the generalization of treatment should not be understood as a sort of natural condition for the production of symptoms, but simply as one of the elements which helps to create a distinctive social microcontext together with other variables which include the power relations between psychotherapists and patients, stigmatizing encounters with neighbors and passers-by, family conflicts, drug treatment, and the self-legitimation and delegitimation games embedded in the behavior and speech of the informants. The ethnographic example presented below is one I have chosen for its value as a limiting case; in neo-Kraepelinian psychiatry, schizophrenic discourse is regarded as uninterpretable, disorganized and meaningless speech whose very form is a sign of organic dysfunction. However, as we shall see, it is far from being complete nonsense. In the speech of schizophrenics there is also room for meanings which are open to interpretation. In taking an extreme case as my example, then, I test the power of a hermeneutic approach to the analysis of symptoms.

NERVIOS, SYMPTOMS AND CONTEXT

Nervios is one of those cases in which the boundary between symptom and emic diagnosis is unclear. The expression "I suffer from nerves" may be both a complaint and a sort of self-diagnosis based on folk or lay knowledge. But this is not a problem exclusive to our case. In many other instances symptoms and names of diseases are closely linked, not only in lay contexts but in biomedicine and contemporary psychiatry as well. As Kleinman and Good ask themselves, What is depression? A disease, a symptom or a mood? (1985, p. 2). In fact, "depression" in neo-Kraepelinian psychiatry identifies both a disease and a symptom, to the extent that they become confused, for when symptoms are reified as physical signs it is sometimes impossible to know where one ends and the other begins. However, it is fair to say that psychiatry distinguishes the symptom from the disease as the part is distinguished from the whole. "Depression" is therefore a symptom insofar as it is accompanied by other symptoms which make up a nosologically different grouping.

But how can anthropology differentiate between folk illness and symptom? The existing literature offers no answers to this question. And perhaps it is not so essential for interpretive anthropology to differentiate between symptom and emic diagnosis, since this is a distinction established by biomedical knowledge and not necessarily present in lay knowledge. In the end, whether it is categorized as either self-diagnosis or complaint, the discourse of the informant is still evidence of distress, and for the ethnographer it remains a point of entry into a particular narrative in which the important thing is not the formal differentiation of categories, but the web of meanings behind the expression. However, I would tentatively suggest a distinction between the use of categories, such as "nerves" or "migraine" to define an illness, and forms of expression that convey the immediacy of distress, such as "I'm having a nervous breakdown!" or "I've got a migraine!" This approach seems to be the most appropriate, although it is not without practical problems of the sort I encountered when one of my informants told me: "I have a problem with my nerves. I get so nervous! I have terrible convulsions! It's a symbiosis." Here diagnosis and symptom are nearly impossible to separate. Textualized by ethnographic description, the complaint merges with the diagnostic category.

"I suffer from nerves" or "I'm having a nervous attack!" were symptoms constructed by all the schizophrenic patients of my acquaintance regardless of their different ethnic affiliations. It appears as a constant in many of the narratives I recorded, although because of the variety of cultural and historical traditions which my informants represent, it is risky to equate "I suffer from nerves" with "*narahatiye qalb*." To cite just a few examples from the ethnographic literature on terminologically related symptoms and malaises, the "*ataque de nervios*" of Hispanic North Americans and the Caribbean (Low, 1981, 1994; Guarnaccia, Canino, Rubio-Stipec & Bravo, 1993; Swerdlow, 1992) should be differentiated from the "*nervoso*" of the Brazilian *favela* dwellers (Scheper-Hughes, 1992) and the *nevra* of the emigrant Greek women, which Margaret Lock has related to nostalgia (Lock, 1991; see also Dunk 1988).

Nevertheless, I noticed that *nervios* is a category easily accepted by all my informants. Toward the end of my fieldwork, I even brought it up occasionally in order to find out to what extent it was a shared category, and invariably my expectations were confirmed. *Nervios* was a sort of communicative meeting point, not by chance, but because it was part of the symbolic universe of the kinship and friendship network of the patients, who used expressions such as "J's nerves are in bad shape" or "P had a nervous attack the other day." In these cases it was a veiled way of pointing to affliction and disruptive behavior, which family members associated with madness (*locura* in Spanish, *bogeria* in Catalan) or, when they used psychiatric terms, with "schizophrenia." The language of "nerves," then, was common not only to patients but also to the family universe of interaction: neighbors, workmates, etc. It suggested that the patient's problem was "something normal," just as it was also "normal" for this to have happened in a particular family. When the patient's "illness" was socially normalized, the family, in consequence, was destigmatized. Nevertheless, under some circumstances this protective attitude could give way to its opposite. On these occasions, it was less a question of *nervios* than of a social and moral blemish.

When family members spoke of the patient's affliction in terms of *nervios*, they were expressing understanding and support, but when the situation became critical they tended to appeal to the patient's capacity for self-control, and it was not unusual to hear them say, "Take your medication. You have to take it because you are mentally ill"; or "If you don't take your medication, you'll get sick again;" or "You're crazy and you must listen to what your mother says." *Nervios* emerged, then, as a normalizing category which could be substituted by others—"madness" or "illness"— if the exercise of coercive authority was thought necessary; for example, when the informant refused to "take his medication," or when the public image of the family was at stake.

It should come as no surprise that the question of medication was one of the main causes of conflict between the family and the patient. From the family's point of view, it was one of the few available resources for preventing the sort of behavior that Goffman called transgressive (for instance, storing trash in the bedroom, shouting at night in nearby streets, or behaving publicly in a sexually promiscuous way). Refusing treatment was a principal point of patient resistance, allowing the patient to claim greater personal autonomy by rejecting the diagnosis: "I feel fine. Fourteen years ago my nerves were real bad, but it was just a moment of madness, and it's over now. It's over."

This presents us with a conflict of interests and meanings. Relatives, age mates and workmates consider the patients' behavior to be "dangerous" both to others and to themselves, because they are unaware of what they are doing. This idea comes out quite clearly in family members' narratives but also in other "texts;" for example, the following letter sent by some of Alba's former co-workers sent to the judge in support of her involuntary commitment to a "psychiatric center":

> We, the undersigned, are employed at Bank X...and we have all been Alba's co-workers. We request that a writ be issued for her admission to a psychiatric center so that she can receive treatment for her mental and physical condition. We enclose two photocopies of the diagnosis and confirmation that she has been found unable to work by reason of mental illness.

They go on to say that Alba was diagnosed as having "paranoid schizophrenia," that she had been an inpatient in various "psychiatric centers," and that matters had come to a head because "she isn't taking any medication or seeing a doctor and she is living on the street." But what is most interesting here are the "objective" reasons brought forward to justify her hospitalization:

> Her behavior is typical of this sort of illness—she has a glazed look, and she sings, shouts or weeps in the company's operations room without seeming to mind—or without even noticing—the presence of customers or co-workers. She treats the company as if it were her own home and in the operations room she combs her hair, changes her clothes and spreads her personal possessions (which she carries in baskets or bags) on the floor, etc. She often locks herself in the bathroom, naked, beating the walls and any other object within reach, crying and shouting for long periods of time. She also uses the bathroom to wash her clothes, which are filthy and smell unbearably. She then uses these clothes to wash herself.
>
> It is getting more and more difficult to make her see sense because she is completely crazy and cannot reason or understand. Her mind is split in two and the periods of lucidity are increasingly shorter....She is vulnerable to all kinds of danger, and her health is deteriorating day by day. We are witnesses to her gradual disintegration, but powerless to help because she cannot make decisions for herself and nobody has taken charge of her....We have no wish to wait until it is too late, we must help her before it is no longer possible to do so.

This letter, which recalls the behavior of the Gururumba wild man, expresses a generalized social attitude about the behavior of my informants: mental illness cancels out its victim's self-awareness and personal autonomy ("she cannot make decisions for herself"), creating the conditions for the development of socially inappropriate behaviors (the use of a banking institution as a home), which demand a response from the appropriate social and institutional mechanisms. The cultural context is obviously not that of the Gururumba; here we are dealing with a complex society in which other people and institutions play their roles: the judge; the co-workers; the person suffering from "schizophrenia"; the psychiatric center as a suitable environment for Alba; and the perplexed bank customers only briefly alluded to, but nonetheless also present in the text. What is of real interest here is the shared interpretation of Alba and her inability to act as a conscious social subject. Although the writers of the letter are laypersons, and a small subset of laypersons at that, it is not too much to assume that their demand for Alba's institutionalization is representative of what is regarded as appropriate and inappropriate, normal and abnormal, healthy and pathological in a broader context, or at least in the context formed by banks and psychiatric centers dealing with persons who use "the operations room" as a home.

The medical-psychiatric system not only supports the beliefs of the lay people; it is also used by them to justify their case for Alba's hospitalization. From their litany of arguments—she has been diagnosed as having schizophrenia; she has already been admitted to several psychiatric centers; when she takes medication her crises subside—we can infer (if only within the small universe of the letter) that the judgments of lay people and psychiatrists coincide. It should also be said that this sort of letter is rarely written without the help of a psychiatrist who knows the legal mechanisms required for involuntary commitment; otherwise, where would laypersons get the idea that Alba's behavior "is typical of this sort of illness"? Thus, this letter represents a universe of meanings shared by professionals and lay people defining what is happening to Alba as a disease, and proposing a way to solve the problem.

However, things usually look quite different from the other side. Alba, for example, does not believe that she should be confined to a psychiatric center (otherwise a letter requesting involuntary hospitalization would not have been necessary). Neither does she see her behavior as a problem for either her former co-workers or for herself. She does not even think that she needs psychiatric help to solve her problems, or at least not to the extent suggested by her co-workers' letter to the judge. And although Alba only complains sporadically about her nerves, on the occasions when I was able to converse with her, she expressed opinions not unlike those of another informant, Manel, concerning his admission to a psychiatric center:

> I was fine. Well, my nerves were really bad and I was going around all dirty. I hadn't changed my clothes because I had a very difficult exam. The police brought me here for a shower. I don't really understand it because it's quite normal, isn't it?

Manel went on to explain more clearly that it was "normal" to be "nervous" before such an important exam, just as it was not to have shaved or showered. In this way he rejected the possibility that an illness or disorder might have led to his hospitalization. Having a normal episode of *nervios* delegitimated the attitude of his family and therapists, and their insistence on the need for pharmacological or psychological therapy on an inpatient basis. Even when he had no choice but to admit that he was in a psychiatric hospital and that he was receiving certain drugs, he continued to defend his social position:

> They give medication to everyone. They've given me something which isn't very strong so that I can stay calm in here. I'm really fed up with this place.

Estroff's account of North American "schizophrenics" makes reference to a normalizing discourse stressing the idea that "everybody's got a little mental illness" (Estroff et al., 1991). Here, instead of extending a stigmatizing category to a general context, more polysemic and neutral categories like *nervios* are used to reflect clearly exogenous circumstances—in this case, preparing for an exam.

If we understand that lay people and professionals can agree about the classification of a particular type of behavior, we can also understand that my informants, despite their ethnic diversity, were able to develop more or less common strategies, complaining of nerves instead of illness, madness, schizophrenia or any other category that would involve losing their autonomy as social actors. To what extent this can be seen as the product of a particular subculture of people who share a social position and repertoire of routines is a matter of controversy, especially in light of the way schizophrenia has been regarded as a sort of deculturalization. Unlike shamanic dissociation, which uses cultural patterns to organize the experience, in schizophrenia it is the experience itself that seems to disrupt the cultural tradition (Devereux, 1973, p. 55). It is precisely this rupture which leads to social consensus about schizophrenia, which in turn provokes resistance on the part of some of those affected by it. Responses vary, but complaining about one's nerves, even in the case of those who are obviously ill, is one possible strategy for avoiding social delegitimation. Even the possibility that schizophrenia is caused by a neurochemical dysfunction which leads to irreversible cognitive impairment detracts nothing, at least in this case, from the creative and communicative potential of the afflicted in the face of shared experience. Although Kraepelin saw in this no more than disorganized and uninterpretable speech, my informants evidenced a real need to organize their experience of distress in terms of cultural categories, and here *nervios* became a form of resistance to the threat of social delegitimation.

I want to point out, however, that the meaning of such complaints as "I suffer from nerves" or "my nerves are acting up" is not limited to resistance. "Nerves", in fact, became a symbol which condensed various individualized meanings as well as shared meanings.

DISPARITIES: SYMPTOMS AND NARRATIVES

In an attempt to illustrate the diversity of possible meanings contained in the symptom "I suffer from nerves" or "My nerves are real bad," I present below the narratives of three informants of different ethnic origin who made frequent use of this complaint. All three were extensively interviewed, although the texts vary substantially in length according to the narrative ability of each informant. They were all asked what they meant by "My nerves are real bad" or similar complaints. In all three cases *nervios* was expressed in the symbolic universe of the informants as the core of their affliction, but in the first case the symptom referred primarily to an interpersonal conflict and took on the character of moral self-defense against these situations; in the second, it was a self-reflexive and autobiographical symbol that evoked situations of torture; and in the third case it emerged as an obstacle to the informant's creative aspirations.

Narrative I: "The plaintiff"

Observation: María is an Andalusian woman (from the south of Spain) about 45 years of age who has lived for several decades in Barcelona. When asked "What do you mean by 'nerves'?" she became agitated and responded with a strange story full of contradictory assertions in which multiple meanings referring to family and marital conflicts were linked to the symptom. The interview was recorded on tape, in Spanish.

My nerves are in bad shape. My husband makes me real nervous because he rapes me and calls me a ball of fat...My husband is real big and he hurts me, every time he makes love to me he rapes me. I don't want him to make love to me. The main thing is that I am tired of him because all he does is exploit me. He's had me working for him for nineteen years and he hasn't paid me a nickel and he doesn't give me enough for the food; and when he does give me something it's only a thousand *pesetas* [Spanish currency] and there are the two of us and two kids to feed. And he goes to restaurants and spends five thousand pesetas on a meal, and then drops another ten thousand pesetas playing the slot machines. I don't want to hate him. And my husband hates my mother. And my mother hates her...my husband. And on top of everything he got mad at me because I went off with my father and he said that that was the last straw and he took our apartment which is worth 12 million pesetas away from me and my children and I'm waiting for the trial because I don't have enough money to hire a lawyer. Doctor J.A.M.will back me up. He's a psychometrist and he lives in G, on X Street, telephone...well, I don't remember the telephone number. But J.A.M. will back me up and he's been on television as a commentator. And Mr. A.O.P. will also back me up which shows that he's right... And now I'm here because I went to the bank, I wanted to leave the house and I stole fifty thousand pesetas from my mother and I gave her back twenty and I wanted to live my own life because I've been handicapped all my life. At home they make my life impossible. I've got no say in things at home. I'm a nobody. Only David [her son] loves me. Everybody else orders me around. The house is filthy and he does nothing around the house. Off he goes to the slot machines to lose ten thousand pesetas.My son is the only one who loves me. He was born on day x of y, Saint C's day, at four o'clock in the afternoon. I was eating a slice of melon. It was really hot, thirty-two degrees [Celsius].

   I'm handicapped. I'm shortsighted. I have 1.75 in each eye. I wear orthopedic shoes. I'm handicapped and now I'm applying to see if they'll give me some money. They have asked me for a certificate to show I'm living with my husband but he doesn't know that I've reported him, that I've filed a complaint... I was going to write direct to the Pope so that they would annul the marriage but because I have two kids he won't do it. Because I was married by the Roman, Catholic, and Apostolic Church and I received Christ in the grace of God. I have received all the sacraments, the first baptism, the second confirmation, the third penitence, the fourth Eucharist, the fifth extreme unction, the sixth holy orders and the seventh matrimony. I'm a poetess:

My God does not move me to love you
nor the heaven that He has promised me.
Neither does the Hell which we fear

move me to stop offending you

My husband makes me a nervous wreck because every time he rapes me I go out of my mind, and since my little girl was born four years ago we haven't made love. I haven't made love with anybody for a year and I never have.

Narrative II: "The son of the tiger hunter who never killed a tiger"

<u>Observation</u>: Babu is a Konkan about 35 years of age. He complains constantly of being "a nervous wreck", which he traces back to an episode of torture to which he was subjected as a child. He also feels "depressed," and constantly revisits his past and his relationships with his family. Here the symptom acts as a reflexive symbol which allows him to make sense of his affliction through the interpretation of biography. The text combines material from several interviews, in Spanish and English.

I was born in the south of India. My parents are from there from Misoré [Mangalore]. It's a simple town, more agricultural than industrial. It has long, wide beaches. There is plenty of fish, tropical fruit and a lot of rice. It's surrounded by the jungle which is full of coconuts, mangos and wild animals. When I was a few months old my parents took me to Bombay, but I started going back to Misoré to spend some time with my mother when I was four. Both my father and my mother had houses there. I remember that in my mother's house there was a garden where the servants used to make bracelets with flowers. There was a water well in the middle of the garden. In those days people were very simple. They speak Tulu there. I was in love with one of our servants. She was very beautiful and had long hair. I used to sit in her lap and caress her breasts. She told me that I was a very jealous boy. One of my first disappointments was when she left. She got married to an Englishman who was the general manager of a big company, and went to live in Scotland. Everybody at home was against that marriage, specially my mother who said that a "*hariya*" couldn't get married to a white man.

My father liked coming to Misoré as well. Both my mother and my father came to be alone and not have to put up with each other. My father had many friends there and he would go with them to the jungle to hunt tigers and boars. After the hunt he would play cards, drink and argue with them until a fight started. When he was drunk he got very violent, he was very independent and took a lot of risks. In fact, he ruined us by betting on the horses. He was capable of driving for ten or fifteen hours to go to the race track and put down some bets. I was a cowardly child, though. I was frightened of the jungle. I was terrified that the snakes would fall on my bed at night.

One day when I was 7 or 8 years old my father took me out of Bombay and, without saying anything to my mother, took me hunting in the South. I had to follow him around the jungle. Sometimes we couldn't see anything. We cut the thick vegetation with machetes and at night we waited for the tigers. He said that I had to lose my fear. He gave me a rifle to shoot our dog that had just broken one of its back legs but I couldn't do it. He told me that I wasn't a man: 'You are a coward like your mother. Why are you scared of everything?'. He wasn't afraid of anything, though, not even death. He wandered around the jungle at night without a care in the world while I was scared stiff even at home. He picked up snakes with his bare hands and threw them against trees. His friends called him "fearless." To try to make me lose my fear he used to put dolls and fruit on my head and then shoot them off. He was a good shot. I can't understand why he never shot a tiger. His friends had shot several.

My father was a middle-ranking executive with Company X. He took the gasoline and fuel to the planes. He was in charge of 15 or 20 people and he did their work for them to show that he was the best. Some nights I went with him to his office at the airport to see the foreigners and the airplanes arriving in Bombay. The bosses of the company wanted to throw him out because he defended the workers, but he had a lot of prestige in the company. The workers used to come home and drink with him. Then they would start fighting. They used to bow down at his feet so that he wouldn't hit them. He said that they were like women. My grandfather was very authoritarian. In the south of India the landowners controlled everything, even the lives of their workers. My father admired generals like Rommel, Napoleon and Gandhi. He didn't know how to be diplomatic with anybody. He didn't trust people who didn't drink. He didn't trust anybody who didn't drink with him because he thought they might be trying to take advantage of him.

One night, when I was nine, I saw my father make love to one of my aunts. She was a cousin of his who was also married but who he had sexual relations with, so it seems. At that moment I felt a burning desire to kill my aunt. My father was a great ladies' man, but I never managed to attract a single one. I was a sickly child and always had bronchitis. My father used to say that my ears were like a rabbit's and so he called me *dobo-soso* which in Konkani means "white rabbit." He told my uncles and aunts that I looked more like a woman than a man and that I was skinny and frail like someone with tuberculosis. He wanted me to be strong and brave and I was afraid of disappointing him. He got furious when I cried. For him, crying was one of the most contemptible things. It was a sissy thing and not something that a man should do. I only saw him cry once: the day my mother died.

My grandmother was an old Konkani who had once been very rich. Both she and my grandfather were of the landowning Brahmin caste (*smartha*). She was always telling us stories about the past, like the time she was invited by Queen Victoria when she visited India. For her my father could do no wrong. She never reproached him for anything, even for coming back drunk every night and beating my mother and the rest of us. He was always right and everything he did was correct. When she was staying with us in Bombay she was the boss. She argued with my mother and wouldn't let her run the household. I hated my grandmother. She poisoned our lives. Sometimes I played tricks on her, like pulling her hair when her back was turned and then running off. Because she was old and ailing she took ages to turn round and she never realized who it was.

My mother took real good care of me. At night she sang songs and told me the story of 'Little Red Riding Hood.' She called me *re*, which in Hindustani means 'dear' and in Konkani 'king.' During the monsoon season she carried me to school so that I wouldn't catch a cold and when I was ill she would go to school and take notes for me. She was a primary-school teacher, but had stopped working when she got married. I was a good student until I was 15 which is when I had typhus. From then on I began to lose my intelligence. I was very used to being spoiled by my mother. I think she treated me better than my sisters. In India women are still regarded as something of a problem. When they get married they have to be given a dowry. Many marriages in India are arranged by the parents. When my mother left me at school I always thought about her. I always used to sleep with her because she didn't sleep with my father. She was afraid of him. Once I saw my father hit her so hard that the whip broke.

One night my father arrived home. My mother was pregnant and he made her lift a lump of granite above her head. It was a stone that we used to grind spices. She was crying and I was beating my father, but then he beat us both. It was like this every day. He laid down rules for my mother: 'first rule, when I speak about something you have to respond correctly to the question I ask you on the same subject; second rule, you have to speak slowly without raising your voice because the women who raise their voices are the ones who sell fish in the market, with no class, pariahs; third rule, when you make a mistake, apologize.'

He often came back drunk at night. Whenever he got drunk he picked fights with people. He woke us up. My mother slept with me in one bed and my sisters slept in another. He used to wake us up and beat us. Then he would pick up a gun, put it to my head and fire. It wasn't loaded, but I could never be absolutely sure. This happened night after night. We all cried. The next day he would behave as if nothing had happened. We were all afraid of speaking to him. Our nerves were in shreds. My mother had periods of depression and nervous breakdowns. She got frightened and began to tremble. My eldest sister, R, also has 'nervous disorder.' My other sister who lives in Y [an Arab country] also suffers from her nerves and her hands shake. My mother said that her mother [the grandmother] had gone crazy because her boyfriend got married to someone else. She started drinking and walking around the streets naked. But my mother said nothing about this outside the house, because in India mental diseases are taboo. In the psychiatric hospitals in India they beat the patients. Indian society hasn't accepted mental illness. If one of the family has a mental illness, they are treated very badly, and everybody is against them. This happens when a person has *pagal*, but not when they have depression or nerves. *Pagal* cannot be cured and it's for the poor people, the *shudras* and the *pariahs*.

I loved my mother very much. I slept with her until I was 21 or 22 when I went to England. This is normal in India. Later I hated her because she didn't divorce my father. She said that there was nothing to be done. In India it is not considered proper for a woman to get divorced.

When I was eleven I began to masturbate. Almost every day. I used to do it slowly thinking about my schoolteacher, who was very pretty. My father used to say that sex was normal. He was always surrounded by women. He looked like David Niven. He was tall. I had no luck with women, though... My father liked this and told me that I was a coward and that I was like a woman. He said that I looked queer but I was never attracted to men. One day a boy of about twenty years old invited me to go to the cinema and started to touch me. He was a neighbor of ours. I didn't stay to watch the film and ran out. Later, at university, I fell in love with a girl in my class. She rejected me. She said she loved me as a friend. At this point I began to drink. I arrived home drunk every night. This went on for two years. Sometimes my father asked me to drink a liquor called *daru* with him. I told him that I didn't like drinking spirits, but when I went out drinking I did drink it as well. The thing was that I didn't want to drink with my father because he always got violent when he was drunk.

One night before I went to England I hit my father and broke his teeth because he was going to hit my mother. I had to run out of the house because he wanted to shoot me. I had to spend six days in the country. When I went back he behaved as if nothing had happened. Then I went to England where one of my sisters lived. There I worked part-time as a shoe salesman and a waiter while I did my degree. I started going to a club for foreigners. I wanted to find myself a girlfriend, but it was difficult for me to find an English girlfriend because the English are very colonial and the Indians have an inferiority complex with them. It was also difficult to find an Indian girl because I spoke little Hindustani. Religion was also a barrier because I am Catholic. In India, the Hindus look down on the Catholics because we eat pork. What's more, the Catholic Indian girls wanted to marry English men and not me. I began to hate the English because I wasn't having any luck with the women. There, in the club, I met my wife. She is a teacher and had gone to London to study English. By that time I had finished my degree and was working in a multinational corporation. I didn't get on too well with some of my colleagues. I felt that I was losing my capacity for knowledge. My colleagues noticed this and I had to work a lot of hours. I began to get nervous. Then I got married and I came to Spain.

When I was working here [in Barcelona] my nerves got very bad. I was depressed and I didn't want to leave the house. I remembered those nights of torture with my father, when he whipped my brother on his penis and when he pretended to shoot me in the head and I was always expecting him to kill me.

But he never did. I thought that, because I had suffered so much, I was Jesus Christ. When I was a child I had sometimes had fantasies about being a famous soccer or tennis player, acclaimed by the people. Or that I was a great scientist and I had made an important discovery, or I was really Swedish and had been adopted by some dirty Indians. Now I also thought that I was very important. Work was going badly. I was feeling very nervous and had cerebral paralysis, I couldn't work and always had to stay after everyone else had gone home. I knew they wanted to get rid of me but before this happened my nerves got bad and I took some sick leave. The last days that I worked I began to think stupid things, for example, the American bosses were going to come to Barcelona and promote me to director. My boss would then bow and scrape and beg forgiveness. Everybody praised me. And the truth is that when I walked through the office I seemed to hear people cheering and hailing me as their new boss. Then I began to think that I was the president of all the foreign multinational companies in Barcelona and they would come to ask me for work and favors. When I was walking down the street I thought that the women who were wearing blue and white wanted to be my lovers, and the men who were wearing the same colors were my collaborators. President Bush had stepped down to give me a chance because I was more intelligent. When I watched American television, by satellite, I thought they were speaking about me because they had installed an electronic device in my house to protect me from assassination attempts. But by this time being President of the USA was not enough and I wanted to be king of the whole world, and as I had suffered so much as a child it was as if I had been crucified by my father, because I have never heard a story like mine anywhere. It was terrible, a continuous torture. Then I had come back to life to help all the people. I had stopped being Babu to become Jesus Christ.

Narrative III: "The artist"

Observation: Rafael is a thirty-year-old Catalan. He complains of "being nervous" and of "having a turn." In his case the symptom refers to the unwanted effects of his medication, which prevent him from developing his creativity. Here, "being nervous" becomes a way of expressing his desire to negotiate his treatment.[2] This interview was recorded on tape, in Catalan.

When I have a turn it's terrible. The medication makes me real nervous and stops me from being creative. It's a real bad case of nerves, because being a painter you may see one thing and you see two, three or four possibilities in it, and you work on them as they grab your interest. I work as they grab my interest, and they do grab my interest. The artistic perception of things sometimes keeps you from leading a practical life, eh! My problem is one of social order, undoubtedly of social and personal order. The problem is being marginalized, and medication doesn't help at all. The only solution is to talk it over, put our cards on the table and talk.

I had a turn, I had a crisis but I'm getting over it now. I don't want to label it as schizophrenia or anything like that. My partner left me and I started drinking heavily. A liter of wine a day, plus the beers I drank in the bars. I began to hear voices and I thought everyone was looking at me. My body began to slow down. I heard the kids [of one of the neighbors] saying things like, 'Do you want some coffee?' or 'Tell us a story' and I would tell them a story while I sketched whatever came to mind. I was studying science then and I kept my calculations and concepts hidden in a cupboard. I was afraid someone might come and take them for their own purposes. You know, copy my ideas or something like that. These things were really important because they were the guidelines for my creative process. They were the guidelines that I wanted to use to direct my creative or artistic process. It's embarrassing to speak about this, eh! [...] Well, I'll tell you about it as well as I can because it's the first time I've talked about this. It's the most vulnerable point of my ability to understand things.

Well look, in a nutshell, I had tried to be a mathematician and a physicist at the same time. Then I saw that by studying science I could see through the molecular structure of neurons or of anything else I chose to study. They had a particular form and I used this form to create art. Just the way a mathematical form could derive into particular signs or a scientific experiment could have a special image. Well, I used it to create symbolic forms such as, I don't know, an upside-down wineglass. Subtle details, but they say a lot about active things in science. I was interested in relating science to art. I chose science because we artists emulate what we want science to be and so science rides on what we have tried to express in art. Just think of Leonardo, or so many other painters who perhaps have provided answers for postindustrial society, who have tried to understand science so that, through their work, a whole series of abstract concepts that people don't understand will become viable. Painting, cubism for instance, was an expression of spatial geometry that got to be really productive, or the spectrometry that Dalí used. I believe that science should be subordinate to art, to the creative spirit, but now science is trying to function by itself, without art and this hurts people. Scientists aren't creative.

Artists have worked on all these things and that is why I was involved. I liked being creative and I liked the way things were. I didn't want things to be public because I am very shy. And that's what I wanted to do, relate science and art. I know I was a bit crazy [Catalan, *pirat*] but it's all over now. It was a crisis but that doesn't mean that I can't continue to be creative, but with my feet more firmly on the ground [Catalan, *seny*]. The problem now is not that I'm crazy. The problem is the medication. It's nasty because it's wrecking my nerves. I can't think or do anything. This is the problem I have now. The tension building up in me is causing my creativity to stagnate. I believe that there are interesting things in science that I can make use of for art, even if it's only on the level of images and forms. But my nerves won't let me. Look, it starts so slow I don't even realize it, and then suddenly it hits me, I go all funny and I can't do anything for the rest of the day, man! I can't keep on being creative when I'm like this. Couldn't you give me something that isn't as strong?

Apart from the pathological meanings which can be derived from a psychiatric and/or psychoanalytic reading, these narratives are meaningful in ways that organize the speakers' experiences of affliction, make sense of their individual situations, and outline strategies for negotiation. Cultural and religious values come into play, and life events and circumstances or intellectualized discourses are evoked. But the important thing here is that the complaints about *nervios* do not refer to an exclusively literal meaning, such as being upset, disturbed, irritated, etc., but condense a complex range of meanings, experiences, emotions, conflicts and events which acquire their meaning in the context of individual biography and social life. I turn now to a more empirically precise examination of these ideas.

In the first case, the symptom "My nerves are in bad shape" condenses a family problem as well as a conflict of experiences and loyalties in which the possibility of a separation is in conflict with Catholic religious values. Nor does one need great powers of interpretation to see that the speaker's expository style is, particularly in the second half, that of a personal defense in which the legal process of separating from her husband and her request for a disability pension seem not only to coincide, but to merge. The fact that she presents herself as a "practicing Catholic" who has received all the sacraments (including extreme unction and holy orders) or that she introduces supposed guarantors, about whom she provides complete information, lends her story a tone of defense against such misfortunes as losing her "twelve-million-peseta" home and the custody of her children. Oddly, "nerves" is not used to justify her application for a disability pension. Instead, she uses the argument of being handicapped, not mentally but physically: "I'm short-sighted. I have 1.75 in each eye. I wear orthopedic shoes." But why doesn't she use the argument of *nervios* here? The answer in this case, from an emic viewpoint, is that *nervios* do not reflect an organic abnormality or pathological impairment but "damage" caused by her husband, and this enables her to base her claim on having been harmed. She is a plaintiff who possesses all the requisite moral and social characteristics ("I have received all the sacraments," "I am a poetess," "... will back me up") while her husband has practically none ("he rapes me," "he plays the slot machines," "he calls me a ball of fat"). Here the symptom is also the symbol of a moral defense grounded in the identification between *nervios* and the "damage" that the defendant (her husband) caused the litigant.

The second case is clearly the richest in content, since the symptom condenses a biographical self-reflection and introduces a story filled with details about caste and gender differences; social institutions such as dowry; expectations about marriage and ethnic hierarchies; and multicultural scenarios in which these forms of organization acquire meaning. Of course, there are many possible interpretations. We may think that when Babu says that "his nerves are in shreds" he is referring to the episodes of torture, and that these experiences re-emerge when he is about to be fired, a strange symbolic death which returns him to a universe of childish fantasy in which, like his father's employees, his co-workers and former boss throw themselves on his mercy. We may consider, without forcing the narrative too much, that his boss represents his father, who pretended to shoot him night after night with an unloaded gun. The presence of certain elements also lends itself to a psychoanalytical interpretation: for instance, the phenomenon known as "the neurotic's family romance" (being a Swedish child) (see Freud, SE, IX, p. 238), or Babu's relationship with his mother and the curious succession of women in his life (his mother is a schoolteacher, he masturbates thinking about his schoolteacher, and finally he marries a schoolteacher). The torture situations can be interpreted as the result of behavior that can easily be understood in Oedipal terms: Babu sleeps with his mother until he is 21 or 22, the father tortures Babu because he sleeps with his wife, and the mother does not want to sleep with her husband because she prefers to be with Babu. The fact that Babu sleeps with his mother until such an advanced age then becomes the reason why he has problems in his relationships with women and, as was indicated in the psychiatric reports, is the source of his "pathological" personality and an evident Oedipus complex.

However, to introduce Oedipal models and pathological personalities at this point could be a serious error of interpretation stemming from an excess of *intentio lectoris*. In Babu's narrative, it is not the son who wants to kill his father, but the father who wants to kill his son. This inversion of the standard psychoanalytical narrative is not a matter of chance, but is firmly rooted in the cultural tradition in which Babu lived. Ramanujan tells us that in the mythology and folktales of South India, an image that appears repeatedly sheds light on situations of the kind described by Babu:

> There is a recurrent motif in folktales in South India and elsewhere: A father returns from a long exile or journey and enters his bedroom to find a strange young man sleeping next to his wife. He draws his sword to kill them both, when either his waking wife or a remembered precept (Don't act when angry) stays his hand. The young man is really his son grown to manhood during his

long absence but still sleeping innocently in the same bed as his dear mother.
(cit. in Obeyesekere, 1990, p. 77).

Here, as in Babu's narrative of affliction, it is filicide and not parricide
that is at stake, and any attempt at psychoanalytic interpretation cannot un-
derestimate the importance of evidence from the cultural context of both the
victim and his torturer. The restitution of an *intentio auctoris* and *operis*
becomes a requirement for any attempt at interpretive rigor. For instance,
when Babu says that it is normal for a son to sleep with his mother until the
age of twenty-one, he is not saying that this is pathological, but simply a
cultural institution representative of his local world. To disregard this is simply to be carried away by the intention of the reader without examining the
intention of the author or of the work to verify our conjectures. That is to say,
it is a misreading that resembles the one parodied by Eco when he writes
that some people read *Oedipus Rex* as if it were a detective story in which
the only interest is to find out whodunit (1996, p. 32).

But let us not wander from the point. When Babu complains that his nerves
are in shreds, he evokes not only a literal sense of discomfort and distress,
but also images of torture that give meaning to his biography. Continuities
appear and take on meaning through the category of *nervios*. The *nervios* are
the result of the nightly behavior of his father who, according to Babu, was
simply modeling himself on his own father, a pattern of absolute authority to
which Babu sees no limits. However, the nerves may also have their origin
in his grandmother on his mother's side, who ran naked through the streets,
and who he defines as a case of *pagal*. All his sisters and his younger brother,
who was whipped on his penis when still a little boy, are also affected by
nerves. Likewise, his mother's reaction to her husband's threats is to tremble.
Thus, *nervios* become a meaningful construction which permits Babu to reflect on a series of family events in which he is involved. But this is not all.
When Babu says "my nerves got very bad" he is also safeguarding his social
position. Babu denies that his affliction is a case of *pagal* and prefers to call
it "fantasies," "nerves," and "depression." Recall that Babu identifies *pagal*
as an incurable disease that only affects individuals of the lower castes. Here
the symptom not only facilitates self-reflection, but also has a symbolic nature which evokes strategies of resistance to loss of social position.

Finally, there is the case of the "artist" who gives us a different version of
what "suffering from nerves" means. From an emic viewpoint, the symptom
in his narrative clearly refers to a "tension" induced by "medication" that
hampers his "creative process." But the second meaning, implicit and sym-

bolic, is of a different order. When Rafael says that he suffers from nerves, he is complaining about a particular psychopharmacological treatment and also, more importantly, arguing that his problem cannot be solved by drugs but by "talking it over" and "putting all our cards on the table." Thus the expression also acquires the meaning of negotiating the medical treatment, and Rafael, in order to strengthen his position, explains that science should be subordinate to art and the creative spirit. Here, science is represented by a supposed therapist while he represents art, so that while seeming to speak of other things, Rafael is also saying that his proposal for ending the treatment is more valid than the opinion of his interlocutor who, of course, is not "creative" and is causing irreparable "damage" (nerves) in the same way that "science is trying to function by itself, without art, and this hurts people."

CONFLUENCES: *NERVIOS* AS A SYMBOL OF RESISTANCE

We have seen that various meanings can emerge from a complaint such as "I suffer from nerves" or "my nerves are very bad." So far, it seems that these kinds of symptoms are *passe-partout* expressions, empty vessels which each informant fills with his or her own autobiographical and experiential meanings. However, behind this great diversity, we have also seen that "nerves" also consistently expresses resistance to the stigma generally associated with categories such as "madness" or "schizophrenia," or to the authority represented mainly by psychiatrists, psychologists and family members. María herself, the author of the first narrative, pointed out that her mother, when angry, said: "You're crazy, you're going to stay crazy forever," to which María replied that she was "suffering from nerves" because of her husband. Likewise Babu, in an attempt to maintain his social position by complaining of nerves, resisted accepting a label that would affect his capacity for personal autonomy. And finally Rafael, who spoke of his "turns" and "crises" in a manner so strongly associated with nerves that they can be considered interchangeable, also said: "I had a turn, I had a crisis which is now being cured. I don't want to label it as 'schizophrenia' or anything like that."

On other occasions *nervios* was used either as a symptom or as an alternative diagnosis, or as both simultaneously. For instance, it was not unusual to hear the following:

> I have schizophrenia, or at least that's what they say. It's nerves, nerves and a lot of fear. I'm afraid of nerves and not belonging. The blood rushed to my

head. I believed in witches and saw microphones. Now I think that such things exist and that they can harm me. I have no intelligence left. After so much thinking and agonizing I've become simple-minded.

Here nerves as a diagnostic category and as a symptom converge to refute the judgment of the psychiatrists. Also:

I feel healthy. Fourteen years ago I had an attack of nerves. I had a moment of momentary and transitory madness, but it passed. I felt stabbed to the heart and my head became unbalanced. I felt mentally ill.

In this last case, the informant refused to let anybody change the phrase "moment of momentary and transitory madness," to such an extent that she screamed or became aggressive if anyone changed the order of the words even slightly. What had happened belonged to the past and no longer affected her, and although she was able to define her affliction as "madness" the stigma was reduced by introducing a temporal dimension and by specifying its "momentary" nature.

Xavier expressed himself in a similar way when he spoke about his past: "Everything's fine, nothing's wrong with me, absolutely nothing. That was just a small crisis of nerves." When I attempted to probe his present feelings, *nervios* became not only a diagnosis but also a symptom:

Sometimes I scream, I get real nervous, I say all the nonsense that comes into my head and then it disappears [...]. It's all because of the medicine and my nerves, and also because I'm worried about my mother. Medicine isn't good for anybody, that's why I'm going to stop taking it. The doctor should reduce my medication, he should reduce it. Then I'd be pleased, I'd be happy. I wouldn't be nervous and I would lead a normal life.

It is not difficult to see that *nervios* and "medication" appear here as parallel meanings which prevent him from leading a "normal life," although in a different way than in Rafael's case.

The complaints about medicine were generalized, and with good reason, because the side effects of anti-psychotic medicines are not easily alleviated. In the course of her fieldwork Estroff (1981, 1982), in order to show the discrepancies between the therapists' view of medication and the psychomotor disturbances that such drugs produced in the patients, ignored Weber's maxim that "one need not have been Caesar in order to understand Caesar" (1968, p. 5) and voluntarily experienced the effects of this type of drug.

Although I did not go to quite the same lengths in my own work, I was able to confirm that in many cases the complaints about the effects of medication are well founded, although this is not to say that the symptoms involving nerves invariably refer only to this universe of meanings. On occasion, nerves and medication, although present, are not associated quite so closely in the narratives of the informants. For instance, Abel told me:

> I have dysentery. Seven years ago something happened that made me real nervous. The doctor prescribed me a strong dose of *Etumina* [a drug] and I masturbated and that gave me dysentery. I can't defecate normally. I don't enjoy eating. I'm worried and my nerves are so bad I'm going to pieces. It could lead to a tumor or a cancer. I'm fed up with telling people but nobody's taking any notice.

Gil said the following:

> I have terrible convulsions, nerves, agitation, pains that tear me apart. It's a symbiosis. In the long term it's fatal. In the long term it's fatal.

In these cases, when the affliction is a physical disease such as dysentery or what Gil calls a "symbiosis," the informant rejects the possibility of a mental disorder or, more specifically, of schizophrenia or related pathologies.

But "nervios" is not always associated with a physical disease. On other occasions patients flatly refuse to accept the existence of a physical disease, and only very grudgingly do they concede that they do have some form of distress that amounts to *nervios*, but they regard it as independent of any treatment or hospitalization:

> I do not have an illness. My parents want to control me and so they've sent me here. I feel perfectly healthy. Well, I'm lazy. I was born bone idle. Sometimes just doing nothing makes me nervous. I've always been nervous but that's quite normal.

Here, "to get nervous" is on a par with other defects like laziness or being "born bone idle," but it is not an illness that should require treatment or prevent him from being at home with his parents.

It is also common for patients to use parents as referents for their present *nervios*. Siro says:

> I'm always very nervous ...The doctors say that it is schizophrenia. I don't know. I don't think so. My father had bad nerves. When he was young he was in an asylum and he couldn't finish his military service, and because his nerves were bad he used to hit me.

Here "nervous" contrasts with a diagnosis like "schizophrenia," and Siro resorts to family history to present an image of normality and, at the same time, to justify the way he had been mistreated. In fact, *nervios* are composed of clusters of meanings in which numerous interpretants constitute a narrative of unlimited potential, full of second, third and fourth meanings, but an opposition between "schizophrenia" and *nervios* emerges consistently as an attitude of resistance to delegitimation.

In 24 of the 27 cases that I analyzed in depth, *nervios* as a central complaint or symptom stood in opposition to the categories used by professionals and family members, regardless of the variety of other possible meanings captured in the expression. But since my purpose here is to illustrate an approach to the symptom, I will return now to the four points outlined at the beginning of this chapter in light of the ethnographic data.

First, I pointed out that the polysemy present in a symptom could be understood using Ricoeur's idea of the two dimensions of signification: an apparent meaning and a symbolic meaning. On one level, "nervios" clearly has a literal meaning—emotional tension, worry, agitation, unease, distress, etc.—which is not problematic, since in many cases these states are side effects of psychopharmacological treatment. On another level, we can see that in different narratives "nervios" acquires a second meaning of resistance to stigmatization and the loss of social position. Unlike metaphor, however, this second meaning is not produced at the expense of the semantic coherence of the literal meaning, but superimposes itself on it, giving the symptom a symbolic dimension that may be several layers deep, given the range of other possible meanings.

Second, I proposed analyzing symptoms as texts. Here, for obvious reasons, it has been necessary to textualize symptoms, which I have even represented as condensed forms of a broader narrative. But how far apart are the intention of the author and the intention of the work? As ethnographers we are not interested in the psychology of the informants, only in what they talk about and what we inscribe. The case of *nervios*, for example, offers us an example of shared meaning which can be understood as the result of a game of delegitimation and resistance. If we examine individualized cases, however, the intention of the work and the intention of the author are more closely imbricated, as we saw in the narratives of "the plaintiff," "the son of the tiger hunter" and "the artist," although this does not necessarily mean that these narratives cannot be subject to structural analysis, a sort of *explication de texte* that removes the sender from his or her own message and substitutes the intention of the work in a way that annuls its author. This is what Geertz has ironically called the discovery of "the Continent of Meaning" and the "mapping out" of its bodiless landscape (1973, p. 20). Nevertheless, we should not forget that our textualizations are the product of ethnography, and not a given. This allows us to maintain that a symptom is *not* a text, but should be interpreted *as* a text in response to certain descriptive requirements.

Third, I then took up Turner's approach to dominant ritual symbols, in which their multiplicity of meanings can be structured around two poles, one sensory and the other ideological. On this point Turner says:

> At the sensory pole are concentrated those *significata* that may be expected to arouse desires and feelings; at the ideological pole one finds an arrangement of norms and values that guide and control persons as members of social groups and categories (1967, p. 28) [italics in original].

Obviously Turner is dealing with a very different social and cultural context. However, if we adapt and broaden Turner's idea of polarized meanings, we can recognize that the differences between a literal meaning of *nervios* (anxiety, agitation, distress) and its symbolic meaning of resistance express the sensorial and ideological levels of the symptom. The problem is, though, that in *nervios* these two poles do not necessarily involve an opposition or contradiction such as Turner found between emotions and social values, affections and matrilineal loyalties. In a symptom such as "my nerves are in shreds!" these two types of meaning are not necessarily in opposition but are present in two different guises: physical and psychological sensations, and ideological and cultural constructions. It was basically this dual nature of symptoms that Hokansalo was attempting to resolve by saying that symptoms could be indexical but that they were essentially symbolic. However, if symptoms are constructed linguistically, why bother with indices? Would it not be more appropriate to say that a symptom generally evokes a literal meaning which is also its sensorial pole and a symbolic meaning which is its ideological pole? I believe that it is, because it explains how symptoms may simultaneously refer to physical and/or psychic distress, and also evoke genealogical reflections, legal proceedings, negotiation, moral worlds of affliction and forms of resistance. Moreover, what allows us to define a symptom as an ethnographic object and not something else is the fact that it is a crossroad where feelings of distress and cultural values intersect in semiosic form.

Finally, I suggested the need to investigate the relation between the symptom and its context, because it is here that the polysemic potential of a symptom becomes clear. The symbolic meaning of resistance cannot be understood without locating it in the context of two opposing positions, one of which is superordinate (that of psychiatric professionals and family members, who use words like "schizophrenia" and "inability to manage for themselves") while the other is subordinate (the afflicted, who talk about their *nervios* and deny having "schizophrenia" in an attempt to avoid social delegitimation and loss of personal autonomy). There is a context in which "my nerves are very bad" has a unique meaning which cannot be extrapolated to other contexts where "nerves" might refer to a corporate executive's feelings of stress; to "nerves of steel;" or, stretching our imagination a bit, to a coded message which communicates the capture of a spy. "I suffer from nerves" can, in fact, mean quite different things, but it is context that assists our interpretations and validates our conjectures. The need for context is even greater for symbolic meanings than for literal ones. The meaning of nerves as anxiety, disquiet, distress, etc. is a sort of intercontextual meaning (within certain limits) that permits communication among different microcontexts. However, the symbolic meaning of resistance is much more clearly dependent on its context of meaning. For an interpretation to have any value, it will have to take into account the importance of this link, at least if it wants to avoid confusing winks of complicity with winks of parody, the auditory hallucinations characteristic of Native American mourning with those of psychosis, *mal d'ollo* with delusional disorder, or my informants' "nerves" with those of a Wall Street executive—to mention just a few of the potential relations between symptoms and possible contextual worlds.

NOTES

1. The initial aim of my research was to study the EMs of individuals diagnosed as suffering from schizophrenia in the city of Barcelona and their relation with social networks and with the phenomenon known in social psychiatry as the *revolving door*: frequent relapses and readmissions to psychiatric institutions. Later I modified my approach, because my interest shifted to another type of phenomenon. In the cases that I analyzed it soon became clear that the complaint or symptom of "I suffer from nerves" was sufficiently frequent to attract the attention of any ethnographer. This and other related observations led me to study symptoms as complaints, messages sent from an informant, and to review the literature on the subject. Here I include only a few cases, for purposes of illustration, in which complaints about *nervios* were a constant. The cases were collected during my fieldwork, a period of three years (1990-1993) in different psychiatric institutions in Barcelona: *Hospital Clínic de Barcelona* (4 months),

Institut Frenopàtic (6 months), *Area de Rehabilitación Integral* (ARI) (7 months) and the *Centre d'Assisténcia Primària en Salut Mental de Gràcia* (CAP SM) (9 months). It should be pointed out that the cases were not only monitored and analyzed within these institutional settings, but also in visits to the patients' homes and informal meetings in "neutral" places such as cafés and local restaurants. In some cases I managed to record the narratives of the informants on tape, but on other occasions I had to make do with a written record, reconstructed from notes after the conversation had taken place.

2. Despite my repeated explanations to the contrary, Rafael always identified me as a health professional. For this reason, his complaints about his nerves are inseparable from his attempts to negotiate his treatment.

CHAPTER 11

The Limits of
Ethnographic Interpretation

It is a spring afternoon, and I am in a Barcelona rehabilitation center for "chronic psychotics" chatting with two informants. On my left is Joan Manel (JM), 18 years old, and on my right is Miguel (MG). The former begins to speak about the relationship between humankind and nature. He picks up two pencils ("This is mankind and this is nature") which he arranges on the table in two parallel lines. "In the past they were together," he says, "but now they are separate." According to JM, something will have to happen for "man to return to nature" and for "the survival of the human race." He expresses himself with certainty and conviction. When I question him further, he continues:

> JM: You believe in what is tangible, like this newspaper. It is tangible, but you have to believe in something else. Just think, person X told me what I've just told you. He's proved it and seen it and he told me all about it: Man must stop thinking if he is to return to nature. He must be like he was before; he mustn't think; he mustn't build arms or chemical things. He's got to stop thinking to return to nature.

[We go out into the garden]

> Nature has feelings. Have you ever seen a cherry tree cry? It's quite clear when they're sad. Look at this plant [he points to a bush]. This plant is happy because the wind is blowing.

Ethnographer: And when is it sad?

JM: It's sad when someone cuts a piece off it like this [he points to a mark where a branch had been]. Just look at this hole. It's a scream. You look on plants as if they had no feelings, but they do. Haven't you ever been taught to understand plants? They have feelings just like us!

Ethnographer: Like us?

JM: They want to have feelings like us.

Ethnographer: How do you know?

JM: Someone told me.

Ethnographer: Who?

JM: I can't tell, but ask me anything, just as if you were speaking to him.

Ethnographer: Was it a person who told you?

JM: Yes. A man.

Ethnographer: If it's a man, how does he know?

JM: He knows just like I know [he gets angry]. Look, you've always been told that there's a sun [he draws a sun]. You've also been told that the earth is round, and it isn't. It's oval. And once it was like this [he draws a rounded, misshapen object with one black and one white part]. And now there's only this part left [the black part].

Ethnographer: How do you know?

JM: Someone told me.

Ethnographer: Explain it to me. Give me reasons, because if you don't I can't believe it.

JM: There isn't any reason. It isn't logical. It's cyclical. It's a cycle which has no logic.

Ethnographer: But it follows a process?

JM: Yes, but it's cyclical. It isn't tangible.

Ethnographer: So what is it? Is it like a dream or a poem...?

JM: A dream is also a reality. When you dream you resolve your unconscious problems. You're working. You've been taught that the earth is round, but it's like this [he draws a line through the middle of the circle].

Ethnographer: It's cut in two?

JM: Yes.

Ethnographer: Why?

JM: Because that's how it is, it's divided in two by the satellite and meteorite war, wars and weapons. Look, can you see this line [he draws a line]? You've always been told that it's next to the sun [he draws a sun next to the straight line] but it's next to the sea [he draws a line next to the sea].

Ethnographer: What is this line?

JM: It's life. This line is life.

[MG suddenly joins in]

MG: That's what you think, that's what's in your head and you believe it's true, but it comes from here [he points to his head].

JM: That's how things are! Like this! [shouting] Someone told me. You two don't know who I am. I've got special powers.

This text, remarkable for the surprising nature of "the said," reveals a paradoxical situation. The speaker does not have any symptoms or complaints that show an awareness of illness. Nevertheless, for a psychiatrically trained observer, his speech is the disorganized voice of psychosis, the loss of a sense of reality, the confusion between the intrapsychic and the exogenous, the expression of madness, the index of a disorder revealed in delusional ideas; in short, a type of symptom or sign which is only recognized by the professional because the sufferer is unaware of its significance. And it is through this reading that "what is said" becomes an indication of pathology, and the sender and receiver of a message are more sharply differentiated than in other possible situations.

For the sufferer, there is no need to report an illness, since he does not recognize his experience as such. For the professional, it is precisely this lack of acceptance which gives his speech a heavier pathological charge, the sign that we are faced with a severe mental disorder such as schizophrenia. As we try out a series of different interpretations and approaches, we should ask ourselves, What exactly do we have here, a set of signs or a series of symptoms?

If we accept that symptoms are constructed linguistically, we can tentatively say that we are in fact dealing with symptoms. So far we have argued that, in general, symptoms are expressed and physical signs are revealed naturally or by technical means (for example, CAT scans, X-rays, or laboratory tests). However, what the informant says does not seem to be a report of being unwell or a complaint about pain, suffering or affliction. Despite being linguistic, then, it does not constitute a symptom (subjective evidence of illness), in contrast to a sign discovered by the professional. Instead, we are dealing with a phenomenon which is a symptom in the eyes (and ears) of others, defined as a symptom by the social context in which it is uttered. Here, the ethnographer's approach will be similar to Goffmann's (see above), attempting to untangle the meanings imposed on madness by its social context.

The fact is that JM's speech is not intended to communicate illness or affliction. So what is it? An unintentional symptom, the meaning of which lies in it being recognized as such in a social context? If so, we should ask ourselves to what extent, although we are dealing here with language, we are faced with a wink or a twitch. In fact, the content of JM's speech seems to escape his control. He seems trapped in its logic, forced to think and talk in a bizarre, although—as Kraepelin pointed out in *Die Erscheinungsformen des Irreseins* (The Manifestations of Insanity)—not completely incoherent fashion.

In the previous chapter, we saw how persons diagnosed as schizophrenic did not speak only nonsense; they also expressed opinions others would find reasonable. It was not a question of total incomprehensibility, but of apparently impenetrable zones closed to exegesis, as when María ("the plaintiff") associated her tendency to speak in verse with her religious beliefs and her divorce; or when Rafael ("the artist") told us about auditory experiences in which some children offered him coffee or asked him to tell them a story. However, on the other hand, they spoke of intelligible situations in connection with interpersonal conflicts and experiences of torture and delegitimation. Their speech was not completely incoherent, although some idiosyncratically associated dysentery with onanism. Babu ("the son of the tiger hunter"), for instance, spoke in a measured and even self-critical way about his previous auditory experiences and his past certainty that he was Jesus Christ.

Likewise, JM's speech is not completely distorted. When he speaks of the arms race, of how humanity has been separated from nature, of the earth being oval and of plants having feelings, his speech is coherent. Nevertheless, an excessive certainty in his arguments hints at the presence of a supposed "someone else," incomprehensible to the observer, who tells him what things are really like. On other occasions, JM said that this "someone" spoke to him from far away, sending him messages that he could hear with his "special powers." And it is precisely his uncompromising certainty that his "knowledge" is special, the conviction with which he defends arguments so out of keeping with the context of meaningful conventions in which he finds himself, which makes JM's speech more impenetrable to ethnographic understanding.

It certainly seems that JM speaks in a code that is different from the conventional one, or that this other code takes possession of him, making him speak in a certain way. But the code, if it exists, is idiosyncratic because it is not accessible to anyone else; and we may even consider the possibility that there is in fact no code, no intention, only an irremediable confusion that leads JM to mistake his thoughts for reality. The second informant, MG, cleverly introduces this possibility when he makes the following criticism: "That's what you think, that's what's in your head and you believe it's true, but it's from here [he points to his head]."

JM reacts angrily to this by telling both the ethnographer and MG that things really are as he sees them and that his interlocutors do not appreciate his faculties and powers. And it is at this moment, which he fills with convictions, mysterious powers and uncompromising positions when, curiously, any possible intention seems to disappear, leaving in its wake a confusion that seems to be a twitch rather than a wink. A twitch in the true sense of the word, for it overtakes the speaker in mid-utterance; this is why, instead of a clearer argument or even a more confusing one which is still subject to a coherent and culturally contextualized order of meanings, we find a certain incoherence in his speech. It is a curious and complex sign which seems to be less a red spot on the skin, a scar or an abdominal mass than a deformation of "what is said." We are now in a position to recognize a paradox opposite to the one arising out of the neo-Kraepelinian interpretation that took winks for twitches. Now the dilemma is the reverse: to what extent can ethnographic interpretation treat twitches as winks, the disorganized speech of aphasia as a sort of cultural code, and the distortion of delirium as an intentional narrative with a communicative goal?

Whether the special way in which JM speaks is a natural manifestation or not, we must first determine to what extent "the said"—like a movement of the eyelid—can be considered a wink. Otherwise, we may find ourselves face to face with a conundrum such as the one mentioned in Chapter 1, in which the delusional ideas of "harm" and "reference" observed by the psychiatrist had an unexpected coherence when placed within their Galician cultural context. Moreover, there is nothing to prevent us from first exhausting the possible ethnographic interpretations before we resort to identifying the phenomenon as a sort of twitch. However, as a self-critical exercise, we should note that interpretation is stretched here to its limits, because the semiosic becomes confused with the physical.

It seems clear that, from the emic point of view, the conversation with JM is simply a discussion in which the informant possesses knowledge to which the ethnographer wishes to gain access. This situation is very different from the clinical one in which the professional guides the interview and establishes a diagnosis and a course of treatment which do not take the patient's beliefs into account. From an ethnographic and interpretive perspective, however, it is a question of defining not the underlying pathological processes, but the meaning of "the said" at a level beyond what is immediately apparent; that is to say, its symbolic, deep or implicit meaning. I have already argued that ethnographic interest lies not in the psychology of the informant but in the moral and cultural worlds of meaning reflected in his speech. So in this case the ethnographer's problem is the difficulty of making an exegesis based on a relationship between "the said" and the context of meaning which it reflects, because it is likely that this context simply does not exist. Nonetheless, let us make an interpretive effort based on a series of conjectures which will help us to delve into the possible intention of our informant.

To do so, we must first be aware of the difficulties involved in verifying or corroborating an interpretation. It is true that in the domain of interpretation we have no experimental methodologies or causal inferences which, as in the procedure of explanation, enable us to corroborate our hypotheses. Even so, this does not mean that "anything goes." Eco has very cleverly shown that it may not be possible to verify an interpretive conjecture, but it is at least possible to discount the worst interpretations by placing them side by side with the text as a whole:

> Even the most radical deconstructionist accepts the idea that there are interpretations which are clearly unacceptable. This means that the text to be interpreted imposes restrictions on its interpreters. (1996, p. 19).

More optimistically, Ricoeur has observed that although an interpretation cannot be verified, it can be validated according to procedures similar to legal interpretation. He states:

> In conclusion, if it is true that there is always more than one way of construing a text, it is not true that all interpretations are equal and may be assimilated to so-called "rules of thumb" (1979, p. 91).

And also:

> An interpretation must not only be probable, but more probable than another. There are criteria of relative superiority which may easily be derived from the logic of subjective probability (1979: 91).

Bearing these principles in mind, let us attempt for a moment to test some of the following conjectures about JM's speech:

1. It may be a rather sophisticated way of speaking, using rhetorical

devices which include metaphor, symbolism and allegory.

2. JM may simply be playing a role, and therefore it may not be a question of hidden meanings but of sustaining a pretense.

3. We may also consider the possibility that the informant in question comes from a particular cultural context, historical tradition or subculture in which split planets and weeping cherry trees have a socially recognized meaning.

THE FIRST READING: FIGURATIVE LANGUAGE

Let us suggest that the peculiarities in what JM says are an artifact of the ethnographer's misreading, because he is really using rhetorical devices to express himself. From this point of view, the literal interpretation would simply be a mistaken approach, since JM's intention is to speak of something without naming it. In short, everything that he says about weeping cherry trees, sad plants, planets broken by the meteorite war or lines next to the sun or the sea should be understood on the symbolic or even metaphoric level.

The conjecture may be revealing. We can see that JM's narrative is reminiscent of metaphor as a rhetorical strategy ("Have you ever seen a cherry tree cry?") that makes literal interpretation impossible. We may also conjecture that the whole discourse about split planets, lines representing life, and plants that have feelings like humans has a symbolic meaning which enables the informant to speak about himself, a way of speaking through which a personal situation acquires a figurative dimension. So we shall have to formulate interpretive hypotheses that will give us access to the speaker's intention and help us understand what he really means. We may imagine the following:

1. When JM says "planet," he means himself, and when he says that it is split in two he is telling us that he feels divided for some reason, perhaps in his family loyalties, the ambivalence of his feelings, or the conflict between who he is and who he wants to be. (This last hypothesis is not as outlandish as it may seem. On other occasions, JM told us that his life seemed to be routine and monotonous, but he actually led a double life as a detective and had uncovered one of the best-kept secrets of international politics; this, he said, was

the reason why he was being persecuted and locked up in a variety of psychiatric institutions).

2. The "meteorite war" and the "arms race" are his own problems and interpersonal conflicts, so that the planet broken up by meteorites is himself in relation to certain important events. In this context, the meteorites may be electroshock treatments or admissions to psychiatric hospitals, or (why not?) the expansion of the arms industry may mean the pharmacological industry; so, as in the case of the artist, we are dealing with symbolic forms which articulate private meanings through broad and general references.

3. What is more, when he states that life is next to the sea and not next to the sun, he may be speaking rhetorically about himself and his relation with his parents, and therefore he is providing us with a coded message which reveals his affective preferences: life (JM) is on the side of the sea, which he uses as a symbol for his mother, and not on the side of the sun, which is his father.

4. Likewise, when he says that cherry trees cry he is also using a metaphor. They don't cry like humans; the withered leaves simply hang down because they haven't been watered. He may also be speaking metaphorically when he states that plants scream; that is, a bush suffers when one of its branches is broken off. For the same reason he argues that plants can be happy, and enlarges on his explanation: "this plant is happy because the wind is blowing."

Of course, stretching the imagination somewhat, there may be people who habitually express themselves in a highly rhetorical manner, whether because they derive a sort of aesthetic pleasure from it, or use it to command the attention of their interlocutors. Nevertheless, it is rather difficult to take conjectures of this type to the point where the text as a whole confirms our interpretations. To begin with, we quickly begin to doubt whether JM's style really has to do with figurative forms of self-expression. Is JM really creating metaphors (or even an allegory) about himself and his intrapsychic sensations and experience? When he says that the earth is split by a meteorite storm, is JM speaking literally, or does he really mean something else?

Our suspicions are not without foundation, most importantly because this figurative language, rather than being the product of intention, seems to be taking place at JM's expense. Something tells us that the metaphors are not a source of aesthetic pleasure, not an allegory for something else. And this something is nothing less than the uncompromising certainty with which JM defends his positions. His certainty, moreover, prevents complicity with his interlocutor because, when questioned, JM responds not by explaining the hidden meaning of what he has said, but only with a defense of its literal meaning. For JM, the images of weeping cherry trees, sad plants, and planets split in two are not part of an aesthetic strategy, but are in fact a reality, even though it is an intangible, cyclical, inexplicable reality accessible only to him and to "someone else," the interior voice that tells him what things are really like. Here there is no rhetorical strategy, only the staunch defence of a literal meaning. He is not constructing metaphors; rather, the metaphors seem to be speaking through him.[1]

THE SECOND READING: DECEIT

Another interpretation we may explore is that JM is either lying or acting, pretending to believe or trying to make us think he believes things that, in reality, he does not. There are many possible reasons for this, ranging from the practical joke to stranger motives such as, for example, an adolescent desire to seem important by claiming supernatural powers. In favor of this possibility there is the small clue of his attempting to gain a position of superiority when he asks, "Haven't you ever been taught to understand plants?" We cannot completely exclude this possibility, even though it is only hypothetical. But a certain interpretive economy suggests to us that JM's speech is neither a lie nor a performance, but the incoherent reflection of demented beliefs. We can imagine the possibility of a deliberate lie or a theatrical performance (which, after all, have the same implication: an intention behind the bizarre speech), but this interpretation ultimately does not serve us. JM may have been playing a role for four months and this may have gone unnoticed by all the people around him during this time (the ethnographer included), but it is not very likely that someone would take this performance to extremes that result in psychiatric confinement, treatment with drugs, or losing his independence as a social (and legal) person. And the fact is that JM is capable of defending his beliefs even at this price. This is why JM's speech suggests to us something other than mere showing off, or a theatrical performance out of context. JM believes in his role. What is more, even without having to resort to exogenous information, we can appreciate that the text of the interview itself raises obstacles to this interpretation: the violence of JM's response to questioning surprises both MG and the ethnographer. Not only does the interview text fail to give us clues that could support this interpretation; the very absence of such clues practically invalidates it.

THE THIRD READING: THE TRUTH

What if everything JM told us were true? Not a metaphysically grounded truth, or even a universal one, but simply a set of beliefs, conceptions and knowledge within a specific cultural framework. This would be, of course, a possibility of the same order as a Nigerian claiming that ants are running around his brain, or Michiko speaking of the fox's spirit, or "the son of the hunter" asserting that in India it was normal for a son to sleep with his mother until he was quite old. In this hypothesis, the strange quality of JM's speech would clearly be the result of a problem of communication in which the receiver of the message is ignorant of the sender's code, and therefore his understanding is limited to what his own categories enable him to grasp. However, this is not the case. Just as a wink can convey shared meanings such as complicity or parody depending on the context, the meaning of JM's speech is not anchored in any historico-cultural tradition or even in a microcontext such as one in which sufferers complain of "nerves" in order to avoid the delegitimation of being categorized as schizophrenic or mentally ill. In contrast, JM's statements—not all of them, but most importantly his certainty about the nature of things—drift aimlessly away from his cultural context of reference. He seems to have created a cosmogony all his own, as well as a language or special code with keys that are inaccessible to others. In this he finds pleasure or enjoyment, since in the few moments in which he was capable of self-criticism, he concluded with *"o allò o res"* ("that or nothing"):[2] that is to say, either his world of weeping cherry trees and misshapen planets; or a void, probably death. ·

Nevertheless, there is a small truth here; not a shared or social truth, only an individual one, a discursive form partially susceptible of interpretation or textualization as a narrative. The ethnographer may be able to reconstruct from it an experience-near or emic perspective. But there are also impenetrable zones that resist any attempt at interpretation, where the metaphors are not even metaphors, the lies are not lies, and the truths do not form part of a shared reality. We already know why this is the case: JM's speech is often incomprehensible because he is less the sender of a message than the mouthpiece of his interior voices.

This does not mean that we should, as Kraepelin suggested, suspend our capacity for surprise and perplexity at what our informants tell us. Even managing to discern that, in a certain context, a movement of the eyelid may be a sort of twitch is by no means an insignificant advance, and recognizing it as such requires exegesis, even though the limits of ethnographic interpretation are all too obvious: 1) a sometimes fruitless search for autochthonous meaning; 2) a lack of interest in the search for pathological meaning; and 3) an unwillingness, at least for the time being, to attempt an explanation that goes beyond "the said" and, therefore, beyond the hermeneutic circle.

These three limitations are present in the above interpretation of JM. All three readings come up against areas which admit of no interpretation of autochthonous meaning. Any such interpretation founders on obstacles in, though not of, the informant's speech, obstacles not of meaning but of unknown processes (emotional, neurochemical, organic, etc.) which distort the flow of discourse. It is at this point that interpretive anthropology reaches the limits of its capacity to account for the ways in which meaning may be both constructed and warped. This should not prevent us from devising other approaches for explaining JM's disordered speech. One of these is classical psychoanalysis which, as we have seen, resolves the problem of interpretation by using a model combining a hermeneutics of meaning with an explanatory theory of drives in order to account not only for the meaning of the text but also the meaning of the abnormalities present in it. As we saw in the analysis of Devereux's approach, this was the direction taken by classical psychoanalytic anthropology, and is also characteristic of some of the new contributions in this field such as Obeyesekere's search for a synthesis, albeit more hermeneutic and less energetic than the Freudian one, between emotions and meanings based on a concept analogous to dream work: the work of culture. More specifically, and in Obeyesekere's own words: "The work of culture is the process whereby symbolic forms existing on the cultural level get created and recreated through the minds of the people" (1990, p. XIX). In short, it is the process which links the public and the private, culture and private fantasies, meanings and deep motivations.[3] It is precisely this process that has broken down in JM's speech.

In processual approaches, which are also explanatory, neither symptoms nor their possible meanings nor illness narratives are construed in terms of their context of meaning, but as the products of processes which may conceal drives and, in some cases, also cognitive mechanisms and/or neurochemical reactions. This is alien territory for interpretive anthropology if we bear in mind the declaration of principles with which Geertz ended his essay "Thick Description" more than twenty years ago:

> The essential vocation of interpretive anthropology is not to answer our deepest questions, but to make available to us answers that others.... have given,

and thus to include them in the consultable record of what man has said (1973, p. 39).

Nevertheless, as in JM's case, there may be circumstances in which this access to the answers given by others is, if not unfeasible, at least uncertain, situations in which it is difficult to separate the semiosic from the physical, winks from twitches, signs (natural) from symptoms (symbolic). Here a hermeneutic approach to symptoms reaches limits of a sort opposite to those encountered by neo-Kraepelinian attempts to reify and naturalize the sufferer's speech, symptoms and cultural categories. There is now the danger of culturalizing the natural, of mistaking the physical for the semiosic, signs for symptoms—but there is also the possibility of pausing to linger, although not passively, on this threshold.

NOTES

1. The informant in question not only denies expressing himself figuratively, but has considerable difficulty understanding that metaphorical or metonymic discourse can be used in everyday circumstances. Once JM asked me about an expression which his father often used and which he found completely incomprehensible: "Women are a real headache." When I explained to him that something was missing from the expression and—quite apart from the falsity of the assertion—it should be understood to mean: "Women create problems and, therefore, cause headaches," he simply was not able to understand the key to the hidden meaning. Here it seems that his twitch or physical sign consists of taking literally that which is figurative.
2. In Catalan, the language of Catalonia (northeastern Spain).
3. Attempts have also been made to analyze the process of constructing meanings using cognitive anthropology. See especially the work of Shore (1991), in which the author attempts to combine hermeneutics and cognitivism.

Epilogue: Open Work

In this book I have analyzed two approaches: 1) the symptom as organic manifestation and 2) the symptom as symbolic construction. At this point, it has been established that the first approach closes the symptom off from interpretation by denying the semiosic nature of its production, while the second opens it up to interpretation by restoring the existence of the human sender of the message. By way of conclusion, I want to make these arguments explicitly.

My aim in the first part of this book was to show how neo-Kraepelinism stresses the passivity of the sender of the message to such an extent that his or her creative and expository ability is annulled. It is certainly true that psychiatry distinguishes between signs and symptoms in such a way that the former are regarded as signals or observable physical indications, and the latter as statements or subjective evidence. Moreover, the diagnostic exercise remains a semiology for deciphering a code consisting of physical and nonphysical signs. However, neo-Kraepelinian approaches seem to restrict the interpretation of meaning to clinical inference. The symptom has no native meaning, but is rather evidence of pathology. In this reification we can observe the lack of interest in the symptom as a message, or in its sender; the symptom is presented as a natural fact.

Central to neo-Kraepelinism is the precedence the reader's intention takes over the meaning of the work and the intention of the author. The symptom and its disease are defined in organic terms, with the aim of prescribing a treatment. By way of analogy, it may be said that symptoms are observed rather than interpreted in the same way that an art restorer analyzes the texture and pigmentation of *Las Meninas* in order to prevent it from deteriorating. In the case of symptoms, however, the author is present, and while she speaks, complains or otherwise expresses her suffering, she dynamically constructs and reconstructs her statements with a communicative purpose.

I have already pointed out that for most mental disorders, organic etiologies remain hypothetical. Given this situation, what the patient says is of primary importance for defining such diagnostic criteria as "auditory hallucinations" or "feelings of hopelessness"—a whole range of phenomena accessible only through the patient's speech. In contrast to the observational capacity of biomedicine, with its technological ability to penetrate the universe of the organs, contemporary psychiatry is limited to dealing more with symptoms than with physical signs. On many occasions, for instance in JM's hermetic narrative, signs become indistinguishable from speech itself, because manifestations of psychosis such as "delusions" or "disorganized speech" present not as biological evidence, but emerge from the speaker's very words.

But the matter does not end here. If we add to these limitations Canguilhem's observation that symptoms and signs are rarely superimposed (1966, p. 61), the problem gets worse. For example, as Canguilhem himself points out, any good urologist knows that a patient who complains of "my kidneys"[1] is someone who has nothing in his kidneys, because for the patient kidneys are "a muscular and cutaneous territory," not organs (1966, p. 61). Of course, if the technological means exist to produce physical signs, whatever patients say about their kidneys will become less important, because the clinician will have something observable and measurable to rely on. Psychiatry, by contrast, is almost completely limited to the domain of the patient's utterances, to "my kidneys hurt" or "I hear voices" constructed in a narrative of affliction. At this point the paths diverge: psychiatry can either treat symptoms as physical signs reified to make them manageable within a universalist paradigm; or it can recognize that symptoms are not signs and therefore require interpretation.

Neo-Kraepelinism opted for the first of these two possibilities. This involves a political commitment having to do with the corporate and socioeconomic interests of the profession, at the cost of treating winks as twitches.

The clinical relation required by neo-Kraepelinism (and also by biomedicine in general) between professional and patient is rather odd from an ethnographic point of view. The clinician takes the position that Lacan neatly captured as the "subject who supposedly knows" (1973, p. 240). In perfect opposition to this, patients "do not know," and when they feel unwell, they turn to the professional in search of relief, both for their malaise and for the anguish that it causes. Patients describe what they feel, relate their symptoms and tell the story of their affliction. From all this information the professional salvages only a few facts on which to base a diagnosis. This salvage operation involves converting "Oh, my God! Life has no meaning since my husband died" into "feelings of despair." If in the telling the patient's story seems to wander from the subject—"Of course my daughter's grown up now and wants to live by herself"—the professional may listen patiently for a bit, but finally asks, "Do you feel tired in the mornings? Have you lost weight recently?" The patient gets the point, and tries to be more focused. Once again the psychiatrist may interrupt with more questions: "Have you ever thought about suicide?" "Have you ever thought that life just wasn't worth living?" "Do you sleep well at night?" The patient responds to these questions, but generally in biographical and moral terms. Again the clinician tries to narrow it down to "How long have you been feeling like this?" or "Are you taking any medication?"—thus converting the story into an inventory of facts reshaped in terms of diagnostic criteria.

Situations similar to the one outlined above have been defined by Brown (1993) as the opposition between the patient who tells a story (his or her own), and the psychiatrist who follows the story as he would a mystery, in search of clues and evidence (p. 255). At first this idea seems suggestive. Think of the traces of pipe tobacco smoke still floating in the air, the mud on the shoes of Mr. X, the microscopic piece of Persian carpet which gives Sherlock Holmes a vital piece of information for solving the case. In an apparently similar fashion, the clinician untangles the patient's tale, not to take pleasure in it but to convert it into a language of facts: "low energy," "insomnia," and "poor appetite," but also "feelings of hopelessness," "low self-esteem," etc. Symptoms are raised to the same level of reification as the mudstained shoes or the pipe smoke in a process of inference through which what the patient says is transformed into the logic of real facts—traces, clues, natural signs—whose meaning depends on the logical and conceptual processes of the receiver of the message. In this way the autochthonous meaning vanishes because it is inexpert, ignorant of the true code by which facts acquire meaning: loss of weight, feelings of hopelessness, poor appetite, thoughts of suicide and insomnia as manifestations of depression.

However, clinical procedure and criminal investigation are not entirely similar. Like Holmes, the psychiatrist also wants to find out "whodunit," but has the advantage of a ready-made classification. In addition, the signs of interest to a psychiatrist are natural and universalizable, while the detective has to confront a potentially infinite variety of individual situations because human will has intervened, a "motive" which is clearly the intention of an author. This is why, despite Brown's suggestive "Psychiatric Intake as a Mystery Story", the analogy of the clinician and the detective is only apparent, and in fact inverse: the clinician naturalizes the semiosic, while the detective reads human will into footprints and physical evidence.

The problem of disguising symptoms as physical signs is no trivial matter, but one of fundamental practical importance. If an Iranian woman's complaint of heart distress is understood by the clinician to mean only physical sensations, it is a clear misreading. If this same hypothetical clinician continually modifies the treatment because his schizophrenic patients complain unceasingly about their nerves, there is a failure of interpretation and a communication problem. The list of examples is as long as that of possible worlds of affliction, and we do not have to deny the existence of literal meanings that allow a degree of understanding in order to see that widely divergent meanings can make the situation untenable.

Although in different cases the nuances vary, the processes are always the same: the conversion of symptoms into physical signs; the suppression of authorship; avoidance of the message; and the meaningful intention of the complaint. In short, the intention of the reader comes to dominate, limiting the symptom to his own interpretation. The semiosic has become physical, a natural phenomenon that acquires meaning only insofar as the receiver of the message constructs it. The resulting model is unidirectional, with interpretation moving from the clinician to the patient or, more accurately, from the professional to the disease itself. The only variability of any significance here is produced by clinical inference: will the diagnosis be anxiety or depression?

Nonetheless, symptoms can be understood in another way, as they were in psychoanalysis and in the phenomenological-existential school of psychiatry. An interpretive ethnography of symptoms and affliction also plays an important and distinctive role here. Because it has no interest in establishing pathological meanings, it bypasses the debate about whether the causes of mental illness are moral, social, psychological or biological. This is simply not its problem, or at least, not its main preoccupation. Its aim is to understand affliction or, in Geertz's terms, to gain access to (and record) the responses given by others.

Interpretive ethnography, in contrast to neo-Kraepelinism, focuses its attention on recovering the autochthonous meaning of symptoms, both literal and symbolic. The aim here is not therapy but understanding symptoms through their context. In this there is a certain similarity to the approach of the art critic or literary critic, although a symptom is not *Las Meninas*, nor a complaint *Finnegan's Wake*. There is no need to seek aesthetic meaning in symptoms, although some anthropologists have tried this approach (Good, 1994; Devisch, 1991). In any case, aesthetics—a dogmatic science, as Weber characterized it—goes in search of meanings that have little to do with our purposes. These digressions aside, however, the response to a work of art is not so very different from the response to a symptom. Interpretive anthropology seeks in the symptom an intention other than its own, developing conjectures that must be validated by the message of the work. The work and its author therefore take center stage relative to *a priori* etic categories modifiable, as Pike cautions us, by fieldwork. The pigmentation, texture, or other physical aspects of the symptom-as-painting are simply not of interest, and the ethnographer goes straight to the interpretation of "the said." Therapy is not a possibility; yet, curiously, this contemplative stance yields a kind of application, not an uncritically pragmatic one, but a resource which emerges from the ethnographic process itself: it reveals the native meaning of symptoms.

In the clinical interview above, in which the patient spoke of the burden of grief she has carried since the death of her husband, the clinician read into her story a pathological meaning largely alien to the ethnographer's task. Only some of the messages contained in her words caught his interest, particularly those which furnished the basis for a diagnosis. What is important for the ethnographer is precisely what the clinician discards as irrelevant: the meaning of death and loss in a specific cultural context, the structures of kinship that give rise to certain tensions between mother and daughter, the spiritual entreaty implicit in her "Oh my God!" What interests the ethnographer are the cultural meanings evoked by the narrative, shared meanings of the sort transmitted by a wink, the hierarchies of meaning expressed in a cultural code; the individual psychology of the winker (or the sufferer) is not the issue here. At this point, the ethnographer goes beyond the informant, as the clinician does with the patient, in search of knowledge that is not limited only to the individual's experience, but with the important difference that in ethnography this does not produce a conflict between naturalist approaches and semiosic realities. It is difficult to imagine an ethnographer trying to discern meaningful intention in red spots on the skin, because physical signs, in and of themselves, do not communicate anything. This is not to say, however, that patients, observing their spots, may not subsequently use them to construct symptoms that are fully semiosic. Here it is possible to carry out the ethnographic task of investigating the meaning of the spots for the suf-

ferer as a representative of a cultural tradition or social group that shares
certain ideas about such occurrences. The aim then becomes an understanding of the terms in which the natural can become the object of a particular
cultural construction, without losing sight of the fact that "the said" is said
by someone.

To the extent that the symptom refers to a physical or psychological condition that produces distress, the approach of the clinician who reifies symptoms is not the same as that of the hypothetical ethnographer who semioticizes
physical signs. It is the difference between locating the referent of a word,
and searching for an intentionally constructed message where there are only
natural signs. In both cases, although in opposite ways, what is ultimately
neglected is the existence of language: the clinician converts symptoms into
a language of facts and natural signifiers, while our hypothetical ethnographer robs language of meaning by reducing everything to a linguistic phenomenon.

The image of the ethnographer seeking some hypothetical original meaning for physical signs is, of course, absurd. In our conceptual world there is
no confusion between the universe of facts and the symbolic order which
would permit unlimited derivations of meaning. However, it is also a mistake to see symptoms as a mere natural facts, not because clinical psychiatry
should abandon its therapeutic intent, but because, in the absence of well-
founded etiological knowledge, we run a greater risk of confusing the culturally specific with the universally pathological. The headache and brainache
of a Puerto Rican; the heart distress of an Iranian woman; the auditory hallucinations of a Native American in mourning; the *nervios* of chronic psychiatric patients in Barcelona; the *nervoso* of the Brazilian *favelas*; the diffuse
quality of depression in South Asia; and the culture-bound syndromes which
expose the limitations of universal psychiatric criteria and the pathogenic-
ity/pathoplasticity model—all these are facts that speak for themselves. The
dual task of anthropology here is to provide a critical perspective on contemporary psychiatry, and to open up symptoms to the work of understanding. None of which should prevent us from finding in symptoms not only
culture and language, but also pain, oppression and suffering.

NOTES

1. In the Mediterranean context, to complain of "the kidneys" is a common reference to lower-back pain.

REFERENCES

Ackerknecht, E.H. (1943). Psychopathology, primitive medicine and primitive culture. *Bulletin of the History of Medicine, 14*, 30-67.

Ackerknecht, E.H. (1946). Natural diseases and rational treatment in primitive medicine. *Bulletin of the History of Medicine, 19*, 467-497.

Ackerknecht, E.H. (1947). Primitive surgery. *American Anthropologist, 49*,25-45.

Alvarez-Heidenreich, L. (1987). *La enfermedad y la cosmovisión en Hueyapan, Morelos* [Illness and culture in Hueyapan, Morelos]. Mexico: Instituto Nacional Indigenista.

American Psychiatric Association. (1980). *Diagnostical and statistical manual of mental disorders* (3rd edition). Washington, D.C.: American Psychiatric Association.

American Psychiatric Association. (1987). *Diagnostical and statistical manual of mental disorders* (3rd revised edition). Washington, D.C.: American Psychiatric Association.

American Psychiatric Association. (1994). *Diagnostical and statistical manual of mental disorders* (4th edition). Washington, D.C.: American Psychiatric Association.

Andreasen, N.C. (1985). Positive vs. negative schizophrenia: A critical evaluation. *Schizophrenia Bulletin,11*, 380-9.

Andreasen, N.C., & Carpenter, W.T. (1993). Diagnosis and classification of schizophrenia. *Schizophrenia Bulletin, 19*, 199-214.

Andreasen, N.C., & Grove, W.M. (1986). Thought, language, and communication in schizophrenia: diagnosis and prognosis. *Schizophrenia Bulletin, 12*, 348-59.

Arato, A. (1972). Lukács' theory of reification. *Telos,11*,42-43.

Baer, H, Singer, M. & Johnsen, J. (1986). Toward a critical medical anthropology. *Social Science and Medicine, 23*, 95-8.

Barthes, R. (1985). *L'aventure sémiologique* [The adventure of semiology]. Paris: Éditions du Seuil.

Basaglia, F. (Ed.). (1976). *Che cos'e la psichiatria?* [What thing is psychiatry?]. Turin: Giulio Einaudi Editore.

Bastide, R. (1965). *Sociologie des maladies mentales* [Sociology of mental illnesses]. Paris: Flammariont.

Bateson, G. (1972). *Steps to an ecology of mind: Collected essays in anthropology, psychiatry, evolution and epistemology.* San Francisco: Chandler Publishing Company.

Beer, D. (1992). Introduction to 'The Manifestations of Insanity.' *History of Psychiatry, 12,* 504-508.

Benedict, R. (1974). *The chrysanthemum and the sword. Patterns of Japanese culture.* New York: New American Library.

Berkman, L.F. (1984). Assessing the physical health effects of social networks and Social Support. *Annual Review of Public Health, 5,* 413-32.

Berkman L.F., & Syme, S.L. (1979). Social networks, host resistance and mortality: A nine-year follow-up study of Alameda County residents. *American Journal of Epidemiology, 109,* 186-204.

Berrios, G.E., & Hauser, R. (1988). The early development of Kraepelin's ideas on classification: A conceptual history. *Psychological Medicine, 18,* 813-21.

Bhatia, M.S., Bohra, N., & Malik, S.C. (1989). Dhat syndrome: A useful clinical entity. *Indian Journal of Dermatology, 34,* 32-41.

Bhatia M.S., & Malik S.C. (1991). Dhat syndrome: A useful diagnostic entity in Indian culture. *British Journal of Psychiatry, 159,* 691-5.

Bibeau, G. (1997). Cultural psychiatry in a creolizing world. Questions for a new research agenda. *Transcultural Psychiatry, 34,* 9-41.

Bloom, J.R. (1990). The relationship of social support and health. *Social Science and Medicine, 30,* 635-7.

Bloom, J.R., & Monterrosa, S. (1981). Hypertension labeling and sense of well-being. *American Journal of Public Health, 71,* 1228-32.

Blumhagen, D. (1982). The meaning of hyper-tension. In N.J. Chrisman & T.W. Maretzki (Eds.), *Clinically applied anthropology. anthropologists in health science settings* (pp. 297-323). Dordrecht: Reidel.

Boas, F. (1966) *Race, language and culture.* Chicago & London: University of Chicago Press.

Boroffka, A. (1988). Emil Kraepelin (1856-1926) and transcultural psychiatry: A historical note. *Transcultural Psychiatric Research Review, 25,* 236-9.

Bottéro, A. (1991). Consumption by semen loss in India and elsewhere. *Culture, Medicine and Psychiatry, 15,* 303-20.

Bravo, M., Canino, G.J., Rubio-Stipec, M., & Woodbury-Fariña, M. (1991). A cross-cultural adaptation of a psychiatric epidemiologic instrument: The Diagnostic Interview Schedule's Adaptation in Puerto Rico. *Culture, Medicine and Psychiatry, 15,* 1-18.

Breuer, J., & Freud, S. (1985). *Estudios sobre la histeria*. [Studies on hysteria]. Buenos Aires: Amorrortu editores.

Broadhead, W.E., Kaplan, B.H., James, S.A., Wagner, E.H., Schoenbach, V.J., Grimson, R., Heyden, S., Tibblin, G. & Gehlbach, S.H. (1983). The epidemiologic evidence for a relationship between social support and health. *American Journal of Epidemiology, 117*, 521-37.

Brown, P. (1993). Psychiatric intake as a mystery story. *Culture, Medicine and Psychiatry, 17*, 255-80.

Butler, D.L., & Stieglitz, T.L. (1993). Contagion in schizophrenia: A critique of Crow and Done (1986). *Schizophrenia Bulletin, 19*, 449-454.

Canguilhem, G. (1955). *La formation du concept de réflexe aux XVIIe et XVIIIe siècles* [The formation of reflex concept]. Paris: Presses Universitaires de France.

Canguilhem, G. (1966). *Le normal et le pathologique* [The normal and the pathological]. Paris: Presses Universitaires de France

Canguilhem, G. (1989).*Études d'histoire et de philosophie des sciences* [Studies on history of philosophy of science]. Paris: Librairie Philosophique J. Vrin.

Canguilhem, G. (1992). *La connaissance de la vie* [The knowledge of life]. Paris: Librairie Philosophique J. Vrin.

Cannon, W.B. (1942). 'Voodoo' death . *American Anthropologist, 44*, 169-81.

Cassel, J. (1976). The contribution of the social environment to host resistance. *American Journal of Epidemiology, 104*, 107-23.

Cassidy, C.M. (1982). Protein energy malnutrition as a culture-bound syndrome. *Culture, Medicine and Psychiatry, 6*, 325.

Castel, R. (1980). *L'ordre psychiatrique*. [The psychiatric order]. Paris: Les Editions de Minuit.

Chadda, R.K. (1995). Dhat syndrome: Is it a distinct clinical entity? A study of illness behaviour characteristics. *Acta Psychiatrica Scandinavica, 91*, 136-139.

Chadda, R.K., & Ahuja, N. (1990). Dhat syndrome. A sex neurosis of the Indian subcontinent. *British Journal of Psychiatry, 156*, 577-9.

Chrisman, N.J., & Johnson, T.M. (1990). Clinically applied anthropology. In T.M. Johnson, & C.F. Sargent (Eds.), *Medical anthropology: Contemporary theory and method* (pp. 93-114). New York: Praeger.

Chrisman, N.J., & Maretzki, T.W. (1982) Anthropology in health science settings. In N.J. Chrisman, & T.W. Maretzki (Eds.), *Clinically applied anthropology. Anthropologists in health science settings*. (pp. 1-31). Dordrecht: Reidel.

Clements, F.E. (1932). *Primitive concepts of Disease*. Berkeley: University of California Press.

Clifford, J. (1983). On ethnographic authority. *Representations, 1*, 118-146.

Cohen, A. (1992). Prognosis for schizophrenia in the Third World: A reevaluation of cross-cultural research. *Culture, Medicine and Psychiatry,16*, 53-75.

254   *References*

Comelles, J.M., & Martínez-Hernáez, A. (1994). The dilemmas of chronicity. *International Journal of Social Psychiatry, 40,* pp. 283-295.

Comptom, W.M., & Guze, S.B. (1995). The neo-Kraepelinian revolution in psychiatric diagnosis. *European Archives of Psychiatry and Clinical Neuroscience, 245,* 196-201.

Cooper, J.E., Kendell, R.E., Gurland, B.J., Sharpe, L., Copeland, J.R.M., & Simon, R. (1972). *Psychiatric diagnosis in New York and London.* London: Oxford University Press.

Cooper, J., & Sartorius, N. (1977). Cultural and temporal variations in schizophrenia: A speculation on the importance of industrialization. *British Journal of Psychiatry, 130,* 50-5.

Corin, E.E. (1990). Facts and meaning in psychiatry. An anthropological approach to the lifeworld of schizophrenics. *Culture, Medicine and Psychiatry, 14,* 153-88.

Crapanzano, V. (1992). *Hermes' dilemma and Hamlet's delight. On the epistemology of interpretation.* Cambridge: Harvard University Press.

Crow, T.J., & Done, D.J. (1986). Age of onset of schizophrenia in siblings: A test of the contagion hyphotesis. *Psychiatric Research, 18,* 107-17.

Csordas, T. (1990). Embodiment as a paradigm for anthropology. *Ethos,18,* 5-47.

Csordas, T. (1993). Somatic modes of attention. *Cultural Anthropology, 8,* 135-156.

Csordas, T. (1994). Introduction: the body as representation and being-in-the-world. In T. Csordas (Ed.), *Embodiment and experience. The existential ground of culture and self,* (pp. 1-24). Cambridge: Cambridge University Press.

Csordas, T., & Kleinman, A. (1990). The therapeutic process. In T.M. Jonhson & C.E. Sargent (Eds.), *Medical Anthropology. Contemporary Theory and Method* (pp. 11-25). New York: Praeger.

Davis, J.M. (1992). Terapéuticas orgánicas [Organic therapies]. In H.I. Kaplan, A. Freedman, & B.J. Sadock (Eds.),*Tratado de psiquiatr'a* [Comprehensive textbook of psychiatry]. (pp. 1474-1506). Barcelona: Masson.

Day, R., Nielsen, J.A., Korten, A., Ernberg, G., Dube, K.C., Gebhart, J., Jablensky, A., Leon, C., Marsella, A., Olatawura, M., Sartorius, N., Strömgen, E., Takahashi, R., Wig, N., & Wynne, L.C. (1987). Stressful life events preceding the acute onset of schizophrenia: A cross-national study from the World Health Organization. *Culture, Medicine and Psychiatry, 11,* 123-205.

De Martino, E. (1983) [1959]. *Sud e magia* [South and magic]. Milan: Feltrinelli.

Dean, A. (1986). Social support in epidemiological perspective. In N. Lin (Ed.), *Social support, life events and depression.* (pp. 3-13). Orlando: Academic Press.

Deister, A., & Marneros, A. (1993). Subtypes in schizophrenic disorders: Frequencies in long-term course and premorbid features. *Social Psychiatry and Psychiatric Epidemiology, 28,* 164-71.

Desjarlais, R. (1992). *Body and emotion: The aesthetics of illness and healing in the Nepal Himalayas.* Philadelphia: University of Pennsylvania Press.

Devereux, G. (1941). Mohave beliefs concerning twins. *American Anthropologist, 43*, 573-592.

Devereux, G. (1961). Shamans as neurotics. *American Anthropologist, 63*, 1088-1090

Devereux, G. (1973). *Ensayos de etnopsiquiatría general* [Essays on general ethnopsychiatry]. Barcelona: Barral.

Devereux, G. (1975).*Etnopsicoanálisis complementarista* [Complementary ethnopsychoanalysis]. Buenos Aires: Amorrortu editores.

Devisch, R. (1991). The Symbolic and the physiological. Epigastric patients in family medicine in Flanders. *Curare, Special Volume 7*, 69-86.

Dilthey, W. (1949). *Introducción a las ciencias del espíritu* [Introduction to the human sciences]. Mexico: Fondo de Cultura Económica.

Dubos, R. (1959). *Mirage of health. Utopias, progress and biological change.* New York: Harper & Row.

Dubos, R., & Dubos, J. (1992). *The white plague. Tuberculosis, man and society.* New Jersey: Rutgers University Press.

Dunk, P. (1988). Greek women and broken nerves in Montréal. *Medical Anthropology, 11*, 29-46.

Eco, U. (1968). *La struttura assente* [The absent structure]. Milan: Bompiani.

Eco, U. (1977). *Trattato di semiotica generale* [A theory of semiotics]. Milan: Bompiani.

Eco, U. (1984).*Semiotica e filosofia del linguaggio* [Semiotics and philosophy of language]. Turin: Giulio Einaudi editore.

Eco, U. (1996). *I limiti dell'interpretazione* [The limits of interpretation]. Milan: Bompiani.

Edgerton, R.B., & Cohen, A. (1994). Culture and schizophrenia: The DOSMD challenge. *British Journal of Psychiatry, 164*, 222-231.

Eguchi Shigeyuki (1991). Between folk concepts of illness and psychiatric diagnosis: Kitsune-tsuki (fox possession) in a mountain village of Western Japan. *Culture, Medicine and Psychiatry, 15*, 421-51.

Eisenberg, L., & Kleinman, A. (1981). Clinical social science. In L. Eisenberg & A. Kleinman (Eds.),*The relevance of social science for medicine* (pp. 1-23). Dordrecht: Reidel.

El-Islam, M. F. (1979). A better outlook for schizophrenics living in extended families. *British Journal of Psychiatry, 135*, 343-47.

Engstrom, E.J. (1991). Emil Kraepelin: psychiatry and public affairs in Wilhelmine Germany. *History of Psychiatry, 2*, 111-32.

Erasmus, C.J. (1952). Changing folk beliefs and the relativity of empirical knowledge. *Southwestern Journal of Anthropology, 8*, 411-428.

Erickson, D.H., Beiser, M., Iacono, W.G., Fleming, J.A.E., & Lin, T. (1989). The role of social relationships in the course of first-episode schizophrenia and affective psychosis. *American Journal of Psychiatry, 146*, 1456-1461.

Estroff, S.E. (1981). *Making it crazy*. Berkeley: University of California Press.

Estroff, S.E. (1982). Long-term psychiatric clients in an American community: Some sociocultural factors in chronic mental illness. In N.J. Chrisman & T.W. Maretzki (Eds.), *Clinically applied anthropology. Anthropologists in health science settings* (pp. 369-393). Dordrecht: Reidel.

Estroff, S.E. (1989). Self, identity, and schizophrenia: In search of the subject. *Schizophrenia Bulletin, 15*, 189-96.

Estroff, S.E. (1993). Identity, disability and schizophrenia. The problem of chronicity. In S. Lindenbaum & M. Lock (Eds.), *Knowledge, power & practice. The anthropology of medicine and everyday life* (pp. 247-286). Berkeley: University of California Press.

Estroff, S.E., Lachicotte, W., Illingworth, L., & Johnston, A. (1991). Everybody's got a little mental illness: Accounts of illness and self among people with severe, persistent mental illness. *Medical Anthropology Quarterly, 5*, 331-69.

Ey, H., Bernard, P., & Brisset, C.H. (1978).*Tratado de psiquiatría* [Treatise on psychiatry]. Barcelona: Toray-Masson.

Fabrega, H.Jr. (1970). On the specify of folk illnesses. *Southwestern Journal of Anthropology, 26*, 305-14.

Fabrega, H.Jr. (1974). *Disease and social behavior: An interdisciplinary perspective*. Cambridge: The MIT Press.

Fabrega, H.Jr. (1987). Psychiatric diagnosis. A cultural perspective. *The Journal of Nervous and Mental Disease, 175*, 383-94.

Fabrega, H.Jr. (1989). The self and schizophrenia: A cultural perspective. *Schizophrenia Bulletin, 15*, 277-90.

Fabrega, H.Jr. (1992). Commentary. Diagnosis interminable: Toward a culturally sensitive DSM-IV. *The Journal of Nervous and Mental Disease, 180*, 5-7.

Fabrega, H.Jr. (1993). Biomedical psychiatry as an object for a critical medical anthropology. In S. Lindenbaum & M. Lock (Eds.), *Knowledge, Power and Practice. The anthropology of medicine and everyday life* (pp. 166-188). Berkeley: University of California Press.

Faris, R.E.L., & Dunham, H.W. (1939). *Mental disorders in urban areas. An ecological study of schizophrenia and other psychosis*. Chicago: University of Chicago Press.

Faust, D., Miner, R.A. (1986). The empiricist and his new clothes: DSM-II in perspective. *American Jorunal of Psychiatry, 148*, 962-67.

Ferrater Mora, J. (1988).*Diccionario de filosofía* [Dictionary of philosophy]. (Vols. 1-4). Madrid: Alianza Editorial.

Fletcher, R.H., Fletcher, S.W., & Wagner, E.H. (1988). *Clinical epidemiology: the essentials*. Baltimore: Williams & Wilkins.

Foucault, M. (1964). *Histoire de la folie à l'âge classique* [Madness and civilization]. Paris: Plon.

Foucault, M. (1972). *Naissance de la clinique* [The birth of the clinic]. Paris: Presses Universitaires de France.

Foucault, M. (1990). *La vida de los hombres infames* [The life of infamous men]. Madrid: Las ediciones de la Piqueta.

Frake, C.O. (1961). The diagnosis of disease among the Subanun of Mindanao. *American Anthropologist, 63,* 113-32.

Frake, C.O. (1980). *Language and cultural description.* Stanford: Stanford University Press.

Frankenberg, R. (1988). Gramsci, culture, and medical anthropology: Kundry and Parsifal? Or rat's tail to sea serpent? *Medical Anthropology Quarterly, 2,*454-59.

Freedman, D. (1992). The Search: Body, mind, and human purpose. *American Journal of Psychiatry, 149,* 858-66.

Freud, S. (1953-1974). *Standard edition of the complete psychological works of Sigmund Freud* (Vols. 1-24) (J. Strachey, A. Freud & A. Strachey, Trans.). London: Hogarth Press.

Freud, S. (1985). *Obras completas de Sigmund Freud* [Complete works of Sigmund Freud]. (L. López-Ballesteros, Trans.). (Vols. 1-3). Madrid: Biblioteca Nueva.

Freud, S. (1988). *Escritos sobre la histeria.* [Fragments of an analysis of a case of hysteria]. Madrid: Alianza.

Fried, J. (1982). Explanatory models of black lung: Understanding the health-related behavior of Appalachian coal miners. *Culture, Medicine and Psychiatry, 6,* 3-10.

Gadamer, H.G. (1975). *Wahrheit und Methode* [Thuth and method]. Tübingen: J.C.B. Mohr.

Gastó Ferrer, C., & Vallejo Ruiloba, J. (1991) Biología de los trastornos afectivos [Somatic dimensions of affective disorders]. In J. Vallejo Ruiloba & C. Gastó Ferrer (Eds.),*Trastornos afectivos* [Affective disorders]. (pp. 311-349). Barcelona: Salvat.

Gay, P. (1988). *Freud. A life of our time.* New York: Norton & Co.

Geertz, C. (1973).*The interpretation of cultures.* New York: Basic Books.

Geertz, C. (1983). *Local knowledge. Further essays in interpretive anthropology.* New York: Basic Books.

Geertz, C. (1988). *Works and lives. The anthropologist as author.* Stanford: Stanford University Press.

Givner, D.A. (1962). Scientific preconceptions in Locke's philosophy of language. *Journal of the History of Ideas, 23,* pp. 340-354.

Goldstein, J.M., & Kreisman, D. (1988). Gender, family environment and schizophrenia. *Psychological Medicine, 18,* 861-72.

Goffman, E. (1969). The insanity of place. *Psychiatry, 32,* 357-88.

Good, B. (1977). The heart of what's the matter. The semantics of illness in Iran. *Culture, Medicine and Psychiatry, 1,* 25-58.

Good, B. (1993). Culture, diagnosis and comorbidity. *Culture, Medicine and Psychiatry, 16*, 427-46.

Good, B. (1994). *Medicine, rationality and experience. an anthropological perspective. Lewis Henry Morgan Lectures.* Cambridge: Cambridge University Press.

Good, B., & Good DelVecchio, MJ. (1981). The meaning of symptoms: a cultural hermeneutic model for clinical practice. In L. Eisenberg, & A. Kleinman (Eds.), *The relevance of social science for medicine.* (pp. 165-196). Dordrecht: Reidel.

Good, B., & Good, M.J.D. (1993). "Learning medicine": The constructing of medical knowledge at Harvard Medical School. In S. Lindenbaum & M. Lock (Eds.), *Knowledge, power & practice* (pp. 81-107). Berkeley: University of California Press.

Gordon, D.R. (1988). Tenacious assumptions in Western medicine. In M. Lock & D.R. Gordon (Eds.). *Biomedicine examined* (pp. 19-56). Dordrecht: Kluwer Academic Publishers.

Grinnell, G.B. (1905). Some Cheyenne plant medicines. *American Anthropologists, 7*, 37-43

Grob, G.N. (1985). *The inner world of American psychiatry, 1890-1940. Selected correspondance.* New Jersey: Rutgers University Press.

Grob, G.N. (1991a). *From asylum to community. Mental health policy in modern America.* Princenton: Princenton University Press.

Grob, G.N. (1991b). Origins of DSM-I: A study in appearance and reality. *American Journal of Psychiatry, 148*, 421-431.

Guarnaccia, P., Parra, P., Deschamps, A., Milstein, G., & Argiles, N. (1992). Si Dios quiere: Hispanic families' experiences of caring for a seriously mentally ill family member. *Culture, Medicine and Psychiatry, 16*, 187-215.

Guarnaccia, P., Canino, G., Rubio-Stipec, M., & Bravo, M. (1993). The prevalence of *ataque de nervios* in the Puerto Rico Disaster Study. The role of culture in psychiatric epidemiology. *The Journal of Nervous and Mental Disease, 181*, 157-165.

Guimón, J., Mezzich, J.E., & Berrios, G.E. (1987). *Diagnostico en psiquiatría* [Psychiatric diagnosis]. Barcelona: Salvat.

Guze, S.B.(1977). The future of psychiatry. Medicine or social science? *The Journal of Nervous and Mental Disease, 165*, 225-30.

Habermas, J. (1989). *Erkenntnis und Interesse* [Knowledge and human interest]. Frankfurt: Suhrkamp Verlag.

Hahn, R. (1995). *Sickness and healing. An anthropological perspective.* New Haven & London: Yale University Press.

Hahn, R., & Kleinman, A. (1983). Biomedical practice and anthropological theory. *Annual Review of Anthropology, 12*, 305-33.

Harris, G. (1957). Possession 'hysteria' in a Kenya tribe. *American Anthropologist, 50,* 1046-66.

Harris, M. (1968). *The rise of anthropological theory. A history of theories of culture.* New York: T.Y. Crowell.

Hoenig, J. (1983). The concept of schizophrenia Kraepelin-Bleuler-Schneider. *British Journal of Psychiatry, 142,* 547-556.

Hokansalo, M.L. (1991). Medical symptoms: A challenge for semiotic research. *Semiotica, 87,* 251-68.

Hollingshead, A.B., & Redlich, A.B. (1958). *Social class and mental illness: A community study.* New York: John Wiley.

Hopper, K. (1991). Some old questions for the new cross-cultural psychiatry. *Medical Anthropology Quarterly, 5,* 299-330.

Hopper, K. (1992). Cervantes' puzzle - A commentary on Alex Cohen's prognosis for schizophrenia in the Third World: A reevaluation of cross-cultural research. *Culture, Medicine and Psychiatry, 16,* 89-100.

House, J.S., Landis, K.R. & Umberson, D. (1988). Social relationships and health. *Science, 241,* 540-545.

Hughes, C. (1985a). Glossary of 'culture-bound' or folk psychiatric syndromes. In R.C. Simons & C. Hughes (Eds.), *The culture-bound syndromes. folk illnesses of psychiatric and anthropological interest.* (pp. 469-505). Dordrecht: Reidel.

Hughes, C. (1985b). Culture-bound or construct-bound? The syndromes and the DSM-III. In R.C. Simons & C. Hughes (Eds.), *The culture-bound syndromes. folk illnesses of psychiatric and anthropological interest.* (pp. 3-23). Dordrecht: Reidel.

Jablensky, A., Sartorius, N., Ernberg, G., Anker, M., Korten, A., Cooper, J.E., Day, R., & Bertelsen, A. (1992). Schizophrenia: manifestations, incidence and course in different cultures: A World Health Organization ten-country study. *Psychological Medicine Suppl. 20.*

Jablensky, A., Sartorius, N., Gulbinat, W., & Ernberg, G. (1981). Characteristics of depressive patients contacting psychiatric services in four cultures. A report from the WHO collaborative study on the assessment of depressive disorders. *Acta Psychiatrica Scandinavica, 63,* 367-383.

Jackson, S.W. (1992). The listening healer in the history of psychological healing. *American Journal of Psychiatry, 149,* 1623-1632.

Jakobson, R. (1980) . *Dialogues.* Paris: Flammarion.

Janes, C.R., Stall, R., & Gifford, S.M. (Eds.). (1985). *Anthropology and epidemiology. Interdisciplinary approaches to the study of health and disease.* Dordrecht: Reidel.

Jilek, W.G. (1995). Emil Kraepelin and comparative sociocultural psychiatry. *European Archives of Psychiatry and Clinical Neurosciences, 245,* 231-238.

Johnson, M.K. (1994). Symptom, sign, and wound: Medical semiotics and photographic representation of Hiroshima. *Semiotica, 98,* 89-107.

Johnson, T.M. (1995). Critical praxis beyond the ivory tower: A critical commentary. *Medical Anthropology Quarterly, 9,* 107-110.

Kahn, J.Y. (1978). A diagnostic semiotic. *Semiotica, 22,* 75-106.

Karasek, R., Baker, D., Marxer, F., Ahlbom, A., & Theorell, T. (1981). Job decision latitude, job demands, and cardiovascular disease: A prospective study of Swedish men. *American Journal of Public Health, 71,* 694-705.

Karno, M., Burnam, A.A., Escobar, J.I., Hough, R.L., & Eaton, W.W. (1983). Development of the Spanish language version of the National Institute of Mental Health Diagnostic Interview Schedule. *Archives of General Psychiatry, 40,* 1183-1188.

Karno, M., Jenkins, J.H., De la Selva, A., Santana, F., Telles, C., Lopez, S. & Mintz, T. (1987). Expressed Emotion and schizophrenia outcome among Mexican-American families. *Journal of Nervous and Mental Disease, 175,* 143-151.

Katz, M.M., Marsella, A., Dube, K.C., Olatawura, M., Takahashi, R., Nakane, Yu., Wynne, L.C., Gift, T., Brennan, J., Sartorius, N., & Jablensy, A. (1988). On the expression of psychosis in different cultures: Schizophrenia in an Indian and in a Nigerian community: A report from the World Health Organization project on determinants of outcome of severe mental disorders. *Culture, Medicine and Psychiatry, 12,* 331-55.

Kessler, R.J. (1990). Models of disease and the diagnosis of schizophrenia. *Psychiatry, 53,* 140-7.

Kiev, A. (1972).*Transcultural psychiatry.* London: Penguin Books.

Kinzie, J.D., Manson, S.M., Vinh, D.T., Tolan, N.T., Anh, B., & Pho, T.N. (1982). Development and validation of Vietnamese-language Depression Rating Scale. *American Journal of Psychiatry, 139,* 1276-1281.

Kirmayer L. (1992). The body's insistence on meaning: Metaphor as presentation and representation in illness experience. *Medical Anthropology Quarterly, 6,* 323-346

Kirmayer, L. (1997). Editorial. *Transcultural Psychiatry, 34,* 1-7.

Kleinman, A. (1977). Depression, somatizacion and the new cross-cultural psychiatry. *Social Science and Medicine, 11,* 3-10.

Kleinman, A. (1980). *Patients and healers in the context of culture.* Berkeley: University of California Press.

Kleinman, A. (1986). *Social origins of distress and disease. depression, neurasthenia and pain in modern China.* New Haven: Yale University Press.

Kleinman, A. (1988a).*The illness narratives. Suffering healing and the human condition.* New York: Basic Books.

Kleinman, A. (1988b). *Rethinking psychiatry: from cultural category to personal experience.* New York: The Free Press.

Kleinman, A. (1992). Pain and resistance: The delegitimation and relegitimation of local worlds. In M. Good, P.E. Brodwin, B. Good & A. Kleinman (Eds.) *Pain as human experience. An anthropological perspective* (pp. 169-197). Berkeley: University of California Press.

Kleinman, A. (1995). *Writing at the margin. Discourse between anthropology and medicine.* Berkeley: University of California Press.

Kleinman, A. (1997) "Everything that really matters": Social suffering, subjectivity, and the remaking of human experience in a disordering world. *Harvard Theological Review, 90,* 315-335.

Kleinman, A., & Good, B. (Eds.). (1985). *Culture and depression. Studies in the anthropology and cross-cultural psychiatry of affect and disorder.* Berkeley: University of California Press.

Kleinman, A., Eisenberg, L., & Good, B. (1978). Culture, illness, and care: Clinical lessons from anthropological and cross-cultural research. *Annals of Internal Medicine, 88,* 251-258.

Kleinman, A., & Kleinman, J. (1991). Suffering and its professional transformation: toward an ethnography of interpersonal experience. *Culture, Medicine and Psychiatry, 15,* 275-301.

Klerman, G.L. (1984). The advantages of DSM-III . *American Journal of Psychiatry, 141,* 539-42

Klerman, G.L. (1986). The National Institute of Mental Health—Epidemiological Catchment Area (NIMH-ECA) Program. *Social Psychiatry, 21,* 159-66.

Kraepelin, E. (1909). *Psychiatrie. Ein Lehrbuch für Studierende und Ärzte.* (8th ed.). Leipzig: Verlag Von Johann Ambrosius Barth.

Kraepelin, E. (1988) [1904]. *Lectures on clinical psychiatry* (T. Johnston Trans. 1905) New York: William Wood & Company.

Kraepelin, E. (1992a) [1920]. The manifestations of insanity. *History of Psychiatry, 12,* 509-29.

Kraepelin, E. (1992b). Psychiatric observations in contemporary issues. *History of Psychiatry, 10,* 253-269.

Kriss, E. (1985). Estudio preliminar [Preliminar study]. In *Obras Completas de Sigmund Freud* [Complete works of Sigmund Freud] Vol. III (pp. 3435-3467). Madrid: Biblioteca Nueva.

Kroeber, A. (1952) [1920]. Totem and taboo: an ethnologic psychoanalysis. In A. Kroeber (Ed.),*The Nature of culture* (pp. 301-309). Chicago: Chicago University Press.

Kurtz, S.N. (1991). Polysexualization: A new approach to Oedipus in the Trobriands. *Ethos, 19,* 68-101.

Kurtz, S.N. (1993). A Trobriand complex. *Ethos, 21,* 79-103.

Lacan, J. (1966). *Écrits* [Writings]. Paris: Editions du Seuil.

Lacan, J. (1973). *Les quatre principes fondamentaux de la psychanalyse* [The four principles of psychoanalysis]. Paris: Editions du Seuil.

Lacan, J. (1981). *Les psychoses* [Psychosis]. Paris: Editions du Seuil.

Laín Entralgo, P. (1947). *Claude Bernard y la experimentación* [Claude Bernard and the experimentation]. Madrid: Ediciones el Centauro.

Laín Entralgo, P. (1961). Vida y obra de Thomas Sydenham [Life and works of Thomas Sydenham]. In P. Laín Entralgo (Ed.), *Sydenham.* (pp. 9-65). Madrid: CSIC.

Laing, R.D., & Sterson, A. (1965). *Sanity, madness and the family.* New York: Basic Books.

Langness, L.L. (1965). Hysterical psychosis in the New Guinea Highlands: A Bena Bena example. *Psychiatry, 28,* 258-77.

Laplantine, F. (1973). *L'Ethnopsychiatrie* [Ethnopsychiatry]. Paris: Editions Universitaires.

Leach, E. (1976). *Culture and communication. The logic by which symbols are connected.* London: Cambridge University Press.

Leff, J. (1988). *Psychiatry around the globe. A Transcultural view* (2nd ed.). Plymouth: Gaskell.

Leff, J., Wig, N.N., Bedi, H. Menon, D.K., Kuipers, L., Korten, A., Ernberg, G., Day, R., Sartorius, N., & Jablensky, A. (1990). 'Relatives' Expressed Emotion and the course of schizophrenia in Chandigarh: A two-year follow-up of a first-contact sample. *British Journal of Psychiatry, 156,* 351-6.

Leff, J., Wig, N.N., Ghosh, A., Bedi, H. Menon, D.K., Kuipers, L., Nielsen, J.A., Thestrup, G., Korten, A., Ernberg, G., Day, R., Sartorius, N., & Jablensky, A. (1987). Expressed Emotion and schizophrenia in North India: III. Influence of Relatives' Expressed Emotion and the course of schizophrenia in Chandigarh. *British Journal of Psychiatry, 151,* 166-73.

Leff, J., Sartorius, N., Jablensky, A., Korten, A., & Ernberg, G. (1992). The International Pilot Study of Schizophrenia: Five-year follow-up findings. *Psychological Medicine, 22,* 131-145.

Lévi-Strauss, C. (1962a). *Le totémisme aujourd'hui* [Totemism]. Paris: Presses Universitaires de France.

Lévi-Strauss, C. (1962b). *La pensée sauvage* [The savage mind]. Paris: Plon.

Lévi-Strauss, C. (1964). *Mythologiques I. Le cru et le cuit* [The raw and the cooked]. Paris: Plon.

Link, B.G., Dohrenwend, B.P., & Skodol, A.E. (1986). Socio-economic status and schizophrenia: Noisome occupational characteristics as a risk factor. *American Sociological Review, 51,* 242-58.

Linton, R. (1937). *The study of man.* New York: Appleton-Century.

Lisón Tolosana, C. (1983). *Antropología cultural de Galicia* [Cultural anthropology on Galice]. Madrid: Akal.

Littlewood, R. (1990). From categories to contexts: A decade of the 'new cross-cultural psychiatry.' *British Journal of Psychiatry, 156,* 308-327.

Lock, M. (1990). On being ethnic: The politics of identity breaking and making in Canada, or, *nevra* on Sunday. *Culture, Medicine and Psychiatry, 14,* 237-54.

Lock, M. (1991). Nerves and nostalgia. Greek-Canadian immigrants and medical care in Québec. *Curare, Special Volume 7,* 87-103.

Lock ,M., & Scheper-Hughes, N. (1990). A critical-interpretive approach in medical anthropology: Rituals and routines of discipline and dissent. In T.M. Johnson, & C.F. Sargent (Eds.).*Medical anthropology. contemporary theory and method.* (pp. 47-72). New York: Praeger.

Locke, J. (1975).*An essay concerning human understanding.* Oxford: Clarendon Press.

López Piñero, J.L. (1985).*Ciencia y enfermedad en el siglo XIX* [Science and disease in 19th century]. Barcelona: Península.

Low, S.M. (1981). The Meaning of nervios: A sociocultural analysis of symptom presentation in San Jose, Costa Rica. *Culture, Medicine and Psychiatry, 5,* 25-47.

Low, S.M. (1994). Embodied metaphors: Nerves as lived experience. In T. Csordas (Ed.), *Embodiment and experience. The existential ground of culture and self.* (pp. 139-162). Cambridge: Cambridge University Press.

Lukács, G. (1969). *Historia y conciencia de clase* [Hystory and class consciousness]. Mexico: Grijalbo.

Manson, S., Shore, J.H., & Bloom, J. D. (1985). The depressive experience in American Indian communities: A challenge for psychiatric theory and diagnosis. In A. Kleinman & B. Good (Eds.), *Culture and depression. Studies in the anthropology and cross-cultural psychiatry of affect and disorder.* (pp. 331-368). Berkeley: University of California Press.

Marmot, M., Rose, G., Shipley, M., & Hamilton, P.J.S. (1978). Employment grade and coronary heart disease in British civil servant. *Journal of Epidemiology and Comununity Health, 32,* pp. 244-249.

Marmot, M., & Syme, L. (1976). Acculturation and coronary heart disease in Japanese-Americans. *American Journal of Epidemiology, 104,* 225-47.

Marsella, A.J., Sartorius, N., Jablensky, A., & Fenton, F.R. (1985). Cross-cultural studies of depressive disorders: An overview. In A. Kleinman & B. Good (Eds.), *Culture and depression. Studies in the anthropology and cross-cultural psychiatry of affect and disorder* (pp. 305-324). Berkeley: University of California Press.

Marx, K. (1976).*Capital: A critique of political economy.* London: Penguin Books, Vol. I.

Maser, J.D., & Dinges, N. (1992). Comorbidity: meaning and uses in cross-cultural clinical research. *Culture, Medicine and Psychiatry, 16,* 409-25.

Matsuoka E. (1991). The interpretation of fox possession: Illness as metaphor. *Culture, Medicine and Psychiatry, 15,* 453-77.

Mattehws, W. (1888). The prayer of a Navajo shaman. *American Anthropologist, I,* 49-71.

McGue, M. (1989). Genetic linkage in schizophrenia: Perspectives from genetic epidemiology. *Schizophrenia Bulletin, 15*, 453-64.

Mckeown, T. (1976). *The modern rise of population*. New York: Academic Press.

Menéndez, E.L. (1981). *Poder, estratificación y salud* [Power, stratification and health] Mexico: Ediciones de la Casa Chata.

Menninger, K. (1963). *The vital balance*. New York: Viking Press.

Mezzich, J.E., Fabrega, H.Jr., & Kleinman, A. (1992). Editorial.Cultural validity and DSM-IV. *The Journal of Nervous and Mental Disease, 180*, 4.

Michels, R. (1984). First rebuttal. A debate on DSM-III. *American Journal of Psychiatry, 141*, 548-51.

Mischel, W., & Mischel, F. (1958). Psychological aspects of spirit possession. *American Anthropologist, 60*, 249-60.

Mishler, E.G. (1981). Viewpoint: Critical perspectives on the biomedical model. In E.G. Mishler (Ed.) *Social contexts of health, illness and patient care* (pp. 1-23). Cambridge: Cambridge University Press.

Mishler, E.G., & Scotch, N.A. (1963). Sociocultural factors in the epidemiology of schizophrenia. *Psychiatry, 1*, 315-51.

Morgan, L.M. (1990). The medicalization of anthropology: A critical perspective on the critical-clinical debate. *Social Science and Medicine, 30*, 945-50.

Morsy, S.A. (1981). Towards a political economy of health: A Critical note on the medical anthropology of the Middle East. *Social Science and Medicine, 15B*, 159-63.

Mumford, D.B. (1996) The 'dhat syndrome': A culturally determined symptom of depression? *Acta Psychiatrica Scandinavica, 94*, 163-167.

Nathan, T. (1994). *L'influence qui guérit* [The curing influence]. Paris: Éditions Odile Jacob.

Nations, M.K. (1986). Epidemiological researh on intectious disease: Quantitative rigor or rigormortis? Insights from ethnomedicine. In C.R. Janes, R. Stall & Y.S.M. Gifford (Eds.), *Anthropology and epidemiology: Interdisciplinary approaches to the study of health and disease* (pp. 97-123). Dordrecht: Reidel.

Newman, P.L. (1964). 'Wild man' behavior in a New Guinea highlands community. *American Anthropologist, 66*, 1-19.

Nichter, M. (1981). Idioms of distress. Alternatives in the expression of psyhcosocial distress: A case study from South India. *Culture, Medicine and Psychiatry, 5*, 379-408.

Nurge, E. (1958). Etiology of illness in Guinhangdan. *American Anthropologist, 60*, 1158-1172.

Obeyesekere, G. (1985) Depression, buddhism, and the work of culture in Sri Lanka en A. Kleinman & B. Good (Eds.), *Culture and depression. Studies in the anthropology and cross-cultural psychiatry of affect and disorder* (pp. 134-152). Berkeley: University of California Press.

Obeyesekere, G. (1990). *The work of culture. symbolic transformation in psychoanalysis and anthropology.* Chicago: University of Chicago Press.

Oring, E. (1993). Victor Turner, Sigmund Freud, and the return of the repressed. *Ethos, 21,* 273-94.

Ots, T. (1994). The silenced body -the expressive Leib: On the dialectic of mind and life in Chinese cathartic healing. In T.J. Csordas (Ed.), *Embodiment and experience. The existential ground of culture and self* (pp. 116-136). Cambridge: Cambridge University Press.

Palinkas, L.A., Wingard, D.L., & Barret-Connor, E. (1990). The biocultural context of social networks and depression among the elderly. *Social Science & Medicine, 30,* 441-447.

Pandolfi, M. (1990). Boundaries inside the body: Women's sufferings in Southern peasant Italy. *Culture, Medicine and Psychiatry, 14,* 255-273.

Pandolfi, M. (1991). Memory within the body: Women's narrative and identity in a Southern Italian village. *Curare, Special Volume 7,* 59-65.

Parker, A.C. (1909). Secret medicines societies of the Seneca. *American Anthropologist, 11,* 161-85.

Parker, S. (1960). The Wiitiko psychosis in the context of Ojibwa personality and culture. *American Anthropologist, 62,* 603-23.

Parker, S. (1962). Eskimo psychopathology in the context of Eskimo personality and culture. *American Anthropologist, 64,*76-96.

Parsons, A. (1961). A schizophrenic episode in a Neapolitan slum. *Psychiatry, 24,* 109-21.

Parsons, C.D., & Wakeley, P. (1991). Idioms of distress: Somatic responses to distress in everyday life. *Culture, Medicine and Psychiatry, 15,* 111-32.

Pascalis, J.G., Perceau, A., Théret, L., Jarraya, A. & Achich, A. (1988). Les classifications de Kraepelin à la DSM III [From Kraepelin classifications to DSM-III]. *Sociéte Médico-Psychologique, 4,* 359-62.

Peirce, C.S. (1966) *Collected papers of Charles Sanders Peirce (C.P.)* (Vols 1-2). Cambridge: The Belknap Press of Harvard University Press.

Pike, K. (1967). *Language in relation to a unified theory of the structure of human behavior.* Paris: Mouton.

Pinel, P. (1800). *Traité médico-philosophique sur l'alienation mentals ou la manie* [Treatise on insanity]. Paris: Caille et Ravier.

Popper, K. R. (1985). *La lògica de la investigació científica* [The logic of scientific discovery]. Barcelona: Laia.

Prior, L. (1993).*The social organization of mental illness.* London: Sage Publications.

Pugh, J.F. (1991). The semantics of pain in Indian culture and medicine. *Culture, Medicine and Psychiatry, 15,* 19-43.

Reagan, A.B. (1922). Medicine songs of George Farmer. *American Anthropologist, 24,* 332-69.

Rhodes, L.A. (1990). Studying biomedicine as a cultural system. In T.M. Johnson & C.F. Sargent (Eds.), *Medical anthropology: Contemporary theory and method* (pp. 159-173). New York: Praeger.

Rhodes, L.A. (1993). The shape of action: Practice in public psychiatry. In S. Lindenbaum & M. Lock (Eds.), *Knowledge, power and practice. The anthropology of medicine and everyday life* (pp. 129-144). Berkeley: University of California Press.

Ricoeur, P. (1965).*De l'interprétation. Essai sur Freud*] On interpretation. Essay on Freud]. Paris: Éditions du Seuil.

Ricoeur, P. (1969). *Le conflit des interpretations* [The conflict of interpretations]. Paris: Éditions du Seuil.

Ricoeur, P. (1974). Phénoménologie et herméneutique. *Man and World, 7*, 211-30.

Ricoeur, P. (1979). The model of the text: Meaningful action considered as a text. In P. Rabinow, & W.M. Sullivan (Eds.), *Interpretive social science. A reader.* (pp. 73-101). Berkeley: University of California Press.

Ritenbaugh, C. (1982). Obesity as a culture-bound syndrome. *Culture, Medicine and Psychiatry, 6*, 347-64.

Rivers, W.H.R. (1924). *Medicine, magic and religion.* London: Kegan Paul, Trench, Trubner.

Robins, L.N., Helzer, J.E. (1986). Diagnosis and clinical assessment: The current state of psychiatric diagnosis. *Annual Review of Psychology, 37*, 409-32.

Róheim, G. (1955). *Magic and schizophrenia.* New York: International Universities Press, Inc.

Rosen, G. (1947). What is a social medicine. A genetic analysis of the concept. *Bulletin of the History of Medicine, 21*, 674-733.

Rosen, G. (1993). A history of public health. Baltimore & London: The Johns Hopkins University Press.

Rubel, A.J. (1960). Concepts of disease in Mexican-American culture. *American Anthropologist, 62*, 795-814.

Russell, F. (1898). An Apache medicine dance. *American Anthropologist, XI*, 367-72.

Ryle, G. (1960). *Dilemmas. The Tarner Lectures 1953.* Cambridge: Cambridge University Press.

Ryle, G. (1967). *El concepto de lo mental* [The concept of mind]. Buenos Aires: Paidos.

Sartorius, N. (1992). Commentary on prognosis for schizophrenia in the Third World, by Alex Cohen. *Culture, Medicine and Psychiatry, 16*, 81-3.

Sartorius, N. (1993). WHO's work on the epidemiology of mental disorders. *Social Psychiatry and Psychiatric Epidemiology, 28*, 147-55.

Sartorius, N., Gulbinat, W., Harrison, G., Laska, E., & Siegel, C. (1996). Long term follow-up of schizophrenia in 16 countries. A description of the International Study of Schizophrenia conducted by the World Health Organization. *Social Psychiatry and Psychiatric Epidemiology, 31,* 249-257.

Sartorius, N., Jablensky, A., Korten, A., Ernberg, G., Anker, M., Cooper, J.E., & Day, R. (1986). Early Manifestations and First-Contact Incidence of Schizophrenia in Different Cultures. A preliminary report on the initial evaluation phase of the WHO Collaborative Study on Determinants of Outcome of Severe Mental Disorders. *Psychological Medicine, 16,* 909-928.

Sartorius, N., & Janca, A. (1996). Psychiatric assessment instruments developed by the World Health Organization. *Social Psychiatry and Psychiatric Epidemiology, 31,* 55-69.

Saussure, F. (1974). *Cours de linguistique générale* [Course on general linguistics]. Paris: Payot.

Scheper-Hughes, N. (1990). Three propositions for a critically applied medical anthropology. *Social Science and Medicine, 30,* 189-97.

Scheper-Hughes, N. (1992). *Death without weeping. The violence of everyday life in Brazil.* Berkeley: University of California Press.

Scheper-Hughes, N., & Lock, M. (1987). The mindful body: A prolegomenon to future work in medical anthropology. *Medical Anthropology Quarterly, 1,* 6-41.

Schooler, C.,& Caudill, W. (1964). Symptomatology in Japanese and American schizophrenics. *Ethnology, 3,*172-8.

Scotch, N. (1963). Medical anthropology. *Biennial Review of Anthropology,* 30-68.

Sebeok, T.A., & Sebeok, J.U. (1979). You know my method: A juxtaposition of Charles S. Peirce and Sherlock Holmes. *Semiotica, 26,* 203-250.

Segal, J.H. (1989). Erotomania revisited: From Kraepelin to DSM-III-R. *American Journal of Psychiatry, 146,* 1261-6.

Seppilli, T. (Ed.). (1983). La medicina popolare in Italia [Folk medicine in Italy]. *La Ricerca Folklorica, 8,* 3-136.

Seppilli, T. (Ed.). (1989) *Le tradizioni popolari in Italia. Medicine e magie* [The folk tradition in Italy. Medicine and magic]. Milán: Electa.

Sheung-Tak, Ch. (1996). A critical review of Chinese koro. *Culture, Medicine and Psychiatry, 20,* 67-82.

Shore, B. (1991). Twice-born, once conceived: Meaning construction and cultural cognition. *American Anthropologist, 93,* 9-27.

Simons, R.C., & Hughes, C. (Eds.). (1985).*The culture-bound syndromes. Folk illnesses of psychiatric and anthropological interest.* Dordrecht: Reidel.

Singer, M. (1986). Toward a political-economy of alcoholism: The missing link in the anthropology of drinking. *Social Science and Medicine, 23,* 113-30.

Singer, M. (1990). Reinventing medical anthropology: Toward a critical realignment. *Social Science and Medecine, 30,* 179-87.

Singer, M. (1995). Beyond the ivory tower: Critical praxis in medical anthropology. *Medical Anthropology Quarterly, 9,* 80-106.

Singer, M., Baer, H., & Lazarus, E. (1990). Critical medical anthropology in question. *Social Science and Medicine, 30,* V-VIII.

Singh, S.P. (1992). Is dhat culture bound? *British Journal of Psychiatry, 160,* 280-281.

Snowden, L.R., & Cheung, F. K. (1990). Use of inpatient mental health services by members of ethnic minority groups. *American Psychologist, 45,* 347-55.

Sontag, S. (1991). *Illness as metaphor and aids and its metaphors.* Londres: Penguin Books.

Spiro, M.E. (1992). Oedipux redux. *Ethos, 20,* 358-76.

Spitzer, R. (1980). Introduction. In American Psychiatric Association. (1980). *Diagnostical and statistical manual of mental disorders* (3rd edition). Washington, D.C.: American Psychiatric Association.

Spitzer, R., & Williams, J. (1992). Clasificación en psiquiatría [Classification in psychiatry]. In H.I.Kaplan, A. Freedman & B.J. Sadock (eds.), *Tratado de psiquiatría* [Comprehensive Textbook of Psychiatry] (pp. 585-615). Barcelona: Salvat.

Srole, L., Langner, T.S., Michael, S.T., Kirpatrick, P., Opler, M.K., & Rennie, T.A.C. (1962). *Mental health in the metropolis. The Midtown Manhattan Study.* New York: McGraw-Hill.

Staiano, K.V. (1982). Medical semiotics: Redefining an ancient craft. [Review of the book *Symptoms and illness: The cognitive organization of disorder*]. *Semiotica, 38,* 319-346.

Staiano, K.V. (1986). *Interpreting signs of illness: A case study in medical semiotics.* Berlin: Mouton de Gruyter.

Stone, M.E. (1988). *American Psychiatric Glossary.* Washington, D.C.: Am. Psychiatric Press.

Susser, E.S., & Struening, E.L. (1990). Diagnosis and screening of psychotic disorders in a study of the homeless. *Schizophrenia Bulletin, 16,* 133-45.

Swerdlow, M. (1992). 'Chronicity,' 'nervios,' and community care: A case study of Puerto Rican psychiatric patients in New York City. *Culture, Medicine and Psychiatry, 16,* 217-35.

Sydenham, T. (1816) [1666]. *Observationes medicae circa morborum acutorum historiam et curationem* [Medical observations]. (Vols 1-2). Montpellier: Imprimerie de M.me V.e. Picot.

Szasz, T. (1970). *The manufacture of madness.* New York: Harper & Row.

Tan, E.S. (1988). Transcultural aspects of anxiety. In M. Roth, R. Noyes & G.D. Burrows (Eds.), *Handbook of anxiety, Vol 1: Biological, clinical and cultural perspectives* (pp. 305-326). London: Elsevier Science Publishers.

Taussig, M. (1980). Reification and the consciousness of the patient. *Social Science and Medicine, 14B,* 3-13.

Thérien, G. (1985). Santé, maladie, guérison: Apport de la sémiologie [Health, illness and curing]. In J. Dufresne, F. Dumont & Y. Martin (Eds.) *Traité d'anthropologie médicale. L'Institution de la santé et de la maladie* [Treatise on medical anthropology]. (pp. 85-103). Québec: Presses de l'Université du Quebec.

Thornicroft, G., & Sartorius, N. (1993). The course and outcome of depression in different cultures: 10-year follow-up of the WHO Collaborative Study on the Assessment of Depresive Disorders. *Psychological Medicine, 23,* 1023-1032.

Trostle, J. (1986). Early work in anthropology and epidemiology: From social medicine to the germ theory, 1840 to 1920. In C.R. Janes, R. Stall & S.M. Gifford (Eds.), *Anthropology and epidemiology. Interdisciplinary approaches to the study of health and disease* (pp. 35-57). Dordrecht: Reidel.

Trotter, R.T.II. (1991). Ethnographic research methods for applied medical anthropology. In C. Hill (Ed.), *Training manual in applied medical anthropology.* Washington, D.C.: American Anthropological Association.

Tseng, W.S., Kan-Ming, M., Hsu, J., Li-Shuen, L., Li Wah, O.,Guo-Qian, C., & Da-Wei, J. (1988). A sociocultural study of koro epidemics in Guangdong, China. *American Journal of Psychiatry, 145,* 1538-43.

Turner, E. (1985). Prologue: From the Ndembu to Broadway. In V. Turner, *On the edge of the bush. Anthropology as experience* (pp. 1-15). Tucson: University ofArizona Press.

Turner, V. (1967). *The forest of symbols. Aspects of Ndembu ritual.* Ithaca & London: Cornell University Press.

Turner, V. (1985).*On the edge of the bush. Anthropology as experience.* Tucson: The University of Arizona Press

Uexküll, T. von. (1982). Semiotics and medicine. *Semiotica, 38,* 205-15.

Uexküll, T. von. (1991). Are functional syndromes culture-bound? *Curare, Special Volume 7,* 13-22.

Vallejo Ruiloba, J. (1991). Clasificación de los trastornos afectivos [Classification of affective disorders]. In J. Vallejo Ruiloba & C. Gastó Ferrer (Eds.), *Trastornos afectivos.* [Affective disorders] (pp. 155-180). Barcelona: Salvat.

Waitzkin, H. (1981). A Marxist analysis of the health care systems of advanced capitalist societies. In L. Eisenberg & A. Kleinman (Eds.), *The relevance of social science for medicine* (pp. 333-369). Dordrecht: Reidel.

Wallis, W.D. (1922). Medicines used by the Micmac indians. *American Anthropologist, 24,* 24-30.

Warner, R. (1983). Recovery from schizophrenia in the Third World. *Psychiatry, 46,* 197-212.

Warner, R. (1985). *Recovery from schizophrenia: Psychiatry and political economy.* London: Routledge & Kegan Paul.

Warner. R. (1992). Commentary on Cohen, Prognosis for schizophrenia in the Third World. *Culture, Medicine and Psychiatry, 16,* 85-8.

Waxler, N.E. (1974). Culture and mental illness. A social labeling perspective. *Journal of Nervous and Mental Disease, 159*, 379-95.

Waxler, N.E. (1979). Is outcome for schizophrenia better in nonindustrial societies? The case of Sri Lanka. *Journal of Nervous and Mental Disease, 167*, 144-58.

Waxler, N.E. (1992). Commentary on Cohen, prognosis for schizophrenia in the Third World. *Culture, Medicine and Psychiatry, 16*, 77-80.

Weber, M. (1968). *Economy and society*. New York: Bedmeister Press.

Weiner, D.B. (1992). Philippe Pinel's 'Memoir on Madness' of December 11, 1794: A fundamental text of modern psychiatry. *American Journal of Psychiatry, 149*, 725-32.

Widiger, T.A. & Corbitt, E.M. (1995). Antisocial personality disorder. In W. J. Livesley (Ed.), *The DSM-IV personality disorders. Diagnosis and treatment of mental disorders* (pp. 103-126). New York: Guilford Press.

Wilson, M. (1993). DSM-III and the transformation of American psychiatry: A history. *American Journal of Psychiatry, 150*, 399-410.

World Health Organization. (1973). *The International Pilot Study of Schizophrenia*. Geneva: WHO.

World Health Organization. (1976). *Esquizofrenia: un estudio multinacional*. [The International Pilot Study of Schizophrenia]. Geneva: Cuadernos de Salud Pública.

World Health Organization. (1979). *Schizophrenia: An international follow-up study*. New York: Wiley.

World Health Organization. (1992a). *The ICD-10 classification of mental and behavioural disorders: Clinical descriptions and diagnosis guidelines*. Geneva: WHO.

World Health Organization. (1992b). *Décima revisión de la Clasificación Internacional de Enfermedades: Trastornos mentales y del comportamiento: descripciones clínicas y pautas para el diagnóstico* [The ICD-10 classification of mental and behavioural disorders: Clinical descriptions and diagnosis guidelines]. Madrid: Meditor.

World Health Organization. (1993). *Décima revisión de la Clasificación Internacional de Enfermedades: Trastornos mentales y del comportamiento: descripciones clínicas y pautas para el diagnóstico* [The ICD-10 classification of mental and behavioural disorders: Clinical descriptions and diagnosis guidelines] (2nd ed.). Madrid: Meditor.

Ying, Y.W. (1990). Explanatory models of major depression and implications for help-seeking among inmigrant Chinese-American women. *Culture, Medicine and Psychiatry, 14*, 393-408.

Young, A. (1976). Some implications of medical beliefs and practices for social anthropology. *American Anthropologist, 78*, 5-24.

Young, A. (1980). The discourse on stress and the reproduction of conventional knowledge. *Social Science and Medicine, 14b*, 133-146.

Young, A. (1981). When rational men fall sick: An inquiry into some assumptions made by medical anthropologists. *Culture, Medicine and Psychiatry, 5*, 317-335.

Young, A. (1982). The anthropologies of illness and sickness. *Annual Review of Anthropology, 11*, 257-285.

Young, A. (1991). Emil Kraepelin and the origins of American psychiatric diagnosis. *Curare, Special Volume 7*, 175-81.

Young, A. (1993). A description of how ideology shapes knowledge of a mental disorder (posttraumatic stress disorder). In S. Lindenbaum & M. Lock (Eds.), *Knowledge, power and practice* (pp. 108-128). Berkeley: University of California Press.

Young, A. (1995). *The harmony of illusions. An ethnographic account of posttraumatic stress disorder*. Princeton: Princeton University Press.

Zola, I.K. (1975). Culture and symptoms: An analysis of patients' presenting complaints. In C. Cox & A. Mead (Eds.), *A sociology of medical practice* (pp. 23-48). London: Collier-MacMillan.

INDEX

Other titles in Theory and Practice in Medical Anthropology and International Health

This book is part of a series. The publisher will accept continuation orders which may be cancelled at any time and which provide for automatic billing and shipping of each title in the series upon publication. Please write for details.